Differential Diagnosis
in Nuclear Medicine

EDWARD B. SILBERSTEIN, M.D.

Department of Radiology
E. L. SAENGER RADIOISOTOPE LABORATORY
DEPARTMENT OF INTERNAL MEDICINE
DIVISON OF HEMATOLOGY/ONCOLOGY
UNIVERSITY OF CINCINNATI MEDICAL CENTER
CINCINNATI

JOHN G. McAFEE, M.D.

DEPARTMENT OF RADIOLOGY
DIVISION OF RADIOLOGICAL SCIENCES
UPSTATE MEDICAL CENTER
STATE UNIVERSITY OF NEW YORK
SYRACUSE

McGRAW-HILL BOOK COMPANY

*New York St. Louis San Francisco Auckland Bogotá Guatemala Hamburg
Johannesburg Lisbon London Madrid Mexico Montreal New Delhi Panama
Paris San Juan São Paulo Singapore Sydney Tokyo Toronto*

This book is dedicated to Carol, Lisa, and Scott. Thank you

E.B.S.

To Cathy, Joan, all my children, and grandson J.P.

J.G.McA.

DIFFERENTIAL DIAGNOSIS IN NUCLEAR MEDICINE

Copyright © 1984 by McGraw-Hill, Inc. All rights reserved. Printed in the United States of America. Except as permitted under the United States Copyright Act of 1976, no part of this publication may be reproduced or distributed in any form or by any means, or stored in a data base or retrieval system, without the prior written permission of the publisher.

1234567890 KGPKGP 8987654

ISBN 0-07-057530-4

This book was set in Times Roman by York Graphic Services, Inc.; the editors were Joseph J. Brehm and Eileen J. Scott; the production supervisor was Avé McCracken.
Kingsport Press, Inc. was printer and binder.

Library of Congress Cataloging in Publication Data
Main entry under title:

Differential diagnosis in nuclear medicine.

   Bibliography: p.
   Includes index.
   1. Radioisotope scanning. 2. Radioisotopes in medical
diagnosis. 3. Diagnosis, Differential. 4. Nuclear
medicine. I. Silberstein, Edward B. II. McAfee, John G.
[DNLM: 1. Nuclear medicine. 2. Differential diagnosis.
3. Radionuclide imaging. WN 445 D569]
RC78.7.R4D475   1984   616.07′575   84-968
ISBN 0-07-057530-4

Contents

iii

Part II CENTRAL NERVOUS SYSTEM

11 Cerebral Blood Flow

MARIANO FERNANDEZ-ULLOA

12 Brain Scintigraphy (Static)

MARIANO FERNANDEZ-ULLOA

13 Cisternography

MARIANO FERNANDEZ-ULLOA

Part III   ENDOCRINE SYSTEM

24 Stomach

EDWARD B. SILBERSTEIN AND AMOLAK SINGH

25 Ectopic Gastric Mucosa

AMOLAK SINGH, EDWARD B. SILBERSTEIN, AND SUBHASH SAHA

26 Gastric Emptying

EDWARD B. SILBERSTEIN

27 Liver Flow and Blood Pool

EDWARD B. SILBERSTEIN

28 Liver-Colloid Imaging

EDWARD B. SILBERSTEIN AND RUPPERT DAVID

29 Hepatobiliary Imaging

EDWARD B. SILBERSTEIN, RUPPERT DAVID, AND HIROSHI NISHIYAMA

30 Pancreas

AMOLAK SINGH AND EDWARD B. SILBERSTEIN

31 Bile Acid Breath Test

AMOLAK SINGH AND EDWARD B. SILBERSTEIN

32 Gastrointestinal Bleeding

EDWARD B. SILBERSTEIN

Part VII GENITOURINARY SYSTEM

33 The Kidney (Excluding Transplant)

JOHN G. McAFEE AND EDWARD B. SILBERSTEIN

34 Renal Transplant

AMOLAK SINGH AND EDWARD B. SILBERSTEIN

35 Cystography

AMOLAK SINGH

36 Testes

JOHN G. McAFEE AND EDWARD B. SILBERSTEIN

Part VIII   HEMATOLOGY

37 Schilling Test

EDWARD B. SILBERSTEIN AND AMOLAK SINGH

38 Shortened Chromium-51 Red Cell Survival

EDWARD B. SILBERSTEIN AND AMOLAK SINGH

39 Chromium-51 Red Cell Sequestration

EDWARD B. SILBERSTEIN AND AMOLAK SINGH

46 Leukocyte Imaging—Indium-111 (Focal Accumulation at 4–24 Hours)

EDWARD B. SILBERSTEIN

47 Lymph Nodes

EDWARD B. SILBERSTEIN

48 Spleen

JOHN G. McAFEE AND EDWARD B. SILBERSTEIN

Part IX PERI-DIAPHRAGMATIC DISEASE

49 Lung-Spleen Separation

EDWARD B. SILBERSTEIN

50 Lung-Liver Separation

EDWARD B. SILBERSTEIN

Part X PULMONARY SYSTEM

51 Lung Perfusion

AMOLAK SINGH AND EDWARD B. SILBERSTEIN

52   Lung Ventilation—Xenon, Krypton

EDWARD B. SILBERSTEIN

53   Lung Ventilation—Aerosol

AMOLAK SINGH

Part XI   SKELETAL SYSTEM

54   Bone Localization

JOHN G. McAFEE AND EDWARD B. SILBERSTEIN

55 Non-Osseous Uptake

JOHN G. McAFEE AND EDWARD B. SILBERSTEIN

List of Contributors

Numbers in parentheses indicate the pages on which the authors' contributions begin.

RUPPERT DAVID, M.D., (161, 179)
Department of Diagnostic Radiology, University of Texas System Cancer
Center, M. D. Anderson Hospital, Houston, Texas

MARIANO FERNANDEZ-ULLOA, M.D. (46, 52, 64, 70, 73, 120, 122)
Department of Radiology, E. L. Saenger Radioisotope Laboratory, University
of Cincinnati Medical Center, Cincinnati, Ohio

MICHAEL J. GELFAND, M.D. (2, 5, 14, 15, 17, 23, 24, 25)
Department of Radiology, E. L. Saenger Radioisotope Laboratory, and
Department of Pediatrics, University of Cincinnati Medical Center, and
Childrens Hospital Medical Center, Cincinnati, Ohio

MYRON C. GERSON, M.D., (2, 5, 14, 15, 17, 23, 24, 25)
Department of Radiology, E. L. Saenger Radioisotope Laboratory, and
Department of Medicine, Division of Cardiology, University of Cincinnati
Medical Center, Cincinnati, Ohio

JOHN G. MCAFEE, M.D., (112, 113, 196, 215, 230, 238, 248, 281, 300)
Department of Radiology, Division of Radiological Sciences, Upstate Medical
Center, State University of New York, Syracuse, New York

HARRY R. MAXON III, M.D. (92)
Department of Radiology, E. L. Saenger Radioisotope Laboratory, and
Department of Medicine, Division of Endocrinology and Metabolism,
University of Cincinnati Medical Center, Cincinnati, Ohio

HIROSHI NISHIYAMA, M.D. (179)
The National Center for Devices and Radiological Health, Division of Physical Sciences, Nuclear Medicine Laboratory (F.D.A.), and Department of Radiology, E. L. Saenger Radioisotope Laboratory, University of Cincinnati Medical Center, Cincinnati, Ohio

SUBHASH SAHA, M.D. (150)
Director of Nuclear Medicine, Department of Radiology, Lonesome Pine Hospital, Big Stone Gap, and Lee County Community Hospital, Pennington Gap, Virginia; Former Fellow, Department of Radiology, E. L. Saenger Radioisotope Laboratory

EDWARD B. SILBERSTEIN, M.D. (110, 113, 125, 145, 149, 150, 152, 158, 161, 179, 187, 190, 191, 196, 208, 215, 219, 221, 222, 223, 225, 227, 230, 239, 242, 246, 248, 260, 261, 264, 274, 281, 300)
Department of Radiology, E. L. Saenger Radioisotope Laboratory, and Department of Medicine, Division of Hematology/Oncology, University of Cincinnati Medical Center, Cincinnati, Ohio

AMOLAK SINGH, M.D. (110, 150, 187, 190, 208, 213, 219, 221, 222, 223, 225, 227, 264, 277)
Nuclear Medicine Department, Harry S. Truman Memorial Veterans Hospital, Columbia, Missouri

D. G. VARMA, M.D. (92)
Department of Radiology, Tulane University Medical Center, New Orleans, Louisiana

Preface

This book was written to assist the physician using nuclear medicine in his daily image and in vitro test interpretations. We have provided a wide scope of differential diagnoses for the many patterns that he or she must keep in mind in the major areas of clinical nuclear medicine. Sensitivities, when known, appear in parentheses. With a few exceptions, noted where they occur, we have only listed conditions that have been cited in the literature. The exceptions are entities that have been observed by one of the authors but for which no case report has been published. We have avoided, whenever possible, references to review articles that do not provide an original source. Each entry is referenced to permit rapid location of a source in the literature for the particular finding.

We also hope to assist the physician searching for specific references as he or she writes for the scientific literature. If a potential cause of a scintigraphic pattern has not been found by one of the authors in the nuclear medicine literature it has not been added to the differential diagnosis listed in the book.

We have attempted to review the literature through mid-1983 to provide as complete a listing of referenced diagnoses as possible. We trust that our colleagues will inform us of our omissions.

Edward B. Silberstein
John G. McAfee

Part I

Cardiovascular System

First-Pass Angiography (Non-Quantitative) of the Heart and Great Vessels

MICHAEL J. GELFAND

MYRON C. GERSON

I. First-pass radionuclide angiography (non-quantitative) of the heart and great vessels

    A. Abnormal great vessel flow patterns and morphologic abnormalities

        1. Superior vena cava

            a. obstruction with collateral flow

                (1) common

                    (a) superior vena cava syndrome (59, 166, 190, 301, 302)

                (2) rare

                    (a) baffle obstruction after Mustard procedure for transposition of the great vessels (302)

            b. other patterns

                (1) persistent left superior vena cava (bilateral superior vena cava) (95, 126, 168, 280)

                (2) absence of the right superior vena cava with persistent left superior vena cava (122, 280)

                (3) patent Glenn (superior vena cava to right pulmonary artery) anastomosis (122, 140, 143, 301)

                (4) abnormal right atrial situs (86, 126)

                (5) drainage of right superior vena cava to left atrium (85, 214)

                (6) aneurysmal dilation of superior vena cava (99)

                (7) drainage of left superior vena cava to left atrium (163)

2. Inferior vena cava
    a. filling defect or non-filling
        (1) inferior vena cava thrombosis (70, 195, 294, 312)
        (2) obstruction due to abdominal mass (195)
        (3) collateral flow due to iliofemoral phlebothrombosis (27)
    b. other patterns
        (1) bilateral inferior vena cava (27, 95)
        (2) absence of right inferior vena cava with persistent left inferior vena cava (95, 108)
        (3) deviation of course of inferior vena cava due to large abdominal mass (301)
3. Pulmonary artery
    a. absence (best seen as absence of an anterior vessel on lateral view)
        (1) pulmonary atresia (122, 325)
    b. dilatation
        (1) cor pulmonale (31)
        (2) pulmonic stenosis (59, 168, 301, 302)
        (3) atrial septal defect (166, 167, 168)
4. Thoracic and abdominal aorta
    a. tortuosity
        (1) tortuous thoracic aorta (39)
    b. non-visualization
        (1) thrombosis of abdominal aorta (92)
    c. localized narrowing
        (1) coarctation of aorta (168)
    d. dilatation or focally increased activity
        (1) aortic stenosis (166, 301, 302)
        (2) thoracic aortic aneurysm (167, 168)
        (3) abdominal aortic aneurysm (35, 254, 261, 275)
        (4) sinus of Valsalva aneurysm (167, 168)
    e. photon deficient area adjacent to area of dilatation
        (1) clot in abdominal aortic aneurysm (35)
    f. extravasation
        (1) ruptured abdominal aortic aneurysm (58)
B. Abnormal sequence of great vessel, lung, and cardiac chamber visualization (curves derived from regions of interest may have been used)
    1. Normal antegrade flow with early recirculation to:
        a. right atrium
            (1) atrial septal defect (59, 167, 300)
            (2) partial anomalous pulmonary venous return above the diaphragm (302)
        b. right ventricle, but not right atrium
            (1) ventricular septal defect (300, 302)
        c. both lungs, but not right ventricle
            (1) patent ductus arteriosus (302)

  d. right lung only
  - **(1)** patent right Blalock-Taussig (right subclavian artery to right pulmonary artery) anastomosis[1] (301, 302)
  - **(2)** patent Waterston (ascending aorta to right pulmonary artery) anastomosis[1] (301, 302)

  e. left lung only
  - **(1)** patent left Blalock-Taussig (subclavian to left pulmonary artery) anastomosis[1] (301, 302)
  - **(2)** patent ductus arteriosus (302)

2. Visualization of blood flow below diaphragm after right heart and lung visualization
  - **a.** total anomalous pulmonary venous return below the diaphragm (6, 126)

3. Portion of lung visualized after aorta, but not visualized immediately after pulmonary artery
  - **a.** bronchopulmonary sequestration (120)

4. Visualization of inferior vena cava after right ventricle
  - **a.** tricuspid regurgitation (201)

5. Early visualization of the left heart
  - **a.** right atrium then left atrium before the left ventricle
    - **(1)** pulmonary atresia without ventricular septal defect (300, 301, 325)
    - **(2)** patent foramen ovale with right-to-left shunt (143, 302)
    - **(3)** tricuspid atresia (300, 301)
    - **(4)** Ebstein's anomaly (59, 300, 301)
    - **(5)** critical pulmonic stenosis (300, 301)
  - **b.** right ventricle then left ventricle and/or aorta before the left atrium
    - **(1)** tetralogy of Fallot (143, 168, 300)
    - **(2)** pulmonary atresia with ventricular septal defect (300)
    - **(3)** complex anomalies with ventricular septal defect (300)
    - **(4)** Eisenmenger's syndrome (301)
  - **c.** early visualization of the right heart and aorta before the lungs
    - **(1)** transposition of the great vessels with intact ventricular septum (143, 301, 302, 325)
  - **d.** visualization in sequence of atrium, left ventricle, lungs, right ventricle, and aorta
    - **(1)** transposition of the great vessels after correction by Mustard procedure (167)

6. Left-to-right shunt analysis (C2/C1, area-ratio, or gamma-variate methods)
  - **a.** early increased recirculation more readily detected by quantitative methods
    - **(1)** atrial septal defect (9, 16, 90, 262, 322)

---

[1] As these patients are cyanotic, there will also be early visualization of the left heart and/or systemic vessels

      (2) ventricular septal defect (9, 14, 16, 90, 262, 322)
      (3) patent ductus arteriosus (9, 16, 90, 262)
      (4) partial anomalous pulmonary venous return (14, 322)
      (5) atrial septal defect (post-operative) and transposition of great vessels (16)
      (6) ventricular septal defect (post-operative) and tetralogy of Fallot (16)
      (7) ventricular septal defect (post-operative) (108, 322)
      (8) endocardial cushion defect (16)
      (9) ventricular septal defect after acute myocardial infarction (134)
      (10) systemic arteriovenous fistula (200A)
C. Increased size of cardiac chambers
    1. See blood pool and first-pass heart studies
D. Filling defects in cardiac chambers
    1. See blood pool and first-pass heart studies

References for this chapter may be found at the end of Chapter 10, page 27.

Chapter 2

Gated Blood Pool and Quantitative First-Pass Studies

MICHAEL J. GELFAND

MYRON C. GERSON

I. Gated blood pool and quantitative first-pass studies of the heart
  A. Chamber dilatation
    1. Left ventricle dilated, right ventricle normal
      a. common
        (1) anterior myocardial infarction (240)
        (2) inferior myocardial infarction without right ventricular infarction (264A)
        (3) ischemic cardiomyopathy (57)
        (4) aortic insufficiency (166, 167, 206, 274)
        (5) mitral insufficiency (206, 274)
      b. less common

        (1) idiopathic cardiomyopathy (57)

        (2) myocarditis (290)

  2. Right and left ventricles dilated

    a. common

      (1) idiopathic cardiomyopathy (57)

      (2) right ventricular and inferior wall myocardial infarction (240)

      (3) left ventricular pressure overload with congestive heart failure (206)

      (4) left ventricular volume overload with congestive heart failure (206)

    b. less common

      (1) ischemic cardiomyopathy (57)

  3. Right ventricle dilated, left ventricle normal

    a. right ventricular infarction with posterior or inferior wall infarction (240)

    b. mitral stenosis with pulmonary hypertension (206)

    c. tricuspid insufficiency (274)

    d. pulmonary hypertension (274)

    e. pulmonic valvular insufficiency (274)

    f. primary pulmonary hypertension (166)

  4. Both atria dilated, both ventricles normal or small

    a. restrictive cardiomyopathy (287)

  5. Both atria dilated, both ventricles dilated

    a. congestive cardiomyopathy (287)

  6. Dilated left atrium

    a. mitral stenosis (59, 166, 167, 191)

    b. mitral insufficiency (59, 167, 191, 274)

    c. atrial septal defect (167, 191)

    d. left atrial myxoma (166)

    e. congenital aneurysmal dilatation of the left atrium (194)

  7. Dilated right atrium

    a. atrial septal defect (34, 166)

    b. primary pulmonary hypertension (166)

B. Wall thickness

  1. Increased left ventricular wall thickness (separation of the left ventricle from lung or other cardiac chambers or organs)[1]

    a. left ventricular hypertrophy (274, 290)

  2. Increased right ventricular wall thickness (separation of right ventricle from other cardiac chambers or organs)

    a. pulmonic stenosis (274)

    b. pulmonary hypertension (274)

    c. right ventricular hypertrophy (274)

  3. Increased septal thickness

---

[1] Increased ventricular wall thickness must be differentiated from increased separation of ventricular blood pools and lung due to pericardial disease.

         a. idiopathic hypertrophic subaortic stenosis (218)

    4. Increased thickness of the upper septum during diastole

         a. idiopathic hypertrophic subaortic stenosis (218)

    5. Absence of ventricular septum

         a. single ventricle (290)

C. Filling defects in cardiac chambers

    1. Left ventricular filling defect

         a. left atrial myxoma (60, 167, 217)

         b. left ventricular fibroma (108)

         c. left ventricular clot (119, 234, 274, 288)

         d. left ventricular papillary muscle (hypertrophic) (308)

         e. left ventricular rhabdomyoma (277)

         f. left ventricular outflow obstruction in idiopathic hypertrophic sub-aortic stenosis (218)

    2. Obliteration of the left ventricular cavity during systole

         a. idiopathic hypertrophic subaortic stenosis (218, 286)

         b. valvular aortic stenosis (218)

    3. Left atrial filling defect

         a. left atrial myxoma (60, 167, 217)

         b. left atrial clot (274)

    4. Right ventricular filling defect

         a. metastasis (carcinoma of colon) (279)

    5. Right atrial filling defect

         a. right atrial myxoma (38, 144, 199)

         b. right atrial sarcoma (109)

         c. tumor thrombus from renal carcinoma (278)

D. Abnormal shape

    1. Left ventricle

         a. left ventricular aneurysm (49, 83, 291)

         b. pseudoaneurysm of the left ventricle (49, 83, 291)

    2. Right ventricle

         a. right ventricular aneurysm (31)

         b. infundibular dilatation of the right ventricle with normal pulmonary artery due to Uhl's anomaly (31)

E. Abnormal wall motion—rest

    1. Focal decrease in left ventricular wall motion

         a. common

             (1) acute myocardial infarction (232, 239, 260)

             (2) prior myocardial infarction (238)

             (3) ischemic myocardiopathy (57)

             (4) unstable angina pectoris (205)

         b. less common

             (1) idiopathic congestive cardiomyopathy (anteroapical region) (57)

             (2) due to left ventricular vent at cardiac surgery (109)

             (3) idiopathic hypertrophic subaortic stenosis (septum) (218)

        (4) following blunt chest trauma (290A)

        (5) left bundle branch block with normal coronary arteries (252A)

    c. uncommon

        (1) thalassemia (174)

        (2) after removal of left ventricular fibroma (109)

2. Paradoxical left ventricular free wall motion

    a. left ventricular aneurysm (96, 206)

    b. previous myocardial infarction (206, 260)

    c. acute myocardial infarction (330)

    d. pseudoaneurysm of the left ventricle (83)

3. Paradoxical septal motion

    a. post-cardiac surgery

        (1) following coronary artery bypass surgery (33A)

        (2) following aortic valve replacement (197)

    b. ventricular conduction defect

        (1) left bundle branch block without significant coronary artery disease (139A)

    c. coronary artery disease

        (1) left ventricular aneurysm (111)

    d. right ventricular volume overload

        (1) secundum atrial septal defect (139A)

4. Decreased motion of the right ventricular free wall

    a. right ventricular infarction (264A)

    b. following blunt chest trauma (290A)

    c. atrial septal defect (pre-operative and post-operative) (178)

5. Asynchronous left ventricular wall motion

    a. coronary artery disease (132A)

    b. ventricular pacing (111)

F. Abnormal wall motion—intervention at rest

    1. Intra-aortic balloon pumping

        a. decrease in left ventricular wall motion abnormalities

            (1) complicated myocardial infarction (205)

            (2) unstable angina pectoris (205)

    2. Atrial pacing

        a. induction of decreased septal motion

            (1) aortic insufficiency (292)

            (2) transposition of the great vessels (292)

            (3) restrictive cardiomyopathy (292)

    3. Nitroglycerin (sublingual)

        a. decrease in left ventricular wall motion abnormalities

            (1) coronary artery disease (257)

            (2) coronary artery disease with prior myocardial infarction (257)

    4. Nitroprusside (intravenous)

     a. decrease in left ventricular wall motion abnormalities

       (1) acute myocardial infarction (263)

G. Abnormal wall motion induced by exercise

  1. Left ventricle

     a. coronary artery disease (40, 207, 235)

     b. mitral valve prolapse with coronary artery disease (4)

     c. mitral valve prolapse with normal coronary arteries (4)

     d. left bundle branch block with normal coronary arteries (252A)

     e. sickle cell disease (70A)

H. Abnormal wall motion induced by exercise-effect of interventions

  1. Coronary artery bypass graft surgery

     a. left ventricle—improvement of exercise-induced wall motion abnormalities

       (1) coronary artery disease (154)

  2. Propranolol (oral)

     a. left ventricle—improvement of exercise-induced wall motion abnormalities

       (1) coronary artery disease (186)

  3. Nitroglycerin (sublingual)

     a. left ventricle—improvement of exercise-induced wall motion abnormalities

       (1) coronary artery disease (44)

I. Ejection fraction—rest

  1. Decreased left ventricular ejection fraction with normal right ventricular ejection fraction

     a. common

       (1) acute myocardial infarction (especially anterior) (232)

       (2) three hours after coronary artery bypass surgery (182)

  2. Decreased left ventricular ejection fraction, right ventricular ejection fraction not specified

     a. acute myocardial infarction (232, 239, 260) especially anterior acute myocardial infarction (224, 264)

     b. prior myocardial infarction (260)

     c. ventricular aneurysm (238)

     d. doxorubicin cardiotoxicity (13, 247)

     e. cardiomyopathy (unspecified types) (57, 139)

     f. alcoholic cardiomyopathy (138)

  3. Decreased left and right ventricular ejection fraction

     a. atherosclerotic heart disease and cor pulmonale (23)

     b. atherosclerotic heart disease (198)

     c. idiopathic congestive cardiomyopathy (287)

     d. inferior myocardial infarction with right ventricular involvement (232, 297)

     e. cystic fibrosis (65)

     f. Eisenmenger's complex (144A)

  4. Increased left ventricular ejection fraction

    a. idiopathic hypertrophic subaortic stenosis (42, 218)

    b. severe valvular aortic stenosis (43, 218)

    c. scleroderma (266A)

5. Decreased right ventricular ejection fraction with normal left ventricular ejection fraction

    a. chronic obstructive lung disease (23)

    b. cor pulmonale (23)

    c. cystic fibrosis (65)

6. Decreased right ventricular ejection fraction, left ventricular ejection fraction not specified

    a. mitral valve disease (198, 328A)

    b. aortic valve disease (325A)

    c. pulmonary hypertension or increased right ventricular end diastolic pressure (163A)

    d. severe adult respiratory distress syndrome (172A)

    e. atrial septal defect (178)

7. Decreased right atrial ejection fraction

    a. obstructed outflow of right atrium after Fontan procedure for tricuspid atresia (107)

J. Ejection fraction—interventions at rest

  1. Coronary artery bypass graft surgery

    a. increase in left ventricular ejection fraction, right ventricular ejection fraction not specified

      (1) coronary artery disease (28)

  2. Mitral valve replacement

    a. increase in right ventricular ejection fraction, left ventricular ejection fraction not specified

      (1) mitral valve disease with pulmonary hypertension (175)

  3. Atrial pacing

    a. decrease in left ventricular ejection fraction, right ventricular ejection fraction not specified

      (1) organic heart disease (292)

      (2) coronary artery disease (17)

    b. increase in left ventricular ejection fraction, right ventricular ejection fraction not specified

      (1) normal subjects[2] (17, 292)

  4. Cold pressor test

    a. decrease in left ventricular ejection fraction, right ventricular ejection fraction not specified

      (1) coronary artery disease (319)

      (2) cardiomyopathy (319)

    b. increase in left ventricular ejection fraction, right ventricular ejection fraction not specified

---

[2] Some subjects in this group may have had no change in ejection fraction with intervention.

    (1) normal subject[2] (319)

5. Nitroglycerin (sublingual)

    a. increase in left ventricular ejection fraction, right ventricular ejection fraction not specified

        (1) coronary artery disease (257)

6. Nitroprusside (intravenous)

    a. increase in left and right ventricular ejection fraction

        (1) acute myocardial infarction (263)

7. Digitalis (oral)

    a. increase in left ventricular ejection fraction, right ventricular ejection fraction not specified

        (1) coronary artery disease with left ventricular dysfunction (231)

8. Propranolol (oral)

    a. left ventricular ejection fraction unchanged, right ventricular ejection fraction not specified

        (1) coronary artery disease (185)

        (2) normal subjects (329)

9. Isoproteronol (intravenous)

    a. increase in left and right ventricular ejection fraction

        (1) normal subjects (23)

10. Aminophylline (intravenous)

    a. increase in right and left ventricular ejection fraction

        (1) normal subjects (193)

        (2) chronic obstructive lung disease (193)

11. Angiotensin (intravenous)

    a. decrease in left ventricular ejection fraction, right ventricular ejection fraction not specified

        (1) normal subjects (32)

        (2) coronary artery disease (32)

12. Medical therapy of alcoholic cardiomyopathy

    a. increase in left ventricular ejection fraction, right ventricular ejection fraction not specified

        (1) alcoholic cardiomyopathy (138)

13. Hemodialysis

    a. increase in left ventricular ejection fraction, right ventricular ejection fraction not specified

        (1) cardiomyopathy in uremia (139)

14. Terbutaline

    a. increase in right and left ventricular ejection fraction

        (1) chronic obstructive pulmonary disease (133A)

15. Atrial pacing

    a. increase in left ventricular ejection fraction

        (1) coronary artery disease (270A)

16. Surgery for left ventricular aneurysm

      a. no change in left ventricular ejection fraction
         (1) coronary artery disease (98A)

  17. Induction of anesthesia for coronary artery surgery
      a. decrease in left ventricular ejection fraction, right ventricular ejection fraction not specified
         (1) coronary artery disease (113A)

  18. Oral amrinone
      a. increase in left ventricular ejection fraction, right ventricular ejection fraction not specified
         (1) coronary artery disease (173A)
         (2) idiopathic cardiomyopathy (173A)

K. Ejection Fraction—exercise-induced changes
  1. Decrease in left ventricular ejection fraction with exercise, right ventricular ejection fraction not specified[3]
      a. coronary artery disease (40, 45, 53)
      b. coronary artery disease—handgrip exercise (37, 273)
      c. aortic insufficiency—symptomatic or asymptomatic (41)
      d. aortic stenosis—severe (43)
      e. mitral valve prolapse with coronary artery disease (4)
      f. sudden exercise in normal subjects (94)
      g. mitral insufficiency (47)
      h. idiopathic hypertrophic subaortic stenosis without obstruction (42)
      i. mitral valve prolapse without coronary artery disease (uncommon) (4, 121A)
      j. transfusion dependent congenital anemia and chronic iron overload (174)
      k. cystic fibrosis (65)
      l. prior myocarditis (74)
      m. asymptomatic subjects with age > 60 years (220A)
      n. untreated hypertensive patients (325A)
      o. left bundle branch block without coronary artery disease (252A)
      p. sickle cell disease (70A)

  2. Decrease in left ventricular ejection fraction with exercise, abnormal response of right ventricular ejection fraction[3]
      a. ventricular septal defect ($Q_p/Q_s > 2{:}1$) (144A)
      b. Eisenmenger's complex (144A)
      c. following repair of ventricular septal defect (144A)
      d. proximal right coronary artery disease (24, 148, 270)

  3. Decrease in left ventricular ejection fraction with exercise, increase of right ventricular ejection fraction[3]
      a. left anterior descending coronary artery disease (26)

---

[3] Bicycle exercise (supine or erect) was used unless specified. In some series, failure to increase the left ventricular ejection fraction during exercise is considered abnormal. In most references, an abnormal response of right ventricular ejection fraction to exercise is defined as a failure to increase ejection fraction by a specified absolute percentage.

4. Increase in left ventricular ejection fraction with exercise, decrease in right ventricular ejection fraction with exercise[3]
   a. chronic hypoxic lung disease (211)
   b. tetralogy of Fallot after total correction (233)
5. Increase in left ventricular ejection fraction with exercise, right ventricular ejection fraction not specified[3]
   a. normal subjects (40, 45)
   b. aortic insufficiency—asymptomatic (41)
   c. mitral valve prolapse without coronary artery disease (4)
   d. coronary artery disease—not limited by angina (in some patients) (25)
   e. primary cardiomyopathy (in some patients) (261A)
6. Increased left and right ventricular ejection fraction with exercise[3]
   a. common
      (1) normal subjects (26)
   b. uncommon
      (1) coronary artery disease (26)
7. Abnormal response of right ventricular ejection fraction with exercise, left ventricular ejection fraction not specified[3]
   a. common
      (1) proximal right coronary artery disease (181)
      (2) chronic hypoxic lung disease (211)
L. Ejection fraction-effect of interventions on exercise-induced changes
   1. Coronary artery bypass surgery
      a. increase in left ventricular ejection fraction at exercise, right ventricular ejection fraction not specified
         (1) coronary artery disease (154)
   2. Aortic valve replacement
      a. increase in left ventricular ejection fraction at exercise, right ventricular ejection fraction not specified
         (1) severe aortic stenosis (43)
         (2) aortic insufficiency (46)
   3. Propranolol (oral)
      a. increase in left ventricular ejection fraction at exercise, right ventricular ejection fraction not specified
         (1) coronary artery disease (186, 230)
      b. decrease in left ventricular ejection fraction at exercise, right ventricular ejection fraction not specified
         (1) normal subjects (329)
   4. Digitalis (oral)
      a. no change in left ventricular ejection fraction at exercise
         (1) coronary artery disease with left ventricular dysfunction (88A, 231)
      b. increase in left ventricular ejection fraction at exercise
         (1) coronary artery disease with normal resting left ventricular function (88A)

    5. Nitroglycerin (sublingual)
        a. increase in left ventricular ejection fraction at exercise, right ventricular ejection fraction not specified
            (1) coronary artery disease (44)
    6. Oxygen
        a. increase in left ventricular ejection fraction, left ventricular ejection fraction not specified
            (1) chronic hypoxic lung disease (211)
M. Stroke volume ratios (regurgitant index)
    1. Increased ratio of left ventricular to right ventricular stroke volume
        a. aortic insufficiency (170, 241, 273A)
        b. mitral insufficiency (170, 241, 273A)
        c. ventricular septal defect (241A)
        d. patent ductus arteriosus (241A)
        e. mitral valve prolapse with trivial mitral insufficiency and frequent ventricular extrasystoles (170)
        f. severe left ventricular dysfunction (170)
    2. Decreased ratio of left ventricular to right ventricular stroke volume
        a. atrial septal defect with left-to-right shunt (241A)
        b. anomalous pulmonary venous return (241A)
        c. tricuspid insufficiency (111)
N. Pulmonary blood volume—effect of exercise
    1. Increase in pulmonary blood volume with exercise
        a. coronary artery disease (except single vessel right coronary artery disease) (207)

References for this chapter may be found at the end of Chapter 10, page 27.

Chapter 3

Pericardial Imaging with Blood-Pool Agents

MICHAEL J. GELFAND

MYRON C. GERSON

I. Pericardial imaging
    A. Halo surrounding heart (separation of heart from lungs and liver)
        1. Pericardial effusion (any cause) (62, 133, 234, 317, 327)

    2. Constrictive pericarditis (caseous material filling pericardium) (327)
    3. Lipoma within pericardium (317)
    4. Cholesterol pericarditis (136)
    5. Malignant pericardial effusion (267)
B. Asymmetric or focal separation of heart from lungs and liver
    1. Loculated pericardial effusion (176)
    2. Pericardial cyst (176)
    3. Pericardial clot (234)
    4. Pericardial tumor (unspecified) (317)
    5. Fibrosarcoma of pericardium (80)
    6. Pericardial mesothelioma (328)
C. Separation of heart from left lung
    1. Left ventricular hypertrophy (166)

References for this chapter may be found at the end of Chapter 10, page 27.

Chapter 4

^{99m}Tc-pyrophosphate Imaging

MYRON C. GERSON
MICHAEL J. GELFAND

I. ^{99m}Tc-pyrophosphate imaging
  A. Area of increased uptake smaller than cardiac blood pool
    1. Acute myocardial infarction (72)
  B. Focal uptake
    1. Common
      a. acute left ventricular transmural myocardial infarction (1A, 189, 220)
    2. Less common
      a. acute right ventricular myocardial infarction (265, 315)
      b. acute left ventricular subendocardial myocardial infarction (189, 220)
      c. prior myocardial infarction—persistent activity due to myocardial necrosis or fibrosis (50, 183, 209, 220)
      d. unstable angina pectoris with myocardial necrosis or fibrosis (145, 220, 326)
    3. Rare or unknown frequency
      a. left ventricular aneurysm (3)

    b. pericarditis (91, 210, 268)

    c. calcified aortic or mitral valve (147, 236, 320)

    d. myocardial contusion (78, 116)

    e. penetrating wounds of the heart (78)

    f. after cardioversion (without myocardial injury) (78, 79, 223)

    g. accidental electrical injury (78)

    h. after open heart surgery

        (1) aortic-coronary bypass (from the left ventricular vent or acute myocardial infarction) (158, 236)

        (2) valve replacement (332)

        (3) congenital heart disease (unspecified types and procedures) (332)

    i. alcoholic cardiomyopathy (132)

    j. unstable angina pectoris without myocardial injury (145)

    k. stable angina pectoris (188)

    l. malignancy with direct myocardial invasion (127)

    m. pericardial calcification (320)

    n. aortic aneurysm (59A)

    o. endocarditis

        (1) enterococcal (154A)

    p. calcified costal cartilage (77)

    q. infection after removal of costal cartilage (212)

    r. rib fracture (78)

    s. mechanical soft tissue trauma to the chest wall (86A)

    t. normal breast tissue (78)

C. Diffuse uptake

    1. Common

        a. acute left ventricular subendocardial myocardial infarction (1A, 29)

        b. stable angina pectoris (1A, 189)

        c. unstable angina pectoris (1A)

        d. congestive cardiomyopathy (1A, 215)

        e. ischemic heart disease without clinical acute myocardial infarction (29, 220)

        f. no evidence of acute myocardial infarction (persistent blood pool activity, including patients referred for routine bone imaging) (72, 222)

    2. Rare or unknown frequency

        a. acute left ventricular transmural myocardial infarction (1A)

        b. post-cardioversion (1A)

        c. doxorubicin cardiotoxicity—with or without therapeutic irradiation (61, 171)

        d. malignant pericardial effusion—breast carcinoma (228, 306)

        e. after surgery for valve replacement (332)

        f. amyloidosis (203A)

        g. Chagas' disease (117A)

      h. prior left mastectomy (artefact) (222)

      i. prior in-vivo red cell labeling (artefact) (214A)

D. Doughnut pattern

    1. Acute left ventricular transmural myocardial infarction, extensive (2, 77, 253)

    2. Acute left ventricular nontransmural myocardial infarction, (2, 189)

    3. Acute left ventricular myocardial infarction in a patient with no angiographically significant coronary stenosis (111)

    4. Calcified costal cartilage (artefact) (78)

E. Entire myocardium (without heart blood pool activity)

    1. Hyperparathyroidism

      a. secondary (111, 146)

    2. Perimyocarditis (2A)

    3. Renal failure with elevated serum phosphate (111)

F. Uptake—unspecified pattern

    1. Therapeutic irradiation (272)

References for this chapter may be found at the end of Chapter 10, page 27.

Chapter 5

^{201}Tl-Thallium Myocardial Perfusion Imaging

MYRON C. GERSON

MICHAEL J. GELFAND

I. ^{201}Tl-Thallium myocardial perfusion imaging

  A. Left ventricle including septum

    1. Focal area of decreased uptake

      a. rest

        (1) acute myocardial infarction (313, 314)

        (2) prior myocardial infarction (112, 314)

        (3) ischemic myocardopathy (57)

        (4) idiopathic congestive cardiomyopathy (uncommon) (57, 314)

        (5) sarcoid (56, 156)

        (6) peri-infarction ischemia (313)

        (7) mitral valve prolapse without coronary artery disease (uncommon) (124, 276)

          (8) stable angina pectoris (22)
          (9) unstable angina pectoris
             (a) during chest pain (271)
             (b) while free of chest pain (316)
          (10) left ventricular fibroma[1] (227)
          (11) after resection of left ventricular fibroma (109)
          (12) thalassemia (130)
          (13) Chagas' disease (21)
          (14) mucocutaneous lymph node (Kawasaki) syndrome (304A)
     b. specific location (at rest)
          (1) apex—normal variant (69)
          (2) septum (high septum)—normal variant (69)
          (3) septum (entire septum)—single ventricle (204, 286, 290)
          (4) inferior wall—normal variant (left anterior oblique view, 30°) (69)
          (5) anteroseptal wall—left bundle branch block[2] (196)
          (6) anteroseptal wall—aberrant left coronary artery (114, 125)
          (7) anterolateral wall—anomalous origin of the left coronary artery from the pulmonary artery (87, 229)
          (8) inferoposterior wall—positional artifact (left lateral view with patient supine) (121, 152)
          (9) apex—after placement of left ventricle to aorta conduit (109)
     c. rest or exercise and reperfusion[2]
          (1) common
             (a) prior myocardial infarction (219)
          (2) uncommon
             (a) mitral valve prolapse without coronary artery disease (124, 276)
     d. specific location
          (1) apex—normal variant (69)
          (2) septum (high septum)—normal variant (69)
          (3) inferior wall—normal variant (30° left anterior oblique view) (69)
          (4) anterolateral wall—aberrant left coronary artery (87)
          (5) inferoposterior wall—positional artifact (left lateral view with patient supine) (152)
     e. reperfusion and exercise
          (1) delayed reperfusion after exercise-induced ischemia due to coronary artery disease (36, 112)
     f. exercise but not at rest or reperfusion
          (1) exercise-induced ischemia due to coronary artery disease (19, 246)

---

[1] ^{131}Cs

[2] Many pathologic entities that have been described as occurring at rest have not been evaluated at exercise.

(2) exercise-induced ischemia due to coronary artery disease plus prior myocardial infarction (in the same location) (310)

(3) hypertrophic cardiomyopathy without coronary artery disease (135)

(4) aortic stenosis without coronary artery disease (18)

(5) mitral valve prolapse

  (a) with coronary artery disease (160)

  (b) without coronary artery disease (uncommon) (124, 276)

(6) exercise-induced ischemia due to myocardial bridges (5)

g. specific locations at exercise

(1) inferior wall—mitral stenosis with pulmonary hypertension (137)

(2) lateral wall and septum—left main coronary artery disease (75)

(3) all locations except base—two or three vessel coronary artery disease (75)

h. reperfusion but not at exercise

(1) exercise-induced ischemia due to coronary artery disease (129, 295)

i. specific location, reperfusion but not exercise

(1) anteroseptal wall—left bundle branch block[3] (196)

j. exercise only (rest or reperfusion study not reported)

(1) coronary artery spasm (283)

(2) cardiomyopathy without coronary artery disease (159)

(3) overlying breast tissue (282)

k. after pharmacologic intervention but not at rest

(1) ergonovine

  (a) coronary artery spasm with and without fixed coronary artery stenosis (54)

(2) dipyridamole

  (a) coronary artery disease (8)

(3) methacholine

  (a) coronary artery spasm without coronary disease (110)

l. rest and reperfusion (sequential imaging at rest)

(1) coronary artery spasm with coronary artery disease (219, 271)

(2) unstable angina pectoris (22)

(3) stable angina pectoris (22, 271)

m. rest but not at reperfusion (sequential imaging at rest)

(1) coronary artery spasm with coronary artery disease (187)

(2) unstable angina pectoris (22)

(3) stable angina pectoris (22, 112)

(4) myocardial sarcoidosis (182A)

n. exercise prior to but not after intervention

---

[3] ^{43}K, ^{81}Rb

        (1) common
            (a) percutaneous transluminal angioplasty in coronary artery disease (131)
            (b) patent coronary artery bypass graft in coronary artery disease (244, 309)
        (2) uncommon
            (a) cardiac rehabilitation (by exercise program) in coronary artery disease (63)
    o. rest prior to but not after intervention
        (1) coronary artery bypass surgery in stable and unstable angina pectoris (22)

2. Global decrease in myocardial perfusion
    a. rest
        (1) transient myocardial ischemia of the newborn (88)
    b. exercise but not at reperfusion
        (1) suspected left main coronary artery spasm (284)
        (2) multiple vessel coronary artery disease[4] (333)

3. Focal increase in wall thickness
    a. rest
        (1) specific locations
            (a) posterolateral wall—normal variant (papillary muscle) (69)
            (b) posterior wall—normal variant (papillary muscle) (69)
            (c) septum—normal variant (papillary muscle) (69)
            (d) inferior wall—normal variant (papillary muscle) (69)

4. Diffuse increase in wall thickness
    a. rest
        (1) left ventricular
            (a) systemic hypertension (55)
            (b) aortic stenosis (55)
         (2) Pompe's disease (290)

5. Septal thickness significantly greater than lateral wall thickness
    a. rest
        (1) idiopathic hypertrophic subaortic stenosis (55)

6. Thinning of myocardium
    a. rest
        (1) cardiomyopathy (unspecified types) (113)
    b. exercise but not rest
        (1) aortic stenosis (18)
        (2) coronary artery disease (18)

7. Dilatation of left ventricular chamber
    a. rest
        (1) idiopathic congestive cardiomyopathy (57)
        (2) ischemic cardiomyopathy (57)

(3) endocardial fibroelastosis (289)
  b. exercise but not reperfusion
    (1) coronary artery disease (52, 285)
B. Right ventricle
  1. Focal area of decreased activity
    a. rest and exercise
      (1) mitral stenosis without coronary artery disease (137)
    b. exercise but not rest
      (1) mitral stenosis without coronary artery disease (137)
    c. after dipyridamole but not at rest
      (1) proximal right coronary artery stenosis (53A)
  2. Visualization at rest
    a. right ventricular free wall thickness less than left ventricular free wall
      (1) normal variant (69)[5]
      (2) tachycardia (69)
      (3) atrial septal defect (162)
      (4) myocardial infarction (162)
      (5) hypertrophic cardiomyopathy (162)
      (6) congestive cardiomyopathy (162)
      (7) ventricular septal defect (162)
      (8) pulmonic stenosis (162)
      (9) mitral stenosis (162)
      (10) cor pulmonale (162)
      (11) mitral valve disease (155)
      (12) tricuspid valve disease (155)
      (13) tetralogy of Fallot (290)
      (14) cystic fibrosis (290)
    b. right ventricular free wall thickness greater than or equal to left ventricular free wall
      (1) atrial septal defect (155, 162)
      (2) ventricular septal defect (162, 290)
      (3) tetralogy of Fallot (162, 204)
      (4) pulmonic stenosis (162)
      (5) primary pulmonary hypertension (155, 162)
      (6) Eisenmenger's syndrome (204)
      (7) mitral valve disease (162)
      (8) tricuspid valve disease (162)
    c. right ventricular wall thickness increased, extent not specified
      (1) pulmonary hypertension (68, 155)
      (2) mitral stenosis (68, 155)
      (3) increased right ventricular pressure (89)
      (4) transposition of the great vessels with ventricular septal defect (286)

---

[5]Right ventricle usually not seen at rest in the left anterior oblique view.

           (5) atrial septal defect (155)

    3. Dilation of right ventricular chamber

        a. rest

           (1) idiopathic congestive cardiomyopathy (57)

           (2) ischemic cardiomyopathy (57)

           (3) pulmonary hypertension (68, 76)

           (4) mitral stenosis (155)

           (5) pulmonary sarcoidosis (286)

           (6) cystic fibrosis (290)

           (7) tetralogy of Fallot (290)

C. Right atrium

    1. Visualization of right atrial myocardium

        a. rest

           (1) right atrial enlargement due to tricuspid atresia (71)

           (2) mitral stenosis (1)

           (3) cor pulmonale (1)

           (4) cardiomyopathy (1)

           (5) tetralogy of Fallot (1)

           (6) atrial septal defect (1, 265)

D. Decreased activity surrounding myocardial uptake

    1. Pericardial effusion (76)

E. Lung

    1. Focal increase in uptake

        a. squamous cell carcinoma of lung (73)

    2. Diffuse increase in uptake

        a. rest

           (1) increased pulmonary transit time—congestive heart failure (33)

           (2) transient myocardial ischemia of the newborn (88)

           (3) acute pulmonary edema (169A)

        b. exercise but not reperfusion

           (1) coronary artery disease with pulmonary venous hypertension at exercise (52)

           (2) double- or triple-vessel coronary artery disease (169)

References for this chapter may be found at the end of Chapter 10, page 27.

Chapter 6

Intracoronary Particle Injection

MICHAEL J. GELFAND

MYRON C. GERSON

I. Intracoronary particle injection for myocardial perfusion imaging

    A. Left ventricle

        1. Focal perfusion defect

            a. myocardial infarction (15, 213, 323)

            b. coronary artery disease (15, 161, 213)

            c. valvular heart disease with normal coronary arteries (117)

            d. primary myocardial disease with normal coronary arteries (117, 243)

            e. no known heart disease (117, 243)

            f. Prinzmetal's angina (during angina; normal in the absence of angina) (30)

        2. Change in size of focal perfusion defect

            a. after successful coronary artery bypass graft surgery (118)

References for this chapter may be found at the end of Chapter 10, page 27.

Chapter 7

Radionuclide Angiography of Medium Sized Arteries

MICHAEL J. GELFAND

MYRON C. GERSON

I. Radionuclide angiography (vascular abnormalities only) of medium-sized arteries

    A. Focal area of increased flow with increased flow in feeding arteries and draining veins

    1. Arteriovenous fistula (202, 252)
B. Focal area of increased flow or pooling
    1. Aneurysm (115, 192)
    2. False aneurysm (173, 221, 252)

References for this chapter may be found at the end of Chapter 10, page 27.

Chapter 8

^{201}Tl-Thallium Imaging of Arterial Insufficiency of the Lower Extremities

MICHAEL J. GELFAND

MYRON C. GERSON

I. ^{201}Tl-thallium imaging of arterial insufficiency of the lower extremities

    A. Decreased or asymmetric thallium uptake
        1. Leg exercise
            a. arterial insufficiency of the lower extremities (66, 266)

References for this chapter may be found at the end of Chapter 10, page 27.

Chapter 9

Radionuclide Venography

MICHAEL J. GELFAND

MYRON C. GERSON

I. Radionuclide venography

    A. Axillary and subclavian veins

    1. Filling defect
       a. thrombosis (59, 255)
       b. hypertrophic valve (255)
       c. extrinsic mass (225)
B. Common iliac vein
    1. Filling defect with collateralization
       a. venous thrombosis of the common iliac vein (20, 70)
    2. Filling defect without collateralization
       a. excessive washout from ovarian and periureteric veins in renal vein thrombosis (20)
       b. excessive washout from functioning renal transplant (20)
       c. normal dilutional effect (20)
C. External iliac and femoral veins
    1. Filling defect with collateralization
       a. iliofemoral venous thrombosis (20, 81, 151, 256, 293, 294, 331)

References for this chapter may be found at the end of Chapter 10, page 27.

Chapter 10

Lung Imaging with Radiolabeled Particles in Heart Disease

MICHAEL J. GELFAND

MYRON C. GERSON

I. Lung imaging with radiolabeled particles in heart disease

  A. Decreased perfusion of the right lung

    1. Right pulmonary artery stenosis (98)

    2. Patent right Blalock-Taussig anastomosis (right subclavian artery to right pulmonary artery) (98, 298)[1]

    3. Patent Waterston (ascending aorta to right pulmonary artery) anastomosis (100)[1]

    4. After repair of Waterston (ascending aorta to right pulmonary artery) anastomosis (10)[2]

---

[1] This may be the most common pattern after this anastomosis when there is pulmonary artery blood flow from the right ventricle. However, patent shunts may result in a decrease in flow to either lung.

[2] The reversed pattern may also be seen after repair of surgical systemic-to-pulmonary anastomosis.

   5. After repair of right Blalock-Taussig (right subclavian artery to right pulmonary artery) anastomosis (10)[2]
   6. Valvular pulmonic stenosis (64, 298)
   7. Tetralogy of Fallot (298)[3]
B. Absent perfusion of the right lung
   1. Glenn (superior vena to right pulmonary artery) anastomosis after lower extremity injection (98)
   2. Right pulmonary artery atresia (100)
C. Decreased perfusion of the left lung
   1. Patent ductus arteriosus (100)
   2. Ventricular septal defect (298)
   3. Ventricular septal defect with pulmonic stenosis or pulmonary artery band (10)
   4. Left pulmonary artery stenosis (98)
   5. Patent left Blalock-Taussig (left subclavian artery to left pulmonary artery) anastomosis (98, 298)[1]
   6. Patent Potts (descending aorta to left pulmonary artery) anastomosis (103)[1]
   7. Transposition of the great vessels (203, 311)
   8. Tetralogy of Fallot (179, 226)[3]
   9. Transposition of the great vessels after the Mustard procedure (311)
   10. After repair of Potts (descending aorta to right pulmonary artery) anastomosis (10)[2]
   11. After repair of left Blalock-Taussig (left subclavian artery to left pulmonary artery) anastomosis (10)[2]
D. Absent perfusion of the left lung
   1. Left pulmonary artery atresia (98)
   2. Thrombosis of left pulmonary artery after left Blalock-Taussig (left subclavian to left pulmonary artery) anastomosis (82, 98)
   3. Patent Glenn (superior vena cava to right pulmonary artery) anastomosis after upper extremity injection (98, 128, 298)
   4. Stricture of the left pulmonary artery after Potts (descending aorta to left pulmonary artery) anastomosis (10, 82)
E. Predominant perfusion of upper lung fields (injected erect)
   1. Combined pulmonary arterial and pulmonary venous hypertension (97)
   2. Mitral stenosis (97)
   3. Mitral regurgitation (97)
   4. Left-to-right intracardiac shunt without pulmonary hypertension (98)
   5. Primary pulmonary hypertension (98)
   6. Left-to-right intracardiac shunt without pulmonary hypertension (98)
F. Organs frequently visualized with right-to-left shunting
   1. Kidneys (142, 251)
   2. Myocardium (180, 324)

---

[3] Branch pulmonary artery stenosis is common and, when present, results in decreased embolization of the side of the stenosis.

3. Brain (102, 298)
4. Spleen (251)
G. Heart visualization without right-to-left shunting
    1. Intracardiac thrombus (153)
H. Predominant visualization of lower one-half of body (excluding lungs)
    1. Right-to-left shunt through patent ductus arteriosus (98)

REFERENCES[4]

1. Adachi H, Torii Y, Kamide T, et al: Visualization of right atrial appendix by thallium-201 myocardial scintigraphy: concise communication. J Nucl Med 21:914–918, 1980.

1A. Ahmad M, Dubiel JP, Logan KW, et al: Limited clinical diagnostic specificity of technetium-99m stannous pyrophosphate myocardial imaging in acute myocardial infarction. Am J Cardiol 39:50–54, 1977.

2. Ahmad M, Logan KW, Martin RH: Doughnut pattern of technetium-99m pyrophosphate myocardial uptake in patients with acute myocardial infarction: a sign of poor long-term prognosis. Am J Cardiol 44:13–17, 1979.

2A. Ahmad M, Dubiel JP: Tc-99m pyrophosphate myocardial imaging in perimyocarditis. J Nucl Med 22:452–454, 1981.

3. Ahmad M, Dubiel JP, Verdon TA, et al: Technetium-99m stannous pyrophosphate myocardial imaging in patients with and without left ventricular aneurysm. Circulation 58:833–838, 1979.

4. Ahmad M, Haibach H: Left ventricular function in patients with mitral valve prolapse: a radionuclide evaluation. Clin Nucl Med 7:562–567, 1982.

5. Ahmad M, Merry SL, Haibach H: Thallium-201 scintigraphy evidence of ischemia in patients with myocardial bridges (abstract). Am J Cardiol 45:482, 1980.

6. Alazraki NP, Ashburn WL: Radionuclide imaging in the evaluation of cardiac disease: the role of myocardial perfusion imaging and radionuclide angiography. J Nucl Biol Med 16:224–230, 1972.

7. Alazraki NP, Ashburn WL, Hage A, et al: Detection of left-to-right cardiac shunts with the scintillation camera: pulmonary dilution curve. J Nucl Med 13:142–147, 1972.

8. Albro PC, Gould KL, Westcott RJ, et al: Noninvasive assessment of coronary stenoses by myocardial imaging during pharmacologic coronary vasodilatation: III. Clinical trial. Am J Cardiol 42:751–760, 1978.

9. Alderson PO, Jost RG, Strauss HW, et al: Radionuclide angiocardiography: improved diagnosis and quantification of left-to-right shunts using area ratio techniques in children. Circulation 51:1136–1143, 1975.

10. Alderson PO, Boonvisut S, McKnight R, et al: Pulmonary perfusion abnormalities and ventilation perfusion imbalance after total repair of tetralogy of Fallot. Circulation 53:332–337, 1976.

11. Alderson PO, Gaudiani VA, Watson DC, et al: Quantitative radionuclide angiocardiography in dogs with experimental atrial septal defects. J Nucl Med 19:364–369, 1978.

12. Alderson PO, Douglass KH, Mendenhall KG, et al: Quantitation of left-to-right intracardiac shunts after deconvolution analysis of pulmonary time-active curves (abstract). J Nucl Med 19:697, 1978.

13. Alexander J, Dainiak N, Berger HJ, et al: Serial assessment of doxorubicin cardiotoxicity with quantitative radionuclide angiocardiography. N Engl J Med 300:278–283, 1979.

---

[4] This list contains references for Chapters 1–10.

14. Anderson PAW, Jones RH, Sabiston DC Jr.: Quantitation of left-to-right cardiac shunts with radionuclide angiography. Circulation 49:512–516, 1974.

15. Ashburn WL, Braunwald E, Simon AL, et al: Myocardial perfusion imaging with radioactive-labelled particles injected directly into the coronary circulation of patients with coronary artery disease. Circulation 44:851–865, 1971.

16. Askenazi J, Ahnberg DS, Korngold E, et al: Quantitative radionuclide angiography: detection and quantitation of left-to-right shunts. Am J Cardiol 37:382–387, 1976.

17. Atlan H, Tzivoni D, Weiss A, et al: MUGA atrial pacing as a test for myocardial ischemia (abstract). J Nucl Med 20:668, 1979.

18. Bailey IK, Come PC, Kelly DT, et al: Thallium-201 myocardial perfusion imaging in aortic valve stenosis. Am J Cardiol 40:889–899, 1977.

19. Bailey IK, Griffith LSC, Rouleau J, et al: Thallium-201 myocardial perfusion imaging at rest and during exercise. Circulation 55:79–87, 1977.

20. Barnes RW, McDonald GB, Hamilton GW, et al: Radionuclide venography for rapid dynamic evaluation of venous disease. Surgery 73:706–713, 1973.

21. Beer N, Kertsnuz Y, Collet H: Diagnosis of Chagas' cardiomyopathy by thallium-201 perfusion imaging (abstract). Am J Cardiol 45:396, 1980.

22. Berger BC, Watson DD, Burwell LR, et al: Redistribution of thallium at rest in patients with stable and unstable angina and the effect of coronary artery bypass surgery. Circulation 60:1114–1125, 1979.

23. Berger HJ, Matthay RA, Loke J, et al: Assessment of cardiac performance with quantitative radionuclide angiocardiography: right ventricular ejection fraction with reference to findings in chronic obstructive pulmonary disease. Am J Cardiol 41:897–905, 1978.

24. Berger HJ, Johnstone DE, Sands MJ, et al: First-pass radionuclide assessment of right ventricular performance during exercise in coronary artery disease: relationship to left ventricular reserve and right coronary stenosis (abstract). Circulation 57–58:II-132, 1978.

25. Berger H, Reduto L, Johnstone D, et al: Global and regional left ventricular performance during graded bicycle exercise: assessment by first-pass radionuclide angiography (abstract). J Nucl Med 19:710–711, 1978.

26. Berger HJ, Johnstone DE, Sands MJ, et al: Exercise right ventricular response in coronary artery disease: critical role of concomitant exercise left ventricular performance (abstract). J Nucl Med 20:624–625, 1979.

27. Berkow AE, Henkin RE: Double inferior vena cava or iliac vein occlusion? a diagnostic problem in radionuclide venograms. Am J Roentgenol 130:529–531, 1978.

28. Berman DS, Salel AF, DeNardo GL, et al: Clinical assessment of left ventricular regional contraction patterns and ejection fraction by high-resolution gated scintigraphy. J Nucl Med 16:865–874, 1975.

29. Berman DS, Amsterdam EA, Hines HH, et al: New approach to interpretation of technetium-99m pyrophosphate scintigraphy in detection of acute myocardial infarction. Am J Cardiol 39:341–346, 1977.

30. Berman ND, McLaughlin PR, Huckell VF, et al: Prinzmetal's angina with coronary artery spasm: angiographic, pharmacologic, metabolic and radionuclide perfusion studies. Am J Med 60:727–732, 1976.

31. Bianco JA, Shafer RB: Abnormal images of right heart disorders. Clin Nucl Med 4:369–384, 1979.

32. Bianco JA, Laskey WK, Makey DG, et al: Angiotensin infusion effects on left ventricular function. Chest 77:172–175, 1980.

33. Bingham JB, Strauss HW, Pohost GM, et al: Mechanisms of lung uptake of Tl-201 (abstract). Circulation 57–58:II-62, 1978.

33A. Bingham JB, McKusick KA, Boucher CA, et al: Paradoxical septal motion. Sem Nucl Med 11:165–167, 1981.

34. Bingham JB, McKusick KA, Strauss HW: Right atrial enlargement: cardiac imaging. Sem Nucl Med 10:195–196, 1980.

35. Birnholz JC: Alternatives in the diagnosis of abdominal aortic aneurysm: combined use of isotope aortography and ultrasound. Am J Roentgenol 118:809–813, 1973.

36. Blood DK, McCarthy DM, Sciacca RR, et al: Comparison of single-dose and double-dose thallium-201 myocardial perfusion scintigraphy for the detection of coronary artery disease and prior myocardial infarction. Circulation 58:777–778, 1978.

37. Bodenheimer MM, Banka VS, Fooshee CM, et al: Detection of coronary heart disease using radionuclide determined regional ejection fraction at rest and during handgrip exercise: correlation with coronary arteriography. Circulation 58:640–648, 1978.

38. Bonte FJ, Curry TS: Tc-99m human serum albumin blood pool scan in diagnosis of an intracardiac myxoma. J Nucl Med 8:35–39, 1967.

39. Bonte FJ, Christensen EE, Curry TS: Tc^{99m} pertechnetate angiocardiography in the diagnosis of superior mediastinal masses and pericardial effusions. Am J Roentgenol 107:404–412, 1969.

40. Borer JS, Bacharach SL, Green MV, et al: Real-time radionuclide cineangiography in the noninvasive evaluation of global and regional left ventricular function at rest and during exercise in patients with coronary artery disease. N Engl J Med 296:839–844, 1977.

41. Borer JS, Bacharach SL, Green MV, et al: Exercise-induced left ventricular dysfunction in symptomatic and asymptomatic patients with aortic regurgitation: assessment with radionuclide cineangiography. Am J Cardiol 42:351–357, 1978.

42. Borer JS, Bacharach SL, Green MV, et al: Obstructive vs nonobstructive asymmetric septal hypertrophy: differences in left ventricular function with exercise (abstract). Am J Cardiol 41:379, 1978.

43. Borer JS, Bacharach SL, Green MV, et al: Left ventricular function in aortic stenosis: response to exercise and effects of operation (abstract). Am J Cardiol 41:382, 1978.

44. Borer JS, Bacharach SL, Green MV, et al: Effect of nitroglycerin on exercise induced abnormalities of left ventricular regional function and ejection fraction in coronary artery disease: assessment by radionuclide cineangiography in symptomatic and asymptomatic patients. Circulation 57:314–320, 1978.

45. Borer JS, Kent KM, Bacharach SL, et al: Sensitivity, specificity and predictive accuracy of radionuclide cineangiography during exercise in patients with coronary artery disease: comparison with exercise electocardiography. Circulation 60:572–580, 1979.

46. Borer JS, Rosing DR, Kent KM, et al: Left ventricular function at rest and during exercise after aortic valve replacement in patients with aortic regurgitation. Am J Cardiol 44:1297–1304, 1979.

47. Borer JS, Gottdiener JS, Rosing DR, et al: Left ventricular function in mitral regurgitation: determination during exercise (abstract). Circulation 59–60:II-38, 1979.

48. Bosnjackovic VB, Bennett LR, Greenfield LD, et al: Dual isotope method for identification of intracardiac shunts. J Nucl Med 14:514–521, 1973.

49. Botvinick EH, Shames D, Hutchinson JC, et al: Noninvasive diagnosis of a false left ventricular aneurysm with radioisotope gated cardiac blood pool imaging: differentiation from true aneurysm. Am J Cardiol 37:1089–1093, 1976.

50. Botvinick EH, Shames DM, Sharpe DN, et al: The specificity of pyrophosphate myocardial scintigrams in patients with prior myocardial infarction: concise communication. J Nucl Med 19:1121–1125, 1978.

51. Boucher CA, Beller GA, Ahluwalia B, et al: Inhalation imaging for detection and quantitation of left-to-right shunts (abstract). Circulation 53–54:II-145, 1976.

52. Boucher CA, Zir LM, Beller GA, et al: Increased lung uptake of thallium- 201 during exercise myocardial imaging: clinical, hemodynamic and angiographic implications in patients with coronary artery disease. Am J Cardiol 46:189–196, 1980.

53. Brady TJ, Thrall JH, Clare JM, et al: Exercise radionuclide ventriculography: practical considerations and sensitivity of coronary artery disease detection. Radiology 132:697–702, 1979.

53A. Brown KA, Boucher CA, Okada RD: Serial right ventricular thallium imaging following dipyridamole and relationship to right coronary artery disease (abstract). Am J Cardiol 47:484, 1981.

54. Buda AJ, Doherty PW, Goris ML, et al: The value of exercise thallium-201 myocardial perfusion imaging in differentiating subgroups of patients with coronary artery spasm (abstract). Circulation 57–58,II-135, 1978.

55. Bulkley BH, Rouleau J, Strauss HW, et al: Idiopathic hypertrophic subaortic stenosis: detection by thallium-201 myocardial perfusion imaging. N Engl J Med 293:1113–1116, 1975.

56. Bulkley BH, Rouleau JR, Whitaker JQ, et al: The use of [201]Thallium for myocardial perfusion imaging in sarcoid heart disease. Chest 72:27–32, 1977.

57. Bulkley BH, Hutchins GM, Bailey I, et al: Thallium-201 imaging and gated cardiac blood pool scans in patients with ischemic and idiopathic congestive cardiomyopathy: a clinical and pathologic study. Circulation 55:753–760, 1977.

58. Bunko H, Seto H, Tonami N, et al: Detection of active bleeding from ruptured aortic aneurysm. Clin Nucl Med 3:276–277, 1978.

59. Burke G, Halko A. Goldberg D: Dynamic clinical studies with radioisotopes and the scintillation camera: IV. 99mTc-sodium pertechnetate cardiac bloodflow studies. J Nucl Med 10:270–280, 1969.

59A. Campeau RJ, Gottlieb S, Kallus N: Aortic aneurysm detected by 99m-Tc-pyrophosphate imaging. J Nucl Med 18:272–273, 1977.

60. Case records of the Massachusetts General Hospital: (Case 14–1978). N Engl J Med 18:834–842, 1978.

61. Chacko AK, Gordon DH, Bennett JM, et al: Myocardial imaging with Tc-99m pyrophosphate in patients on Adriamycin treatment for neoplasia. J Nucl Med 18:680–683, 1977.

62. Charkes ND, Sklanoff DM: Radioisotope photoscanning as a diagnostic aid in pericardial disease. JAMA 186:920–922, 1963.

63. Charuzi Y, Vyden J, Berman D, et al: Myocardial perfusion by thallium-201 scintigraphy before and after cardiac rehabilitation (abstract). Clin Res 27:158A, 1978.

64. Chen JT, Robinson AE, Goodrich JK, et al: Uneven distribution of pulmonary blood flow between left and right lungs in isolated valvular pulmonary stenosis. Am J Roentgenol 107:343–350, 1969.

65. Chipps BE, Alderson PO, Roland JA, et al: Noninvasive evaluation of ventricular function in cystic fibrosis. J Pediatr 95:379–384, 1979.

66. Christenson J, Larsson I, Svensson SE, et al: Distribution of intravenously injected thallium-201 in the legs during walking: a new test for assessing arterial insufficiency in the legs. Eur J Nucl Med 2:85–88, 1977.

67. Clarke JM, et al: Technetium-99m in diagnosis of left-to-right shunts. Thorax 21:79–82, 1966.

68. Cohen HA, Baird MG, Rouleau JR, et al: Thallium 201 myocardial imaging in patients with pulmonary hypertension. Cardiol 54:790–795, 1976.

69. Cook DJ, Bailey I, Strauss HW, et al: Thallium-201 for myocardial imaging: appearance of the normal heart. J Nucl Med 17:583–589, 1976.

70. Cordoba SA, Figureas CN, Garcia FR: Scintiscanning in venous thrombosis of the lower extremities. Surg Gyn & Obst 145:533–538, 1977.

70A. Covitz W, Eubig C, Balfour IC, et al: Exercise-induced cardiac dysfunction in sickle cell anemia. Am J Cardiol 51:570–575, 1981.

71. Cowley MJ, Coghlan HC, Logic JR: Visualization of atrial myocardium with thallium-201: case report. J Nucl Med 18:984–986, 1977.

72. Cowley MJ, Mantle JA, Rogers WJ, et al: Use of blood-pool imaging in evaluation of diffuse activity patterns in technetium-99m pyrophosphate myocardial scintigraphy. J Nucl Med 20:496–501, 1979.

73. Cox PH, Belfer AJ, van der Pompe WB: Thallium-201 chloride uptake in tumours, a possible complication in heart scintigraphy. Br J Radiol 49:767–768, 1976.

74. Das SK, Brady TJ, Thrall JH, et al: Cardiac function in patients with prior myocarditis. J Nucl Med 21:689–693, 1980.

75. Dash H, Massie BM, Botvinick EH, et al: The non-invasive identification of left main coronary artery disease. Circulation 60:276–284, 1979.

76. Daspit SG, Stemple DR, Doherty PW, et al: Unusual findings in ^{201}Tl-myocardium scintigraphy: the "hot heart" sign. Clin Nucl Med 2:1–5, 1977.

77. Datz FL, Gray WR, Lewis SE, et al: Costal cartilage calcification presenting a doughnut appearance on ^{99m}Tc-pyrophosphate myocardial imaging. Clin Nucl Med 9:83, 1979.

78. Datz FL, Lewis SE, Parkey RW, et al: Radionuclide evaluation of cardiac trauma. Sem Nucl Med 10:187–192, 1980.

79. Davidson R. Spies SM, Przybylek J, et al: Technetium-99m stannous pyrophosphate myocardial scintigraphy after cardiopulmonary resuscitation with cardioversion. Circulation 60:292–296, 1979.

80. DeLand FH, Felman AH: Pericardial tumor compared with pericardial effusion. J Nucl Med 13:697–698, 1972.

81. DeLong SR, Gober AE, Fernandez-Ulloa M, et al: Iliofemoral venous thrombosis in an infant: diagnosis by radionuclide venography. J Pediatr 94:91–93, 1979.

82. Draulans-Noe HA, Evenblij H: The value of radioisotope scanning in the study of pulmonary circulation in patients with tetralogy of Fallot and systemic pulmonary anastomosis. J Nucl Med Biol 16:145–149, 1972.

83. Dymond DS, Elliott AT, Banim S: Detection of a false left ventricular aneurysm by first-pass radionuclide ventriculography. J Nucl Med 20:851–854, 1979.

84. Esser PD: Improved precision in the quantitation of left-to-right shunts (abstract). J Nucl Med 19:740. 1978.

85. Ezekowitz MD, Phil D, Alderson PO, et al: Isolated drainage of the superior vena cava into the left atrium in a 52 year old man: a rare congenital malformation presenting in the adult with cyanosis, polycythemia, and an unsuccessful lung scan. Circulation 58:751–756, 1978.

86. Ferrer PL, Gottlieb S. Kallos N, et al: Application of diagnostic ultrasound and radionuclides to cardiovascular diagnosis: part II, Cardiovascular disease in the young. Sem Nucl Med 4:387–416, 1975.

86A. Fetz RC, Stadalnik RC, Matin P: Myocardial "false positive" 99m-Tc-pyrophosphate scintigrams. Sem Nucl Med 11:64–65, 1981.

87. Finley JP, Howman-Giles R, Gilday DL, et al: Thallium-201 myocardial imaging in anomalous left coronary artery arising from the pulmonary artery: applications before and after medical and surgical treatment. Am J Cardiol 42:675–680, 1978.

88. Finley JP, Howman-Giles RB, Gilday DL, et al: Transient myocardial ischemia of the newborn infant demonstrated by thallium myocardial imaging. J Pediatr 94:263–270, 1979.

88A. Firth BG, Dehmer GJ, Corbett JR, et al: Effect of chronic oral digoxin therapy on ventricular function at rest and peak exercise in patients with ischemic heart disease: assessment with equilibrium gated blood pool imaging. Am J Cardiol 46:481–490, 1980.

89. Fischer KC, Rabinowitch M, Treves S: Myocardial uptake of thallium-201 for estimation of right ventricular pressures (abstract). J Nucl Med 19:725–726, 1978.

90. Flaherty JT, Canent RV, Boineau JP, et al: Use of externally recorded radioisotope-dilution curves for quantification of left-to-right shunts. Am J Cardiol 20:341–345, 1967.

91. Fleg JL, Siegel BA, Roberts R: Detection of pericarditis with ^{99m}Tc-pyrophosphate images (abstract). Am J Cardiol 39:273, 1977.

92. Flesh LH, Kihm RH, Ciccio SS: Radionuclide imaging of aortic involvement in Buerger's disease: case report. J Nucl Med 18:125–127, 1977.

93. Folse R, Braunwald E: Pulmonary vascular dilution curves recorded by external detection in the diagnosis of left-to-right shunts. Br Heart J 24:166–172, 1962.

94. Foster C, Anholm J. Hellman C, et al: Left ventricular function during sudden strenuous exercise. Circulation 63:592–596, 1981.

95. Freedom RM, Treves S: Splenic scintigraphy and radionuclide venography in the heterotaxy syndrome. Radiology 107:381–386, 1973.

96. Friedman ML, Cantor RE: Reliability of gated heart scintigrams for detection of left-ventricular aneurysm: concise communication. J Nucl Med 20:720–723, 1979.

97. Friedman WF, Braunwald E: Alterations in regional pulmonary blood flow in mitral valve disease studies by radioisotope scanning. Circulation 34:363–376, 1966.

98. Friedman WF, Braunwald E, Morrow AG: Alterations in regional pulmonary blood flow in patients with congenital heart disease. Circulation 37:747–758, 1968.

98A. Froelich RT, Falsetti HL, Doty DB, et al: Prospective study of surgery for left ventricular aneurysm. Am J Cardiol 45:923–931, 1980.

99. Gabriele AR, North L, Pircher FH, et al: Aneurysmal dilatation of the superior vena cava. J Nucl Med 13:227–229, 1972.

100. Gates GF: Radionuclide Scanning in Cyanotic Heart Disease. Springfield, IL: Charles C Thomas, 1974.

101. Gates GF, Orme HW, Dore EK: Measurement of cardiac shunting with technetium labelled albumin. J Nucl Med 12:746–749, 1971.

102. Gates GF, Orme HW, Dore EK: Cardiac shunt assessment with macroaggregated albumin technetium-99m. Radiology 112:649–653, 1974.

103. Gates GF, Orme HW, Dore EK: The hyperperfused lung: detection in congenital heart disease. JAMA 233:782–786, 1975.

104. Gates GF, Orme HW, Dore EK: Surgical systemic-pulmonic shunt assessment (abstract). J Nucl Med 16:528, 1975.

105. Gates GF, Orme HW, Dore EK: Surgery of congenital heart disease assessed by radionuclide scintigraphy. J Thor Cardiovasc Surg 69:769–775, 1975.

106. Gates GF, Goris ML: Suitability of radiopharmaceuticals for determining right-to-left shunting. J Nucl Med 18:255–257, 1977.

107. Gelfand MJ, Janos GG, Schwartz DC, et al: Post-operative evaluation of the Fontan procedure by radionuclide angiography (abstract). J Nucl Med 22:90, 1981.

108. Gelfand MJ, Breitweser J, Dillon T, et al: Comparison of scintigraphic and echocardiographic methods for estimation of left-to-right shunts (abstract). J Nucl Med 19:597, 1979.

109. Gelfand MJ: Unpublished observation.

110. Gerson MC, Noble RJ, Faris JV, et al: Noninvasive documentation of Prinzmetal's angina. Am J Cardiol 43:329–334, 1979.

111. Gerson MC: Unpublished observation.

112. Gerwirtz H, Beller GA, Strauss HW, et al: Transient defects of resting thallium scans in patients with coronary artery disease. Circulation 59:707–713, 1979.
113. Gilday DL, Howman-Giles RB, Rowe R: Combined thallium-201 myocardial imaging and multiple gated blood pool studies in children (abstract). Am J Cardiol 41:442, 1978.
113A. Giles R, Berger H, Barash P, et al: Profound alterations in left ventricular performance during anesthesia induction for coronary surgery detected with the computerized nuclear probe (abstract). Circulation 62:III-146, 1980.
114. Girod DA, Faris J, Hurwitz RA, et al: Thallium-201 assessment of myocardial perfusion in coronary artery anomalies in children (abstract). Am J Cardiol 41:419, 1978.
115. Glass EC, Hansen SK, Dublin AB, et al: Detection of superior mesenteric artery aneurysm by radionuclide angiography: brief case report. Radiology 129:122, 1978.
116. Go RT, Doty DB, Chiu CL, et al: A new method of diagnosing myocardial contusion in man by radionuclide imaging. Radiology 116:107–110, 1975.
117. Goldman S, Hager WD, Woolfenden JM, et al: Microsphere perfusion defects in patients with valvular and primary myocardial disease and normal coronary arteries (abstract). Am J Cardiol 39:272, 1977.
117A. Goncalves da Rocha AF, Meguerian BA, Harbert JC: Tc-99m pyrophosphate myocardial scanning in Chagas' disease. J Nucl Med 22:347–348, 1981.
118. Goodenow JS, Kolibash AJ, Bush CA, et al: Improved myocardial perfusion and contractility following coronary bypass to areas of apparent old infarction. Circulation 53–54:II-208, 1976.
119. Goolsby J, Steele P, Kirch D, et al: Square left ventricle: angiographic and radionuclide sign of left ventricular thrombus. Radiology 115:533–537, 1975.
120. Gooneratne N, Conway JJ: Radionuclide angiographic diagnosis of bronchopulmonary sequestration. J Nucl Med 17:1035–1037, 1979.
121. Gordon DG, Pfisterer M, Williams R, et al: The effect of diaphragmatic attenuation of ^{201}Tl images. Clin Nucl Med 4:150–152, 1979.
121A. Gottdiener JS, Borer JS, Bacharach SL, et al: Left ventricular function in mitral valve prolapse: assessment with radionuclide cineangiography. Am J Cardiol 47:7–13, 1981.
122. Graham TP, Goodrich JK, Robinson AE, et al: Scintiangiocardiography in children: rapid sequence visualization of the heart and great vessels after intravenous injection of radionuclide. Am J Cardiol 25:387–394, 1974.
123. Greenfield LD, Bennett LR: Comparison of heart chamber and pulmonary dilution curves for the diagnosis of cardiac shunts. Radiology 111:359–363, 1974.
124. Greenspan M, Iskandrian AS, Croll MN, et al: Exercise myocardial scintigraphy in patients with mitral valve prolapse (abstract). Clin Res 27:172A, 1979.
125. Gutgesell HP, DePuey EG: Thallium myocardial perfusion imaging in infants and children: value in distinguishing anomalous left coronary artery from congestive cardiomyopathy (abstract). Am J Cardiol 43:402, 1979.
126. Hagen AD, Friedman WF, Ashburn WL, et al: Further application of scintillation scanning technics to the diagnosis and management of infants and children with congenital heart disease. Circulation 45:858–868, 1972.
127. Harford W, Weinberg MN, Buja LM, et al: Positive ^{99m}Tc-stannous pyrophosphate myocardial image in a patient with carcinoma of the lung. Radiology 122:747–748, 1977.
128. Haroutunian LM, Neill CA, Wagner H: Radioisotope scanning of the lung in cyanotic congenital heart disease. Am J Cardiol 23:387–395, 1969.
129. Hecht HS, Hopkins JM, Blumfield DE, et al: Reverse redistribution: worsening of thallium-201 images from exercise to redistribution (abstract). J Nucl Med 20:650, 1979.
130. Hellenbrand WE, Berger HJ, O'Brien RT, et al: Left ventricular performance in thalassemia: combined noninvasive radionuclide and echocardiographic assessment (abstract).

Circulation 56:III-49, 1977.

131. Hirzel HO, Neusch K, Gruentzig AR, et al: Thallium-201 exercise scintigraphy after percutaneous transluminal angioplasty of coronary artery stenosis. Med Clin North Am 64:163–176, 1980.

132. Holman BL, Chisholm RJ, Braunwald E: The prognostic implications of acute myocardial infarct scintigraphy with ^{99m}Tc-pyrophosphate. Circulation 57:302–326, 1978.

132A. Holman BL, Wynne J, Idoine S, et al: Disruption in the temporal sequence of regional ventricular contraction. I: Characteristics and incidence in coronary artery disease. Circulation 61:1075–1083, 1980.

133. Holmes RA, Silbigen ML, Karmen A, et al: Cardiac scanning with technetium-99m labelled albumin. JAMA 198:67–72, 1966.

133A. Hooper W, Slutsky R, Kocienski D, et al: The effect of terbutaline on right and left ventricular function and size in obstructive lung disease (abstract). Am J Cardiol 47:491, 1981.

134. Hopkins GB, Kan MK, Salel AF: Scintigraphic assessment of left ventricular aneurysms. JAMA 240:2162–2165, 1978.

135. Huckell VF, Staniloff HM, Feiglin DH, et al: The demonstration of segmental perfusion defects in hypertrophic cardiomyopathy imitating coronary artery disease (abstract). Am J Cardiol 41:438, 1978.

136. Huckell VF, Staniloff HM, Feiglin DH, et al: Massive pericardial effusion due to idiopathic cholesterol pericarditis detected during ^{99m}Tc-pyrophosphate imaging. Clin Nucl Med 3:409–410, 1978.

137. Huckell VF, Kinahan PJ, Morrison RT, et al: Abnormal right and left ventricular myocardial perfusion in patients with isolated mitral stenosis, angina and normal coronary arteries (abstract). Clin Res 27:176A, 1979.

138. Hung J, Harris PJ, Kelly DT, et al: Improvement of left ventricular function in alcoholic cardiomyopathy documented by serial gated cardiac pool scanning. Aust N Z J Med 9:420–422, 1979.

139. Hung J, Harris PH, Uren RF, et al: Uremic cardiomyopathy: effect of hemodialysis on left ventricular function in end-stage renal failure. N Engl J Med 302:547–551, 1980.

139A. Hung J, Uren RF, Richmond DR, et al: The mechanism of abnormal septal motion in atrial septal defect: pre- and postoperative study by radionuclide ventriculography in adults. Circulation 63:142–148, 1981.

140. Hurley PH, Strauss HW, Wagner HN: Radionuclide angiocardiography in cyanotic congenital heart disease. Johns Hopkins Med J 127:46–54, 1970.

141. Hurley PH, Strauss HW, Wagner HN: Radionuclide angiocardiography and cineangiography in screening patients for cardiac disease (abstract). J Nucl Med 11:633, 1970.

142. Hurley PJ: Patent foramen ovale demonstrated by lung scanning. J Nucl Med 12:177–179, 1972.

143. Hurley PJ, Wesselhoeft H, James AE, Jr.: Use of nuclear imaging in the evaluation of pediatric cardiac disease. Sem Nucl Med 2:353–372, 1981.

144. Isley JR, Jr, Reinhardt JF: Intracardiac myxoma demonstrated on a vascular scan. Am J Roentgenol 88:70–72, 1962.

144A. Jablonsky G, Feiglin D, Hilton D, et al: A study of ventricular function in ventricular septal defects at rest and after exercise (abstract). J Nucl Med 21:5, 1980.

145. Jaffe AS, Klein MS, Patel BR, et al: Abnormal technetium-99m-pyrophosphate in unstable angina: ischemia versus infarction. Am J Cardiol 44: 1035–1039, 1979.

146. Janowitz WR, Serafini AN: Intense myocardial uptake of ^{99m}Tc-diphosphonate in uremic patient with secondary hyperparathyroidism and pericarditis: case report. J Nucl Med 17:896–898, 1976.

147. Jengo JA, Mena I, Joe SH, et al: The significance of calcific valvular heart disease in Tc-99m pyrophosphate myocardial infarction scanning: radiographic, scintigraphic, and pathological correlation. J Nucl Med 18: 776–781, 1977.

148. Johnson LL, McCarthy D, Sciacca R, et al: Right ventricular ejection fraction during exercise in patients with coronary artery disease (abstract). Circulation 57–58:II-61, 1978.

149. Johnson LL, McCarthy D, Sciacca R, et al: Right ventricular ejection fraction during exercise patients with coronary artery disease. Circulation 60:1284–1291, 1979.

150. Johnson PM, Boxer RA, Esser PD, et al: Quantitative pulmonary radioangiography: a reliable method for measuring left-to-right shunts (abstract). J Nucl Med 197:45, 1978.

151. Johnson WC, Patten DH, Widrich WC, et al: Technetium 99m isotope venography. Am J Surg 127:424–428, 1974.

152. Johnstone DE, Wackers FJTh, Berger JH, et al: Effect of patient positioning on left lateral thallium-201 myocardial images. J Nucl Med 20:183–188, 1979.

153. Jones DM, Winn WR: Diagnosis of intracardiac thrombus by ^{99m}Tc-MAA scintiscanning. Radiology 122:175–176, 1977.

154. Kent KM, Borer JS, Green MV, et al: Effects of coronary-artery bypass on global and regional left ventricular function during exercise. N Engl J Med 298:1434–1439, 1978.

154A. Kerber G, Ryan JW, et al: Enterococcal endocarditis: a rare cause of focal cardiac uptake in infarct and myocardial scintigraphy. Arch Int Med 142:1360–1362, 1982.

155. Khaja F, Alam M, Goldstein S, et al: Diagnostic value of visualization of the right ventricle using thallium-201 myocardial imaging. Circulation 59:182–188, 1979.

156. Kinney EL, Jackson GL, Reeves WC, et al: The prevalence of sarcoid heart disease detected by thallium scanning (abstract). Am J Cardiol 43:437, 1979.

157. Kinoshita M, Nakao K, Nohara Y, et al: Detection of circulatory shunts by means of external counting methods. Jap Circ J 33:815–821, 1969.

158. Klausner SC, Botvinick EH, Shames D, et al: The application of radionuclide infarct scintigraphy to diagnose perioperative myocardial infarction following revascularization. Circulation 56:173–181, 1977.

159. Klein GJ, Kostuk WJ: Diagnostic accuracy of non-invasive stress myocardial perfusion imaging (abstract). Circulation 53–54:II-207, 1976.

160. Klein GJ, Kostuk WJ, Boughner DR, et al: Stress myocardial imaging in mitral leaflet prolapse syndrome. Am J Cardiol 42:746–750, 1978.

161. Kolibash AJ, Call TD, Bush CA, et al: Comparative usefulness of exercise thallium 201 imaging and resting intracoronary particle distribution (abstract). J Nucl Med 19:751, 1978.

162. Kondo M, Kubo A, Yamazaki H, et al: Thallium-201 myocardial imaging for evaluation of right-ventricular overloading. J Nucl Med 19:1197–1203, 1978.

163. Konstam MA, Levine BW, Strauss HW, et al: Left superior vena cava to left atrial communication diagnosed with radionuclide angiocardiography and with differential right to left shunting. Am J Cardiol 43:149–153, 1979.

163A. Korr KS, Gandsman ES, Winkler ML, et al: Hemodynamic correlates of right ventricular ejection fraction measured by equilibrium gated radionuclide angiography (abstract). Circulation 62:III-148, 1980.

164. Kriss JP, Yeh SH, Farrer PA, et al: Radioisotope angiocardiography (abstract). J Nucl Med 7:67, 1966.

165. Kriss JP: Diagnosis of pericardial effusion by radioisotopic angiocardiography. J Nucl Med 10:233–241, 1969.

166. Kriss JP, Enright LP, Hayden WG, et al: Radioisotopic angiocardiography: wide scope of applicability in diagnosis and evaluation of therapy in diseases of the heart and great

vessels. Circulation 43:792–808, 1971.

167. Kriss JP, Enright LP, Hayden WG, et al: Radioisotopic angiocardiography: Pre-operative and post-operative evaluation of patients with diseases of the heart and great vessels. Radiol Clin North Am 9:369–383, 1971.

168. Kriss JP, Enright LP, Hayden WG, et al: Radioisotopic angiocardiography: findings in congenital heart disease. J Nucl Med 13:31–40, 1972.

169. Kushner FG, Okada RD, Kirshenbuam HD, et al: Pulmonary thallium-201 after stress in patients with coronary artery disease (abstract). Clin Res 27:182A, 1979.

169A. Lahiri A, Spencer J, Crawley JW, et al: Pulmonary uptake of thallium 201 in acute pulmonary edema. Br J Radiol 55:460–462, 1982.

170. Lam W, Pavel D, Byrom E, et al: Radionuclide regurgitant index: value and limitations. Am J Cardiol 47:292–298, 1981.

171. Landgarten S, Gordon R: Radionuclide demonstrations of Adriamycin-induced cardiac toxicity. Clin Nucl Med 2:429–430, 1977.

172. Lane SD, Patton DD, Staab EV, et al: Simple techniques for rapid bolus injection. J Nucl Med 12:118–119, 1972.

172A. Laver MB, Strauss HW, Pohost GM: Right and left ventricular geometry: adjustments during acute respiratory failure. Crit Care Med 7:509–519, 1979.

173. Lee KR, Robinson RG, Neff JR: Demonstration of a false aneurysm of the extremity by dynamic radionuclide scintigraphy. AJR 129:931–932, 1977.

173A. LeJemtel TH, Keung E, Ribner HS, et al: Sustained beneficial effects of oral amrinone on cardiac and renal function in patients with severe congestive heart failure. Am J Cardiol 45:123–129, 1980.

174. Leon MB, Borer JS, Bacharach SL, et al: Detection of early cardiac dysfunction in patients with severe beta-thalassemia and chronic iron overload. N Engl J Med 301:1143–1148, 1979.

175. Levine FH: Radionuclide and hemodynamic assessment of pulmonary hypertension and right ventricular function after mitral valve replacement (abstract). Am J Cardiol 43:406, 1979.

176. Lewis RJ, Bogel JM: Emergency cardiac photoscan. JAMA 205:27–30, 1968.

177. Liberthson RR, Pohost GM, Dinsmore RE, et al: Atrial septal defect—pre and postoperative evaluation by gated cardiac scanning (abstract). J Nucl Med 19:750–751, 1978.

178. Liberthson RR, Boucher CA, Strauss HW, et al: Right ventricular function in adult atrial septal defect. Am J Cardiol 47:56–66, 1981.

179. Lin C-Y: Lung scan in cardiopulmonary disease: I. Tetralogy of Fallot. J Thoracic Cardiovasc Surg 61:370–379, 1971.

180. Lisbona R: Myocardial visualization on a lung scan. Clin Nucl Med 3:157, 1978.

180A. Lubell DL, Goldfarb DR: Metastatic cardiac tumor demonstrated by 201-thallium scan. Chest 78:98–99, 1980.

181. Maddahi J, Berman D, Matsuoka D, et al: Right ventricular ejection fraction during exercise in coronary artery disease by multiple gated equilibrium scintigraphy (abstract). Circulation 57–58:II-131, 1978.

182. Maddahi J, Gray R, Berman D, et al: Scintigraphic and hemodynamic demonstration of transient left ventricular dysfunction immediately after uncomplicated coronary artery bypass graft surgery (abstract). J Nucl Med 19:735, 1978.

182A. Makler PT, Lavine SJ, Denenberg BS, et al: Redistribution on the thallium scan in myocardial sarcoidosis: concise communication. J Nucl Med 22:428–432, 1981.

183. Malin FR, Rollo FD, Gertz EW: Sequential myocardial scintigraphy with technetium-99m stannous pyrophosphate following myocardial infarction. J Nucl Med 19:1111–1115, 1978.

184. Maltz DL, Treves S: Quantitative radionuclide angiocardiography: determination of Qp:Qs in children. Circulation 47:1049–1056, 1973.
185. Marshall RC, Berger HJ, Reduto LA, et al: Assessment of cardiac performance with quantitative radionuclide angiocardiography: effect of oral propranolol on global and regional left ventricular function in coronary artery disease. Circulation 58:808–814, 1978.
186. Marshall R, Wisenberg G, Schelbert H, et al: Radionuclide evaluation of the effect of oral propranolol on left ventricular function during exercise in patients with coronary artery disease (abstract). Am J Cardiol 43: 398, 1979.
187. Maseri A, Parodi O, Severi S, et al: Transient transmural reduction of myocardial blood flow, demonstrated by thallium-201 scintigraphy, as a cause of variant angina. Circulation 54:280–288, 1976.
188. Mason JW, Myers RW, Alderman EL, et al: Technetium-99m pyrophosphate myocardial uptake in patients with stable angina pectoris. Am J Cardiol 40:1–5, 1977.
189. Massie BM, Botvinick EH, Werner JA, et al: Myocardial scintigraphy with technetium-99m stannous pyrophosphate: an insensitive test for nontransmural myocardial infarction. Am J Cardiol 43:186–192, 1979.
190. Matin P, Ray G, Kriss JP: Combined superior vena cava obstruction and pericardial effusion demonstrated by radioisotopic angiocardiography. J Nucl Med 11:78–80, 1970.
191. Matin P, Kriss JP: Radioisotopic angiocardiography: findings in mitral stenosis and mitral insufficiency. J Nucl Med 11:723–730, 1970.
192. Matin P, Glass EC, Villarica J: Peripheral radionuclide angiography. JAMA 242:1781–1784, 1979.
193. Matthay RA, Berger JH, Loke J, et al: Effects of aminophylline upon right and left ventricular performance in chronic obstructive lung disease: noninvasive assessment by radionuclide angiography. Am J Med 65:903–910, 1979.
194. McClelland RR: Congenital aneurysmal dilatation of the left auricle demonstrated by sequential cardiac blood-pool scintiscanning. J Nucl Med 19:507–509, 1978.
195. McDaniel MM, Coleman JM, Morton ME: Inferior vena cava obstruction due to plasmacytoma demonstrated on phlebography using ^{99m}Tc macroaggregated albumin. Clin Nucl Med 2:135–136, 1977.
196. McGowan RL, Welch TG, Zaret BL, et al: Noninvasive myocardial imaging with potassium-43 and rubidium-81 in patients with left bundle branch block. Am J Cardiol 38:422–428, 1976.
197. McKusick KA, Bingham JB, Pohost GM, et al: Gated cardiac scan analysis of interventricular septal motion following aortic valve surgery (abstract). Circulation 53–54:II-208, 1976.
198. McKusick KA, Bingham JB, Pohost GM, et al: The gated first pass radionuclide angiogram: a method for measurement of right ventricular ejection fraction (abstract). Circulation 57–58:II-130, 1978.
199. Meyers SN, Shapiro JE, Barresi V, et al: Right atrial myxoma with right to left shunt and mitral valve prolapse. Am J Med 62:308–314, 1977.
200. Mishkin F, Knote J: Radioisotope scanning of lungs in patients with systemic-pulmonary anastomoses. Am J Roentgenol 102:267–273, 1968.
200A. Mishkin FS: Lung curve indicating a left-to-right shunt in an infant with a large heart. Sem Nucl Med 11:161–164, 1981.
201. Mishkin FS, Mishkin ME: Documentation of tricuspid regurgitation by radionuclide angiocardiography. Br Heart J 36:1019–1022, 1974.
202. Miyamae T, Fujioka M, Tsubogo Y, et al: Detection of a large arteriovenous fistula between the internal iliac vessels by radionuclide angiography. J Nucl Med 20:36–38,

1979.

203. Muster A, Paul M, Levin D, et al: Diminished left pulmonary artery flow in transposition of the great arteries (abstract). Am J Cardiol 31:150, 1973.

203A. Muz J, Wizenberg T, Samlowski W, et al: Myocardial uptake of technetium-99m pyrophosphate in patients with amyloidosis (abstract). J Nucl Med 21:49, 1980.

204. Neill C, Kelly D, Bailey I, et al: Thallium-201 myocardial scintigraphy in single ventricle (abstract). Circulation 53–54:II-46, 1976.

205. Nichols AB, Pohost GM, Gold HK, et al: Left ventricular function during intra-aortic balloon pumping assessed by multigated cardiac blood pool imaging. Circulation 58:I-176–I-183, 1978.

206. Nichols AB, McKusick KA, Strauss HW, et al: Clinical utility of gated cardiac blood pool imaging in congestive left heart failure. Am J Med 65:785–793, 1978.

207. Okada RD, Pohost GM, Kirshenbaum HD, et al: Radionuclide-determined change in pulmonary blood volume with exercise: improved sensitivity of multigated blood-pool scanning in detecting coronary-artery disease. N Engl J Med 301:569–576, 1979.

208. Oldham HN, Simpson K, Jones RH, et al: Differential distribution of pulmonary blood flow following aortopulmonary anastomosis. Surg Forum 21:201–202, 1970.

209. Olson HG, Lyons KP, Aronow WS, et al: Prognostic value of a persistently positive technetium-99m stannous pyrophosphate myocardial scintigram after myocardial infarction. Am J Cardiol 43:889–898, 1979.

210. Olson HG, Lyons KP, Aronow WS, et al: Technetium-99m stannous pyrophosphate myocardial scintigrams in pericardial disease. Am Heart J 99:459–467, 1980.

211. Olvey SK, Reduto LA, Deaton WJ, et al: First pass radionuclide assessment of right and left ventricular performance in chronic lung disease: effect of oxygen upon exercise reserve (abstract). Clin Res 27:192A, 1979.

212. Owens WI: Personal communication.

213. Oxley DK, Bolton MR, Shaeffer C, et al: Intracoronary myocardial perfusion imaging: patterns in patients with coronary artery disease. Clin Nucl Med 3:99–102, 1978.

214. Park HM, Smith ET, Silberstein EB: Isolated right superior vena cava draining into the left atrium diagnosed by radionuclide angiocardiography. J Nucl Med 14:240–242, 1973.

214A. Pavel DG, Zimmer AM, Patterson JM: In-vivo labelling of red blood cells with ^{99m}Tc: a new approach to blood pool visualization. J Nucl Med 18:305–308, 1977.

215. Perez LA, Hayt DB, Freeman LM: Localization of myocardial disorders other than infarction with ^{99m}Tc-labelled phosphate agents. J Nucl Med 17:241–242, 1973.

216. Perkins PJ: Radioisotopic diagnosis of false left ventricular aneurysm. Am J Roentgenol 132:117–119, 1979.

217. Pohost GM, Pastore JO, McKusick KA, et al: Detection of left atrial myxoma by gated radionuclide cardiac imaging. Circulation 55:88–92, 1977.

218. Pohost GM, Vignola PA, McKusick KA, et al: Hypertrophic cardiomyopathy: evaluation by gated cardiac blood pool scanning. Circulation 55:92–99, 1977.

219. Pohost GM, Zir LM, Moore RH, et al: Differentiation of transiently ischemic from infarcted myocardium by serial imaging after a single dose of thallium-201. Circulation 55:294–302, 1977.

220. Poliner LR, Buja LM, Parkey RW, et al: Clinicopathologic findings in 52 patients studied by technetium-99m stannous pyrophosphate myocardial scintigraphy. Circulation 59:257–267, 1979.

220A. Port S, Cobb FR, Coleman ER, et al: Effect of age on the response of the left ventricular ejection fraction to exercise. N Engl J Med 303:1133–1137, 1980.

221. Powers TA, Harolds JA, Kadir S, et al: Pseudoaneurysm of the profunda femoris artery

diagnosed on angiographic phase of bone scan. Clin Nucl Med 4:422–424, 1979.

222. Prasquier R, Taradash MR, Botvinick EH, et al: The specificity of the diffuse pattern of cardiac uptake in myocardial infarction imaging with technetium-99m stannous pyrophosphate. Circulation 55:61–66, 1977.

223. Pugh BR, Parkey RW, Bonte FJ, et al: Cardioversion and its potential role in the production of "false positive" technetium-99m stannous pyrophosphate myocardial scintigrams (abstract). Am J Cardiol 37:163, 1976.

224. Pulido JI, Doss J, Blomqvist GC, et al: Submaximal exercise testing after acute myocardial infarction: myocardial scintigraphic and electrocardiographic observations. Am J Cardiol 42:19–28, 1978.

225. Puri S, Spencer RP, Moskowitz H, et al: Partial obstruction of left brachiocephalic vein by a goiter. Clin Nucl Med 1:246, 1976.

226. Puyau FA, Meckstroth GR: Evaluation of pulmonary perfusion patterns in children with tetralogy of Fallot. Am J Roentgenol 122:119–124, 1974.

227. Quaife MA, Wilson WJ: Detection of cardiac tumor by rectilinear imaging with ^{131}Cs. J Nucl Med 11:605–607, 1970.

228. Quaife MA, Boschult P, Baltaxe HA, Jr., et al: Myocardial accumulation of labeled phosphate in malignant pericardial effusion. J Nucl Med 20:392–396, 1979.

229. Rabinovitch M, Rowland TW, Castaneda AR, et al: Thallium 201 scintigraphy in patients with anomalous origin of the left coronary artery from the main pulmonary artery. J Pediatr 94:244–247, 1979.

230. Rainwater JO, Jenson DP, Kirch DL, et al: Improvement in myocardial perfusion images and exercise ejection fraction with propranolol in patients with coronary artery disease (abstract). Circulation 57–58:II-62, 1978.

231. Rainwater JO, Jenson DP, Vogel RA, et al: Effects of chronic digitalis administration on exercise ventricular performance and myocardial perfusion images in coronary disease (abstract). Am J Cardiol 43:433, 1979.

232. Reduto LA, Berger HJ, Cohen LS, et al: Sequential radionuclide assessment of left and right ventricular performance after acute transmural myocardial infarction. Ann Intern Med 89:441–447, 1978.

233. Reduto LA, Berger HJ, Johnstone DE, et al: Radionuclide assessment of exercise right and left ventricular performance following total correction of tetralogy of Fallot. Am J Cardiol 45:1013–1018, 1980.

234. Rejali AM, MacIntyre WJ, Friedell HL: A radioisotope method for the visualization of cardiac blood pools. Am J Roentgenol 79:129–137, 1958.

235. Rerych SK, Scholz PM, Newman GE, et al: Cardiac function at rest and during exercise in normals and in patients with coronary heart disease. Ann Surg 187:449–463, 1978.

236. Righetti A, O'Rourke RA, Schelbert H, et al: Usefulness of preoperative and postoperative Tc-99m (Sn)-pyrophosphate scans in patients with ischemic and valvular heart disease. Am J Cardiol 39:43–49, 1977.

237. Righetti A, Crawford MH, O'Rourke RA, et al: Interventricular septal motion and left ventricular function after coronary bypass surgery: evaluation with echocardiography and radionuclide angiography. Am J Cardiol 39:372–377, 1977.

238. Rigo P, Murray M, Strauss HW, et al: Scintiphotographic evaluation of patients with suspected left ventricular aneurysm. Circulation 50:985–991, 1974.

239. Rigo P, Murray M, Strauss HW, et al: Left ventricular function in acute myocardial infarction evaluated by gated scintiphotography. Circulation 50:678–684, 1974.

240. Rigo P, Murray M, Taylor DR, et al: Right ventricular dysfunction detected by gated scintiphotography in patients with acute inferior myocardial infarction. Circulation 52:268–274, 1975.

241. Rigo P, Alderson PO, Robertson RM, et al: Measurement of aortic and mitral regurgitation by gated cardiac blood pool scans. Circulation 60:306–312, 1979.

241A. Rigo P, Chevigné M: Measurement of left to right shunts by gated cardiac blood pool scans: a new technique, in Radioaktive Isotope in Klinik und Forschung. Vienna; Gasteiner Internationales Symposium, Verlag Egermann, 1980, 337–343.

242. Rihimaki E, Heiskanen A, Tahti E: Theory of quantitative determination of intracardiac shunts by external detection. Ann Clin Res 6:45–49, 1974.

243. Ritchie JL, Hamilton GW, Williams DL, et al: Myocardial imaging with radionuclide-labelled particles: analysis of the normal image, abnormal image and technical considerations. Radiology 121:131–138, 1976.

244. Ritchie JL, Narahara KA, Trobaugh GB, et al: Thallium-201 myocardial imaging before and after coronary revascularization: assessment of regional myocardial blood flow and graft patency. Circulation 56:830–836, 1977.

245. Ritchie JL, Hamilton GW, Wackers FT: Thallium-201 Myocardial Imaging. New York: Raven, 1978.

246. Ritchie JL, Azret BL, Strauss HW, et al: Myocardial imaging with thallium-201: a multicenter study in patients with angina pectoris or acute myocardial infarction. Am J Cardiol 42:345–350, 1978.

247. Ritchie JL, Sorensen SG, Narahara KA, et al: Radionuclide ejection fraction: prediction of Adriamycin cardiotoxicity (abstract). J Nucl Med 19:671, 1978.

248. Ritchie JL, Sorensen SG, Kennedy JW, et al: Radionuclide angiography: noninvasive assessment of hemodynamic changes after administration of nitroglycerin. Am J Cardiol 43:278–284, 1979.

249. Rosenthall L: Nucleographic screening of patients for left-to-right shunts. Radiology 99:601–604, 1971.

250. Rosenthall L, Mercer EN: Intravenous radionuclide cardiography for the detection of cardiovascular shunts. Radiology 106:601–606, 1973.

251. Rosenthall L: Qualitative and quantitative analysis of radionuclide cardiopulmonary histograms. CRC Rev Clin Radiol Nucl Med 5:479–493, 1974.

252. Rosenthall L: Intravenous radionuclide angiography in the diagnosis of trauma. Sem Nucl Med 4:395–409, 1974.

252A. Rowe DW, Depuey EG, Sonnemaker RE, et al: Left ventricular performance during exercise in patients with left bundle branch block (abstract). Circulation 62:III-147, 1980.

253. Rude R, Parkey RW, Bonte FJ, et al: Clinical implications of the ''doughnut'' pattern of uptake in myocardial imaging with technetium-99m stannous pyrophosphate (abstract). Circulation 55:III-146, 1977.

254. Ryo UY, Lee JI, Zarnow H, et al: Radionuclide angiography with ^{99m}Tc-labelled red blood cells for the detection of aortic aneurysm. J Nucl Med 15:1014–1017, 1974.

255. Ryo UY, Lee JI, Pinsky SM: Radionuclide venography in the upper extremity. Clin Nucl Med 1:242–244, 1977.

256. Ryo UY, Qazi M, Srikantaswamy S, et al: Radionuclide venography: correlation with contrast venography. J Nucl Med 18:11–17, 1977.

257. Salel AF, Berman DS, DeNardo GL, et al: Radionuclide assessment of nitroglycerin influence on abnormal left ventricular segmental contraction in patients with coronary heart disease. Circulation 53:975–981, 1976.

258. Samuels LD, Stewart C: Rapid diagnosis of pericardial effusion with Tc-99m pertechnetate. J Pediatr 76:125–128, 1970.

259. Sarreck R, Sham R, Alexander LL, et al: Increased ^{99m}Tc-pyrophosphate uptake with radiation pneumonitis. Clin Nucl Med 4:403–404, 1979.

260. Schelbert HR, Henning H, Ashburn WL, et al: Serial measurements of left ventricular ejection fraction by radionuclide angiography early and late after myocardial infarction. Am J Cardiol 38:407–417, 1976.

261. Schwartz H, Berkow AE: Radionuclide angiography as an adjunct in diagnosis of ruptured aortic aneurysm: case report. J Nucl Med 17:1065–1066, 1976.

261A. Schoolmeester WL, Simpson AG, Saverbrunn BJ, et al: Radionuclide angiographic assessment of left ventricular function during exercise in patients with a severely reduced ejection fraction. Am J Cardiol 47:804–809, 1981.

262. Seward JB, Nolan NG, Tancredi RG: Rapid quantitation of left-to-right intracardiac shunts by use of a computer-interfaced gamma camera, in Proceedings of the Fifth Symposium on Sharing of Computer Programs and Technology in Nuclear Medicine, Salt Lake City, Utah, Jan. 15–16, 1975 (Conf—750124), 66–67.

263. Shah PK, Berman D, Pichler M, et al: Improved global and regional ventricular performance with nitroprusside in acute myocardial infarction (abstract). J Nucl Med 20:641 1979.

264. Shah PK, Pichler M, Berman DS, et al: Left ventricular ejection fraction determined by radionuclide ventriculography in early stages of first transmural myocardial infarction. Am J Cardiol 45:542–546, 1980.

264A. Sharpe DN, Botvinick EH, Shames DM, et al: The non-invasive diagnosis of right ventricular infarction. Circulation 57:483–490, 1978.

265. Sheikh AI, Swiryn SP, Pavel DG: Visualization of atrial myocardium with thallium-201: case report. Clin Nucl Med 6:34–37, 1981.

266. Siegel ME, Siemsen JK: A new noninvasive approach to peripheral vascular disease: thallium-201 leg scans. Am J Roentgenol 131:827–830, 1978.

266A. Siegel RJ, O'Connor B, Mena I, et al: Left ventricular function in scleroderma (abstract). Circulation 62:III-319, 1980.

267. Simpson AJ: Malignant pericardial effusion diagnosed by combined ^{67}Ga-citrate and ^{99m}Tc-pertechnetate scintigraphy. Clin Nucl Med 3:445–446, 1978.

268. Singh A, Usher M, Raphael L: Pericardial accumulation of Tc-99m methylene diphosphonate in a case of pericarditis. J Nucl Med 18:1141–1142, 1977.

269. Slutsky R, Ackerman W, Hooper W, et al: The response of left ventricular ejection fraction and volume to supine exercise in patients with severe COPD (abstract). Circulation 59–60:II-234, 1979.

270. Slutsky R, Hooper W, Gerber K, et al: Assessment of right ventricular function at rest and during exercise in patients with coronary artery disease. Am J Cardiol 45:63–71, 1980.

270A. Slutsky R, Watkins J, Peterson K, et al: The response of left ventricular function and size to atrial pacing, with coronary artery disease. Circulation 63:864–870, 1981.

271. Smitherman TC, Osborn RC, Narahara KA: Serial myocardial scintigraphy after a single dose of thallium-201 in men after acute myocardial infarction. Am J Cardiol 42:177–182, 1978.

272. Soin JS, Cox JD, Youker JE, et al: Cardiac localization of [99m]Tc-(Sn)-pyrophosphate following irridation of the chest. Radiology 124:165–168, 1977.

273. Sonnemaker RE, Floyd JL, Ayerdi E, et al: Ejection fraction response to exercise: a comparative study of isometric and dynamic exercise (abstract). Circulation 57–58:II-7, 1978.

273A. Sorensen SG, O'Rourke RA, Chavohuri TK: Noninvasive quantitation of valvular regurgitation by gated equilibrium radionuclide angiography. Circulation 62:1089–1098, 1980.

274. Sprengelmeyer J, Weisberger CL: Practical Nuclear Cardiology. Hagerstown, MD:

Harper & Row, 1979.

275. Spies SM, Kesala BA, Hetzel KR, et al: Improved dynamic and static imaging of abdominal aortic aneurysms. Radiology 124:505–506, 1977.
276. Staniloff HM, Huckell VF, Morch JE, et al: Abnormal myocardial perfusion defects in patients with mitral valve prolapse and normal coronary arteries (abstract). Am J Cardiol 41:433, 1978.
277. Starshak RJ, Sty JR: Radionuclide angiocardiography: use in the detection of myocardial rhabdomyoma. Clin Nucl Med 3:106–107, 1978.
278. Staub RT: Tumor thrombus of the right atrium displayed by rapid sequence scintiphotography. J Nucl Med 11:559–560, 1970.
279. Steiner R, Bull M, Kumpel F, et al: Intracardiac metastases of colon carcinoma. Am J Cardiol 26:300–301, 1970.
280. Stevens JS, Mishkin FS: Persistent left superior vena cava demonstrated by radionuclide angiography. J Nucl Med 16:469, 1975.
281. Stocker RP, Kinser J, Weber JW, et al: Pediatric radiocardiography: shunt diagnosis. Circulation 42:819–826, 1973.
282. Stolzenberg J, Kaminsky J: Overlying breast as cause of false-positive thallium scans. Clin Nucl Med 3:229, 1978.
283. Stolzenberg J, Pollak RH: Rapid redistribution of thallium-201 post stress testing in a patient with variant angina. Clin Nucl Med 4:283–284, 1979.
284. Stolzenberg J, Pollak RH: Absent myocardial uptake of Tl-201 under stress in spite of anatomically normal coronary arteries (letter). J Nucl Med 20: 900–901, 1979.
285. Stolzenberg J: Dilatation of the left ventricular cavity on stress thallium scan as an indicator of ischemic disease. Clin Nucl Med 5:289–291, 1980.
286. Strauss HW, Pitt B, Rouleau J, et al: Atlas of Cardiovascular Nuclear Medicine: Selected Case Studies. St. Louis: C. V. Mosby, 1977.
287. Strauss HW, Pitt B: Cardiovascular Nuclear Medicine. St. Louis: C. V. Mosby, 1979.
288. Strauss HW, McKusick KA, Boucher GA, et al: Of linens and laces—the eighth anniversary of the gated blood pool scan. Sem Nucl Med 9:296–309, 1979.
289. Sty JR, Babbitt DP, Gallen WJ: Scintigraphy in endocardial fibroelastosis. Clin Nucl Med 3:476–477, 1978.
290. Sty JR: Nuclear Medicine Atlas: Atlas of pediatric nuclear cardiology: part II. Clin Nucl Med 5:424–438, 1980.
290A. Sutherland GA, Driedger AA, Sibbald WJ: Myocardial function assessed by radionuclide angiography following blunt chest trauma (abstract). J Nucl Med 21:65, 1980.
291. Sweet SE, Sterling R, McCormick JR, et al: Left ventricular false aneurysm after coronary bypass surgery: radionuclide diagnosis and surgical resection. Am J Cardiol 43:154–157, 1979.
292. Swiryn S, Pavel D, Byrom E, et al: Left ventricular function during induced paroxysmal supraventricular tachycardia assessed by radionuclide angiography (abstract). Clin Res 27:270A, 1979.
293. Sy WM, Lao RS, Bay R, et al: ^{99m}Tc-pertechnetate radionuclide venography: large-volume injection without tourniquet. J Nucl Med 19:1001–1006, 1978.
294. Sy WM, Lao RS, Nissen A, et al: Occlusion of inferior vena cava—features by radionuclide venography. J Nucl Med 19:1007–1112, 1978.
295. Tanasescu D, Berman D, Staniloff H, et al: Apparent worsening of thallium-201 myocardial defects during redistribution—what does it mean? (abstract). J Nucl Med 20:688, 1979.
296. Tauxe WN, Burchell HB, Black HF: Clinical applications of lung scanning. Mayo Clin Proc 42:473, 1976.

297. Tobinick E, Schelbert HR, Henning H, et al: Right ventricular ejection fraction in patients with acute anterior and inferior myocardial infarction assessed by radionuclide angiography. Circulation 57:1078–1084, 1978.

298. Tong ECK, Liu L, Potter RT, et al: Macroaggregated RISA lung scan in congenital heart disease. Radiology 106:585–592, 1973.

299. Tow DE, Wagner HN Jr, Lopez-Majano V, et al: Validity of measuring regional pulmonary arterial flow with macroaggregates of human serum albumin. Am J Roentgenol 96:664–676, 1976.

300. Treves S, Maltz DL, Adelstein SJ: Intracardiac shunts, in James AE Jr, Wagner HN Jr, Cooke RE, ed: Pediatric Nuclear Medicine. Philadelphia: W.B. Saunders, 1973, 231–246.

301. Treves S, Maltz DL: Radionuclide angiocardiography. Postgrad Med 56:99–107, 1974.

302. Treves S, Collins-Nakai RL: Radioactive tracers in congenital heart disease. Am J Cardiol 38:711–721, 1976.

303. Treves S, Kulprathipanja S, Hnatowich DJ: Angiocardiography with iridium-191m: an ultrashort-lived radionuclide ($t_{1/2}$ = 4.9 seconds). Circulation 54:275–279, 1976.

304. Treves S, Collins-Naki R, Ahnberg DS, et al: Quantitative radionuclide angiocardiography in premature infants with patient ductus arteriosus and respiratory distress syndrome (abstract). J Nucl Med 17:554–555, 1976.

304A. Ueda K, Saito A, Nakano H, et al: Thallium-201 scintigraphy in an infant with myocardial infarction following mucocutaneous lymph node syndrome. Pediatr Radiol 9:183–185, 1980.

305. Uhrenholdt A: Detection of right-to-left shunts by external counting of 133-Xenon. Scand J Clin Lab Invest 28:395–400, 1971.

306. Valdez VA, Jacobstein JG: Visualization of a malignant pericardial effusion with Tc-99m-EHDP. Clin Nucl Med 5:210–212, 1980.

307. VanAnswegen A, Lotter MG, Minaar PC, et al: Die Vassetelling van linker-na-regten kardiale aftakkings met behup van gamma-kamera-flikkergraphie. S Afr Med J 47:1700–1704, 1973.

308. VanTrain K: Letter. Softwhere, Ann Arbor, Michigan: Medical Data Systems 5 (4):6, 1978.

309. Verani MS, Marcus ML, Spoto G, et al: Thallium-201 myocardial perfusion scintigrams in the evaluation of aorto-coronary saphenous bypass surgery. J Nucl Med 19:765–772, 1978.

310. Verani MS, Jhingran S, Attar M, et al: Poststress redistribution of thallium-201 patients with coronary artery disease, with and without prior myocardial infarction. Am J Cardiol 43:1114–1122, 1979.

311. Vidne B, Duszynski D, Subramanian S: Pulmonary flow distribution in transposition of the great arteries (abstract). Am J Cardiol 37:178, 1976.

312. Vlahos L, MacDonald AF, Causer DA: Combination of isotope venography and lung scanning. Br J Radiol 49:840–851, 1976.

313. Wackers FJTh, Sokole EB, Samson G, et al: Value and limitations of thallium-201 scintigraphy in the acute phase of myocardial infarction. New Engl J Med 295:1–5, 1976.

314. Wackers FJTh, Becker, Samson G, et al: Location and size of acute transmural myocardial infarction estimated from thallium-201 scintiscans: a clinicopathologic study. Circulation 56:72–78, 1977.

315. Wackers FJTh, Lie KI, Sokole EB, et al: Prevalence of right ventricular involvement in inferior wall infarction assessed with myocardial imaging with thallium-201 and technetium-99m pyrophosphate. Am J Cardiol 42:358–361, 1978.

316. Wackers FJTh, Lie KI, Liem KL, et al: Thallium-201 scintigraphy in unstable angina pectoris. Circulation 57:738–742, 1978.
317. Wagner HN Jr, McAfee JG, Mozley JM: Diagnosis of pericardial effusion by radioisotope photoscanning. Arch Intern Med 108:679–684, 1961.
318. Wagner HN Jr, Rhodes BA: Radioactive tracers in diagnosis of cardiovascular disease. Progr Cardiovasc Dis 15:1–23, 1972.
319. Wainwright RJ, Brennand-Roper DA, Cueni TH, et al: Cold pressor test in detection of coronary heart disease and cardiomyopathy using Tc-99m gated blood pool imaging. Lancet 2 (8138):302–323, 1979.
320. Wald RW, Sternberg L, Huckell VF, et al: Technetium-99m pyrophosphate scintigraphy in patients with calcification within the myocardial silhouette. Br Heart J 40:547–551, 1978.
321. Watson D, Janowitz W, Kenny P, et al: Detection of left-to-right shunts by inhalation of oxygen-15 labelled carbon dioxide (abstract). Circulation 53–54:II-145, 1976.
322. Watson DD, Kenay PKM, Janowitz WR, et al: Detection of left-to-right shunts by inhalation of oxygen-15 labelled carbon dioxide, in Serafini AN, Gilson AJ, Smoak WM: Nuclear Cardiology: Principles and Methods. New York: Plenum, 1977.
323. Weller DA, Adolph RJ, Wellman HN, et al: Myocardial perfusion scintigraphy after intracoronary injection of ^{99m}Tc-labeled human albumin microspheres: toxicity and efficacy for detecting myocardial infarction in dogs; preliminary results in man. Circulation 46:963–975, 1972.
324. Weissmann HS, Steingart RM, Kiely TM, et al: Myocardial visualization on a perfusion lung scan. J Nucl Med 21:745–746, 1980.
325. Wesselhoeft H, Horley PJ, Wagner HN Jr: Nuclear angiocardiography in the differential diagnosis of congenital heart disease in infants (abstract). J Nucl Med 12:406, 1971.
325A. Wexler JP, Steingart RM, Blaufox DM: Physiologic intervention in vascular nuclear medicine. Sem Nucl Med 11:68–69, 1981.
326. Willerson JT, Parkey RW, Bonte FJ, et al: Technetium stannous pyrophosphate myocardial scintigrams in patients with chest pain of varying etiology. Circulation 51:1046–1052, 1975.
327. Winship WS, Pieterse PJ, Houlder AE, et al: Radioisotope cardiac pool scanning: assessment of its value in clinical practice. Am Heart J 80:3–10, 1970.
328. Winship WS, Houlder AE, Horst RL, et al: Radioisotope cardiac pool scanning in children. Pediatr 45:996–1002, 1970.
328A. Winzelberg GG, Boucher CA, Pohost GM, et al: Right ventricular function in aortic and mitral valve disease. Chest 79:520–528, 1981.
329. Wizenberg G, Marshall R, Schelbert H, et al: The effect of oral propranolol on left ventricular function at rest and during exercise in normals and in patients with coronary artery disease as determined by radionuclide angiography (abstract). J Nucl Med 20:639, 1979.
330. Wynne J, Birnholz JC, Homan BL, et al: Radionuclide ventriculography and two-dimensional echocardiography in coronary artery disease (abstract). Am J Cardiol 41:406, 1978.
331. Yao JST, Henkin RE, Conn J Jr, et al: Combined isotope venography and lung scanning: a new diagnostic approach to thromboembolism. Arch Surg 107:146–151, 1973.
332. Young DJ, Damron JR, Utley JR, et al: Perioperative myocardial injury: comparison of electrocardiogram, creatine phosphokinase and technetium-99m pyrophosphate scan (abstract). Am J Cardiol 37:184, 1976.
333. Zaret BL: Myocardial imaging with radioactive potassium and its analogs. Progr Cardiovasc Dis 20:81–94, 1977.

Part II

Central Nervous System

Chapter 11

Cerebral Blood Flow†

MARIANO FERNANDEZ-ULLOA

I. Entities causing decreased or delayed flow

    A. Common

        1. Primary vascular

            a. acute cerebral infarctions (80, 81, 82, 207, 226)

            b. chronic cerebrovascular disease with infarction (58, 80, 81, 226)

            c. carotid artery atherosclerotic obstruction, unilateral or bilateral (58, 81, 196, 207, 226, 303)

            d. middle cerebral artery, anterior cerebral artery, and posterior cerebral artery atherosclerotic obstruction (58, 226, 260, 265, 303)

            e. transient ischemic attacks (80, 81)

        2. Slow arrival (symmetric)

            a. poor bolus injection (80)

            b. improper radionuclide injection (329)

                (1) injection in cephalic vein

                (2) injection with arm in extreme adduction

        3. Subdural hematomas (57, 58, 82, 102, 138, 267, 288)

    B. Less common

---

†Brain flow is usually subdivided into arterial, capillary, and venous phases. Although convenient during the analysis of a radionuclide cerebral angiogram (RNCA), this separation is not always possible. For the purpose of this list we have divided RNCA into an early and a late phase, recognizing the inherent limitations of this approach stemming from a somewhat artificial subdivision of a dynamic process and from the different flow patterns which the same disease can display. The word ''flow'' will be used to describe the degrees of radionuclide activity noted over time; it does not necessarily imply a true quantitative assessment of cerebral hemodynamics.

    The use of an asterisk* in this chapter indicates that this entity has been observed by the author but the case report has not been published.

1. Normal variant
   a. asymmetric caliber of the internal carotid artery associated with segmental hypoplasia or agenesis of anterior cerebral arteries (10)
2. Primary vascular
   a. vertebrobasilar insufficiency (58, 80)
   b. bilateral carotid thrombosis (209)
   c. bilateral middle cerebral artery occlusions (263)
   d. intracranial arterial vasospasm associated with bleeding arterial aneurysm or subarachnoid hemorrhage (114, 299)
   e. major vessel occlusion in neonates (273)
   f. hypoplastic transverse sinus (154)
3. Tumors
   a. primary brain tumors, cystic or causing mass effect (58, 101, 196, 265, 267)
   b. meningiomas [early decreased flow with or without subsequent increased flow (289)]
   c. secondary brain tumors (265, 266, 267, 303)
4. Brain abscess (58)
5. Fluid collections
   a. intracerebral hematomas (196, 248, 258, 267)
   b. subdural hygroma (102)
   c. epidural hematoma (102, 259)
6. Cortical cerebral atrophy (315)
7. Brain death (112, 113, 215, 228)
8. Artefactual, decreased scalp flow caused by pressure of collimator (333)

C. Rare
   1. Primary vascular
      a. superior sagittal sinus thrombosis (342)
      b. associated with carotid-cavernous sinus fistula (194)
      c. associated with intracerebral aneurysms (66)
      d. steal phenomenon associated with giant arteriovenous malformation*
      e. arterial fibromuscular dysplasia (85)
      f. associated with Sturge-Weber syndrome (171)
      g. following surgical carotid artery occlusion (194)
      h. kinking of the internal carotid artery (320)
      i. moyamoya disease (187, 189)
   2. Porencephalic and congenital cysts (7, 196, 267)
   3. Echinococcal cysts (276)
   4. Hydrocephalus (7, 207)
   5. Infantile cerebral paralysis (20)
   6. Invasion of sinuses by tumors (see Section VI)
   7. Status post craniotomy (58)
   8. Decompression hyperostosis (126)

II. Conditions displaying increased or accelerated brain flow mainly involving the early phases of the radionuclide cerebral angiogram

   A. Common

      1. Normal variant; jugular vein reflux (129, 300, 353)

      2. Arteriovenous malformation (58, 196, 207, 226, 323)

      3. Vascular primary brain tumors (90, 192, 226, 323)

   B. Less common

      1. Meningiomas (196)

      2. Brain infarctions displaying the "luxury perfusion" phenomenon (293, 351)

      3. Arterial aneurysms (31, 66)

      4. Recent seizures, focal and generalized (137, 302)

      5. Superior mediastinal venous obstruction causing jugular and intracranial sinus reflux (231, 243)

   C. Rare

      1. Tumors

         a. hemangiomas (267)

         b. hemangioblastomata of Von Hippel-Lindau syndrome (125)

         c. chemodectoma of the jugular glomus (5)

      2. Carotid-cavernous sinus fistula (321)

      3. Moyamoya disease (187, 189)

      4. Inflammation

         a. herpes simplex encephalitis (155, 219)

      5. Bone related

         a. craniofacial fibrous dysplasia (156)

III. Conditions displaying increased and/or accelerated brain flow mainly involving the late phases of the RNCA

   A. Common

      1. Normal variant, radionuclide retention in mildly dilated cerebral veins (58, 226)

      2. Cerebrovascular disease displaying the "flip flop" phenomenon (58, 80, 226, 303)

      3. Tumors

         a. meningiomas (77, 282, 289)

         b. primary brain tumors (192)

         c. metastatic brain tumors (267)

   B. Uncommon

      1. Brain infarction displaying the "luxury perfusion" pattern (290)

      2. Paget's disease of the skull (192)

      3. Cerebral venous angioma (239)

      4. Congenital dilatation of cerebral veins (294)

      5. Associated with intracranial fibromuscular dysplasia (85)

      6. Following craniotomy (347)
      7. Subdural empyema (69)
      8. Sinus pericranii (304A)

IV. Abnormally increased flow involving all phases of the RNCA

    A. Common
      1. Tumors
        a. meningiomas (58, 82, 90, 207, 267)
        b. primary vascular brain tumors (58, 207, 250, 261, 265, 267, 303, 323)
        c. vascular metastatic brain tumors (102)
      2. Paget's disease of the calvaria (84, 134)
      3. Frontal sinusitis (58)
    B. Uncommon
      1. Vascular
        a. large arterial aneurysms (66)
        b. large arteriovenous malformation (58, 303)
        c. aneurysmal dilation of the vein of Galen (53, 295)
        d. cerebral venous angioma (239)
        e. vertebral artery fistula (262)
        f. carotid-cavernous sinus fistula (61, 194)
      2. Vascular tumors
        a. proliferating trichilemmal cyst of the scalp (271)
        b. carotid body tumor (chemodectoma), extracranial (278)
        c. metastatic cervical lymphadenopathy*
        d. hemangiopericytoma (58)
        e. juvenile nasal angioneurofibroma (101)
        f. multiple myeloma of the skull (128)
        g. ependymoma (214)
      3. Inflammation
        a. inflammatory process of the ear (238)
        b. cervical lymphadenitis (301)
        c. tuberculous meningitis (166)
        d. herpes simplex encephalitis (162)
        e. subdural empyema (270)
      4. Craniofacial fibrous dysplasia (83)
      5. Sturge-Weber malformation (53, 214)
      6. Recent focal seizures (350)

V. Conditions displaying persistent increased flow at the base of the skull, medially located; "the hot nose sign"

    A. Common
      1. Internal carotid artery obstruction, unilateral or bilateral (216)

2. Patient on psychotropic agents (330)
B. Uncommon
  1. Encephalitis
    a. herpes simplex encephalitis (219)
  2. Brain death (215, 216)

VI. Entities causing displacement of major intracranial vessels and/or nonvisualization of intracranial sinuses

  A. Common
    1. Hypoplastic transverse sinus (154)
    2. Fluid collection
      a. epidural hematomas (42, 354)
      b. subdural hematoma (25, 58)
    3. Cystic astrocytomas (58)
    4. Brain death (112, 113, 215)
  B. Uncommon
    1. Abscess (58)
    2. Intracerebral hematomas (248, 258)
    3. Bilateral and unilateral hydrocephalus (58, 207)
    4. Invasion of sinuses by tumor (7)
    5. Thrombosis of major intracranial sinuses, sagittal and lateral (18, 41, 109, 192)
    6. Arterial displacement caused by craniofacial fibrous dysplasia (83)
    7. Displacement caused by Paget's disease (111A)

VII. Entities causing increased radionuclide concentration on blood pool images

  A. Common
    1. Tumors
      a. meningiomas (77, 282)
      b. glioblastoma multiforme (267, 323)
      c. cystic astrocytoma (101)
      d. secondary brain tumors (267)
    2. Inflammatory and traumatic processes of the scalp (50)
    3. Paget's disease of the skull (84, 251)
    4. Large arterial aneurysms (341)
  B. Uncommon
    1. Primary vascular
      a. arteriovenous malformations (323)
      b. hemangiomas (267)
      c. moyamoya disease (187)
      d. cavernous sinus occlusion with dilated draining veins (117)
    2. Sturge-Weber syndrome (171)
    3. Juvenile nasal angioneuroblastoma (101)

   4. Craniofacial fibrous dysplasia (83)
   5. Chemodectomas (5)
   6. Viral meningoencephalitis (162)
   7. Sinus pericranii (304A)

VIII. Conditions causing abnormal flow but normal static brain scintigrams
   A. With increased flow
      1. Jugular vein reflux (341)
      2. Arteriovenous malformation (341)
      3. Arterial aneurysms (341)
      4. Cerebral venous angioma (239)
      5. Moyamoya disease (187)
      6. Traumatic intracranial arteriovenous fistula
         a. meningeal artery—meningeal vein (255)
         b. carotid-cavernous (61)
      7. Low grade astrocytoma (261)
      8. Jugular glomus chemodectoma (5)
   B. With decreased flow
      1. Primary vascular
         a. acute brain infarction with/without "flip flop" phenomenon (264, 341)
         b. cerebrovascular disease involving major extracranial and intracranial arteries (58, 264, 341)
         c. transient ischemic attacks (80, 264)
         d. sinus thrombosis (341)
      2. Subdural hematoma (138, 264)
      3. Brain trauma (264)
      4. Intracranial cysts (7)
      5. Hydrocephalus (7, 341)
      6. Cerebral echinococcal cysts (276)

References for this chapter may be found at the end of Chapter 15, page 75.

Chapter 12

Brain Scintigraphy (Static)

MARIANO FERNANDEZ-ULLOA

I. Causes of single focal areas of increased uptake

  A. Common

   1. Vascular

     a. intracerebral thrombosis (116, 127, 345)

     b. brain hemorrhage and hematoma (50, 57, 236, 248, 284)

   2. Tumors

     a. primary

       (1) meningioma (77, 282, 289, 345)

       (2) glioma (53, 64, 101, 233, 319, 345)

       (3) oligodendroglioma (274, 345)

     b. metastatic (102, 232, 312, 345)

   3. Chronic subdural hematomas (14)

   4. Brain abscess (99, 232, 236, 345)

   5. Brain contusion (57, 100, 236, 345)

   6. Skull lesions

     a. status postcraniotomy and burr holes (50, 100, 130, 195)

     b. Paget's disease of the skull (84, 251)

     c. metastases to the skull (156, 195, 312, 319)

     d. frontal sinusitis (206, 296)

   7. Inflammatory, traumatic, and neoplastic processes of the scalp (50, 57, 100, 130, 138, 312)

   8. Normal variant: "ear sign" (241)

  B. Less common

   1. Fluid collections

     a. subdural hygroma (64, 102)

     b. subdural empyema (64)

     c. epidural hematoma (142, 224)

     d. epidural abscess (312)

     e. cephalohematoma (53, 102)

     f. subarachnoid hemorrhage (337, 345)

     g. subgaleal hematoma (236)

The use of an asterisk* in this chapter indicates that this entity has been observed by the author but the case report has not been published.

    h. acute subdural hematoma (138)

2. Vascular lesions

    a. arterial aneurysms (31)

    b. arteriovenous malformations (31, 50, 283, 345)

    c. cerebellar infarction (335)

    d. childhood brain infarction secondary to carotid obstruction and embolism (2, 273)

3. Other less frequent diseases of the skull

    a. skull fractures (54, 57)

    b. fibrous dysplasia (83, 156, 195, 236)

    c. tumors

        (1) osteoma (319)

        (2) invasive carcinoma of the frontal sinus (195)

    d. osteomyelitis (99, 319)

    e. hyperostosis frontalis (195)

    f. thick occipital squama (50)

4. Tumors

    a. pituitary tumors (233, 345)

    b. lymphoma (167, 232, 317)

    c. acoustic neuroma (23, 44, 221, 233, 345)

    d. glioma of:

        (1) brain stem (78, 236)

        (2) optic nerves (211)

        (3) hypothalamus (211)

        (4) chiasma (236)

    e. pinealoma (232)

    f. tumors of the third ventricle (236)

    g. ependymomas and ependymoblastomas (101, 115, 221, 233, 345)

    h. basal meningeal gliomatosis (173)

    i. craniopharyngioma (17, 101, 144, 233)

    j. medulloblastoma (101, 221, 233, 345)

    k. microglioma (331)

5. Recent focal seizures (252)

6. Anoxic brain infarction in childhood (273)

    a. laminar cortical necrosis

    b. periventricular pattern

7. Focal encephalitis (99)

8. Dural metastases (130)

9. Radiation necrosis (192A)

C. Rare

1. Radionuclide contamination (345, 346)

2. Artefactual: "shine through" phenomenon from gastric technetium uptake (in vertex view) (275)

3. Tumors

    a. choroid plexus papillomas (76, 233, 235, 345)

        b. choroid plexus meningioma (36)
        c. hemangioblastoma (43, 221)
           (1) with Lindau-von Hippel disease (125, 233)
        d. dermoid cyst of the fourth ventricle (35)
        e. teratoma (79, 211)
        f. epidermoid tumor (277)
        g. spongioblastoma (233)
        h. mycosis fungoides (161)
        i. lipoma of the corpus callosum (1, 53, 349)
        j. hemangioendothelioma (314)
        k. granulocytic sarcoma (chloroma) of the brain (169)
        l. hypothalamic histiocytosis (211)
      m. meningeal sarcoma (236, 324)
        n. orbital solid tumors (236)
        o. orbital leukemic deposits (101)
    4. Inflammation-infection
        a. viral
           (1) herpes virus encephalitis (34, 120, 155, 162, 219, 247)
           (2) viral meningoencephalitis (162)
           (3) subacute sclerosing panencephalitis (74)
        b. mycobacterial
           (1) intracranial tuberculoma (11, 206)
           (2) tuberculous meningitis (166, 191)
        c. fungi and parasites
           (1) toruloma (206, 336)
           (2) nocardial brain abscess (327)
           (3) rhinocerebral mucormycosis (355)
           (4) cerebral toxoplasmosis (253)
        d. pyogenic abscess in chronic granulomatous disease of childhood (211)
        e. unilateral pyogenic ventriculitis (179)
        f. mycotic aneurysm (206, 272)
    5. Demyelinating disease
        a. multiple sclerosis (52, 105)
        b. progressive multifocal leukoencephalopathy (164)
        c. adrenal leukodystrophy (49)
    6. Vascular
        a. infarction secondary to thrombosis of intracranial sinuses
           (1) lateral sinus (41)
           (2) sagittal sinus (18, 109)
           (3) cavernous sinus (117)
         b. brain infarction secondary to moyamoya disease (2)
        c. lupus erythematosus cerebritis (26)
        d. normal anatomical variant: fenestrated sagittal sinus (279)
    7. Cysts

      a. dysplastic cysts (233)

      b. porencephalic cysts (252)

  8. Congenital diseases

      a. tuberous sclerosis (87)

      b. Sturge-Weber disease, encephalotrigeminal angiomatosis (48, 53, 171, 214, 345)

      c. arterial dolichoectasia or giant serpentine aneurysm (170)

      d. vein of Galen malformation (53, 295)

      e. cranium bifidum defect and biparietal foramina (53)

  9. Bullet tracks (244)

  10. Scalp and soft tissue abnormality

      a. artefactual: scalp uptake caused by recent electroencephalographic procedures (45)

      b. focal ear cellulitis (238)

      c. scalp lipoma plus underlying skull thickening (50)

      d. proliferating trichilemmal cyst of the scalp (271)

  11. Skull disease

      a. multiple myeloma of the skull (128)

      b. epidermoid tumor of the skull (188)

      c. sutural widening secondary to increased intracranial hypertension (214)

      d. hemangioma (156, 195)

      e. fibrosarcoma (156)

      f. eosinophilic granuloma (29, 156)

  12. Granulomatous disease

      a. cerebral sarcoidosis (206, 326)

      b. chronic granulomatous disease of childhood (211)

      c. hypothalamic histiocytosis (211)

  13. Chronic pachymeningitis of unknown etiology (130)

  14. Juvenile cerebral paralysis (214)

  15. Hydrocephalus (53)

II. Conditions causing *multiple* areas of increased uptake. (This section lists specific references to causes of multiple areas of increased uptake, but virtually any lesion noted in Section I which does not occur in a midline structure, e.g. pituitary, could be listed here.)

  A. Common

    1. Artefactual

      a. bilateral "ear sign" (241)

      b. choroid plexus visualization

        (1) lateral ventricle (343)

        (2) lateral and fourth ventricles (110)

    2. Brain metastases (345)

    3. Multiple brain infarctions (127, 260, 312)

    4. Bilateral subdural collections (14, 54, 309)

    5. Inflammation

        a. meningitis and meningoencephalitis (236)

        b. viral encephalitis (64, 99, 162)

    6. Skull lesions

        a. hyperostosis frontalis interna (195)

        b. skull metastases (195)

        c. post-craniotomy changes; burr holes (195)

B. Less common

    1. Artefactual, scalp trauma caused by recent electroencephalography*

    2. Brain contusions (57)

    3. Inflammation

        a. herpes encephalitis (34, 247)

        b. multiple brain abscesses (53, 214)

    4. Infarction

        a. anoxic brain disease in children, laminar necrosis (214)

        b. watershed infarctions in pediatric and adult populations (159, 273)

    5. Subarachnoid hemorrhage, vasospasm induced (337)

    6. Radiation necrosis (192A)

C. Rare

    1. Sagittal sinus thrombosis with associated brain infarctions (342)

    2. Inflammation-infection

        a. cerebral sarcoidosis (229)

        b. cerebral aspergillomatous abscesses (184, 280)

        c. bilateral ventriculitis (99)

        d. cerebral melioidosis (37)

    3. Tumor

        a. unusual presentations of glioma

            (1) multifocal glioblastoma multiforme (250)

            (2) glioblastoma with bilateral periventricular spread (205)

        b. leukemia

            (1) central nervous system leukemic infiltrates (304)

            (2) granulocytic sarcoma of the brain (169)

        c. Lymphoma (317)

            (1) mycosis fungoides (161)

    4. Following seizures (64)

    5. Cortical cerebral atrophy (315)

    6. Gunshot wound (178)

    7. Demyelinating diseases

        a. subacute sclerosing panencephalitis (74)

        b. leukodystrophy (338)

        c. adrenal leukodystrophy (49, 131)

        d. progressive multifocal leukoencephalopathy (164, 227)

        e. multiple sclerosis (213)

        f. Schilder's disease (227)

    8. Sturge-Weber syndrome (171)
    9. Multiple scalp sebaceous cysts (249)
  10. Craniofacial fibrous dysplasia (83)

III. Conditions causing diffuse radionuclide uptake

  A. Common
    1. Meningitis (99)
    2. Encephalitis and meningoencephalitis (99, 162)
    3. Brain contusion (64)
    4. Chronic subdural hematoma (14, 309)
    5. Leukemic infiltrates (64, 236)
    6. Paget's disease (134, 156)
  B. Less common
    1. Recent seizures (302, 350)
    2. Herpes simplex encephalitis (162)
    3. Intracranial lymphoma (317)
    4. Subdural empyema (270)
  C. Rare
    1. Intracranial hematoma (248)
    2. Epidural hematoma (224)
    3. Decompression hyperostosis (126)
    4. Cortical cerebral atrophy (315)
    5. Juvenile hemiplegias (214)
    6. Sturge-Weber syndrome (214)
    7. Subacute sclerosing panencephalitis (74)

IV. Conditions displaying an area of uptake surrounding a cold area (doughnut or rim configuration). The rim configuration has been associated with superficial intracranial disease whereas the doughnut configuration usually represents deeper disease.

  A. Common
    1. Tumor
      a. primary brain tumors (308, 312)
      b. metastatic brain tumors (312)
    2. Brain abscess (99, 312)
    3. Brain infarctions (308, 312)
    4. Subdural hematoma (135, 245, 288, 308, 312)
  B. Less common
    1. Intracerebral hemorrhage and hematoma (185, 308, 312)
    2. Meningioma (312)
    3. Post-craniotomy changes (308)
    4. Scalp sebaceous cyst (249)
    5. Meningitis with multiple abscesses (308)

C. Rare
    1. Fluid collections
        a. epidural hematoma (39, 42, 102, 140, 257, 354)
        b. cephalhematoma (24)
        c. epidural abscess (312)
    2. Giant aneurysm*
    3. Calvarial metastases (312)
    4. Calvarial osteomyelitis (99)
    5. Demyelination
        a. progressive multifocal leukoencephalopathy (164)
        b. leukodystrophy (338)
    6. Wilms' tumor metastases, meningeal (305)
    7. Ear artefact (252A)
        a. cold area due to hearing aid
        b. hyperemic ear

V. Conditions that cause *peripheral* increased radionuclide uptake, unilateral or bilateral

  A. Common
    1. Artefactual
        a. head rotation (54, 352)
        b. scalp; skull; sinuses; scatter from salivary gland (104)
        c. scalp radionuclide contamination (54, 346)
    2. Cerebrovascular disease
        a. subdural hematoma (14, 54, 57, 100, 309)
        b. infarction (54, 57)
    3. Scalp abnormality
        a. trauma: hematomas, laceration, and surgical incision (54, 57, 100, 130)
        b. scalp intravenous sites in children (54)
        c. scalp infection (54, 99, 100)
    4. Skull disease
        a. calvarial tumors (54, 57)
        b. craniotomy changes and burr holes (54, 100, 130)
        c. thickened cranial vault following shunt procedures (54)
        d. asymmetry of the skull caused by fetal and postural molding (54)
        e. Paget's disease of the skull (54, 251)
    5. Meningitis (54, 99)
  B. Less common
    1. Normal variants, e.g. elongated and triangular skull configurations (54)
    2. Intracranial disease
        a. brain contusion (54, 57, 64)
        b. subdural collections

          (1) empyema (54, 270)
          (2) subdural effusion (54)
          (3) subdural hygroma (54, 102)
      c. meningocerebral metastases and tumor spread (57, 102, 130)
      d. anoxic brain damage, laminar cortical necrosis pattern (127, 273)
      e. cephalhematoma (53, 54, 102)
   3. Skull lesions
      a. skull fractures (54, 57)
      b. osteomyelitis (99)
   4. Scalp lesions
      a. herpes zoster infection of the scalp (30)
      b. scalp metastases (30)
      c. subgaleal hematoma (54, 236)
      d. scalp hematoma (100)
      e. scalp infection (100)
C. Rare
   1. Intracranial
      a. brain abscess (54)
      b. epidural hematoma (54, 102, 142, 224, 257)
      c. pachymeningitis (54, 57, 130)
      d. lymphoma (317)
      e. meningeal sarcoma (54)
      f. cerebral hemiatrophy, infantile cerebral paralysis (20, 54, 316)
      g. cortical cerebral atrophy (315)
      h. unilateral hydrocephalus (54)
      i. vasculitis (54)
      j. Sturge-Weber syndrome (48, 54, 171)
      k. leptomeningeal cysts (54)
      l. subarachnoid cysts (54)
      m. porencephaly (54)
      n. tuberculous meningitis (166)
   2. Skull lesions
      a. decompression hyperostosis (126)
      b. calvarial reticulosis (54)
      c. craniofacial fibrous dysplasia (83)
      d. asymmetric premature closure of cranial sutures (plagiocephaly) (54)
      e. hyperparathyroidism (218)
      f. suture widening secondary to intracranial hypertension (214)

VI. Conditions that cause nonvisualization and/or displacement of intracranial sinuses

  A. Common
   1. Artefactual, poor patient positioning (316)

   2. Normal variant
      a. asymmetric sinuses
         (1) sagittal (50)
         (2) transverse (136)
         (3) occipital (111)
   3. Brain death (112, 113)
B. Less common
   1. Vascular
      a. epidural hematoma (140, 183)
      b. thrombosis of intracranial sinuses
         (1) lateral (192)
         (2) sagittal (109, 192)
      c. cavernous sinus occlusion (117)
   2. Intracranial cysts
      a. arachnoid cysts, posterior fossa, and supratentorial (53, 55, 217)
      b. porencephalic cysts (55, 217)
      c. Dandy-Walker malformation (53, 55, 214)
      d. cystic hygroma (55)
      e. posterior fossa and cerebellar cysts (53, 214)
   3. Other intracranial disease
      a. agenesis of the corpus callosum (53)
      b. cerebral hemiatrophy (53, 316)
      c. Arnold-Chiari malformation (53, 55)
   4. Hydrocephalus (53)
      a. aqueduct of Sylvius stenosis (55)
      b. unilateral obstruction of Monro's foramen (55)
   5. Asymmetry of the cranial vault secondary to premature suture closing (55)

VII. Conditions associated with radionuclide accumulation within the lateral ventricles
  A. Inflammatory etiology
      1. Bacterial meningitis and/or ventriculitis (63, 94, 99, 179)
      2. Tuberculous meningitis (68)
      3. Coccidioidal meningitis (297)
  B. Vascular
      1. Intraventricular bleeding (287)
      2. Associated with ruptured phycomycotic aneurysm (108)
  C. Hyperthermic and/or anoxic brain damage (94)
  D. Choroid plexus papilloma (76)
  E. Chemical: intrathecal methotrexate (190)

VIII. Conditions displaying a scintigraphic pattern characterized by symmetric *midline uptake* or midline crossing
  A. Common

1. Bilateral lateral ventricle visualization (see Section VII above)
2. Vascular
    a. interhemispheric infarctions, bilateral obstruction of the anterior cerebral arteries (165, 260)
3. Tumor
    a. meningioma
        (1) supratentorial (233)
        (2) parasagittal (236)
    b. astrocytoma
        (1) astrocytoma of the corpus callosum (192, 324)
        (2) supratentorial (233)
        (3) hypothalamic glioma (211)
        (4) optic glioma (211)

B. Less common
    1. Tumor
        a. tumors of the corpus collosum
            (1) lipoma (1, 349)
            (2) metastatic melanoma (324)
        b. basal meningeal gliomatosis (173)
        c. craniopharyngiomas (101, 144, 233, 236)
        d. medulloblastoma (101, 233, 236)
        e. teratoma of the third ventricle (79)
        f. oligodendroglioma (233)
        g. ependymoma (233)
        h. brain stem gliomas (78)
        i. dermoid cyst of the fourth ventricle (35)
        j. chiasmatic glioma (236)
        k. choroid plexus papilloma (53, 214, 233)
        l. meningeal sarcoma (324)
        m. spongioblastoma (233)
        n. lymphoma, parasagittal (317)
        o. pituitary adenoma (233)
    2. Vascular
        a. bilateral parasagittal epidural hematoma (183)
        b. bilateral carotid artery aneurysms (66)
        c. bilateral infarctions secondary to superior sagittal sinus thrombosis (342)
        d. arteriovenous malformation (31)
        e. dolichoectasia of the anterior cerebral artery (giant serpentine aneurysm) (170)
        f. vein of Galen malformation (53)
    3. Tuberous sclerosis (87)
    4. Tuberculous meningitis (191)
    5. Bilateral visualization of choroid plexuses of fourth ventricles (110)
    6. Bilateral parasagittal sarcoidosis (229)
    7. Hypothalamic histiocytosis (211)

IX. Entities that cause abnormally decreased radionuclide uptake

A. Common
1. Metal plates of the skull (50, 60)

B. Less common
1. Intracranial avascular areas
   a. brain porencephalic cysts (7, 217)
   b. arachnoid cysts (53, 217)
   c. intracranial teratoma (325)
   d. epidural hematoma (286)
2. Artefact: decreased perfusion to scalp pressing against collimator (on blood pool image only) (333)

X. Causes of false-positive brain scintigrams

A. Common
1. Abnormal scalp activity: these frequently simulate subdural collections
   a. scalp vein injection sites (54)
   b. hematomas (100, 138, 226)
   c. lacerations (54)
   d. infection (100)
2. Mispositioning with head rotation (14, 54)
3. Ear uptake, "ear sign" (241)
4. Normal variants of skull configurations (50, 54)
   a. triangular configuration
   b. postural molding
   c. thickened occipital squama
5. Choroid plexus uptake of free pertechnetate
   a. lateral ventricles (345)
   b. fourth ventricle (110)
6. Benign conditions of the skull causing peripheral radionuclide uptake (see Section IV)
7. Asymmetric sinus
   a. sagittal (50)
   b. occipital (111)
8. Frontal sinusitis (296)

B. Less common
1. Radionuclide contamination of the scalp (54, 345, 346)
2. Skull thickening following shunt procedures (54)
3. Artefactual caused by electroencephalography electrodes (45)
4. Febrile and other recent convulsions (230, 252)
5. "Shine through" phenomenon from free pertechnetate uptake in nasopharynx, salivary glands, or gastric mucosa seen in vertex view (104, 275)
6. Inflammatory diseases of the ear (238)

   7. Anatomical variant: fenestrated sagittal sinus (279)
   8. Scalp lipoma (50)

XI. Causes of false-negative brain scintiscans (usually due to its small size; location; poor vascular supply)

   A. Common
      1. Scintiscans obtained within one hour or less after radiopharmaceutical administration (13, 97, 132, 212, 254, 281, 314, 348)
      2. Scintiscan obtained within the first few days following the initial nervous tissue insult, especially with cerebrovascular disease and subdural hematoma (54, 56, 138, 220, 281)
      3. Transient ischemic attacks (80)
      4. Posterior fossa disease (43)
      5. Small lesions located at the base of the skull or adjacent to intracranial sinuses
         a. craniopharyngioma (17, 101)
         b. meningioma (77, 289)
         c. acoustic neuromas (168)
         d. pituitary adenomas (345)
      6. Lesions located in temporal lobes and midline (168)
      7. Metastases
         a. from colonic carcinoma (38)
      8. Bilateral subdural collections (14, 54, 138)
      9. Low grade astrocytomas (223, 261)
      10. Intracerebral hemorrhage (258, 284)
      11. Acute subarachnoid hemorrhage (54)
   B. Less common
      1. Brain stem infarctions (335)
      2. Brain stem tumors (78, 101)
      3. Arteriovenous malformations (212, 323)
      4. Arteriovenous fistulas
         a. carotid cavernous (61)
         b. meningeal artery-meningeal vein (255)
      5. Corticosteroid effect (193, 298)
      6. Cholesteatoma (115)
      7. Hydrocephalus (7, 214)
      8. Multiple sclerosis (52, 225)

References for this chapter may be found at the end of Chapter 15, page 75.

Chapter 13

Cisternography

MARIANO FERNANDEZ-ULLOA

I. Entities displaying cisternographic patterns characterized by nonvisualization of the subarachnoid spaces (SAS) over the convexities and parasagittal areas: the subarachnoid space block pattern

  A. Common

    1. Unsuccessful radionuclide injection (extra-arachnoid injection) (88, 334)

    2. Obstructive communicating hydrocephalus (86, 313)

    3. Post meningitic cisternal block following shunting for hydrocephalus secondary to Sylvian aqueduct stenosis (313)

    4. Obstructive noncommunicating hydrocephalus of childhood and adulthood with associated cisternal block (4, 88, 95, 149, 236)

    5. Status post-acute meningitis (201)

    6. Subarachnoid hemorrhage, acute phase (149)

  B. Uncommon

    1. Spinal subarachnoid block (see Section VI)

    2. Head trauma (91)

    3. Paget's disease of skull (67)

    4. Posterior fossa cysts and tumors (149, 201)

    5. Following posterior fossa surgery (88)

    6. Communicating hydrocephalus associated with brain tumors (313)

  C. Rare

    1. Dandy-Walker malformation (122, 146, 201)

    2. Normal pressure hydrocephalus (NPH) associated with Huntington's chorea (151)

    3. Normal pressure hydrocephalus (NPH) associated with hypertensive cerebrovascular disease (75)

    4. Noncommunicating hydrocephalus associated with occipital encephalocele (311)

The terms obstructive communicating and obstructive noncommunicating hydrocephalus have been adopted in this chapter since they emphasize two of the main pathophysiologic and scintigraphic characteristics. The first one is the obstructive nature of their pathogenesis and the second is the presence or absence of free communication between the intraventricular system and the subarachnoid space as determined by the visualization (communicating) or nonvisualization (noncommunicating) of the lateral ventricles after a lumbar subarachnoid injection of radiopharmaceutical.

5. Hydrocephalus associated with spina bifida cystica (33)

II. Entities displaying bilateral delay of migration of the radionuclide over the convexities
 A. Common
  1. Cerebral atrophy (67, 148, 149, 150, 313)
  2. Obstructive noncommunicating hydrocephalus (i.e. stenosis of aqueduct of Sylvius) (4, 88, 95, 150, 201, 204)
  3. Inadequate radionuclide administration (epidural injection) and/or post injection leakage (240, 334)
  4. Following head trauma (91)
  5. Acute meningitis (322)
 B. Less common
  1. "Normal variant" (157)
  2. Subdural hematoma, bilateral (19, 256)
  3. Alzheimer's disease (51)
  4. Communicating hydrocephalus (158)
  5. Following subarachnoid hemorrhage, remote (339)
  6. Secondary obstruction in communicating hydrocephalus after patent diversionary shunting (201, 204)
 C. Rare
  1. Hydrocephalus associated with spina bifida cystica (33)
  2. Pseudotumor cerebri (149)
  3. Arnold-Chiari malformation (33, 311)

III. Conditions causing transient or persistent visualization of the lateral ventricles
 A. Common
  1. Compensated obstructive communicating hydrocephalus (122, 201, 204)
  2. Communicating hydrocephalus following head trauma (88, 202)
  3. Following evacuation of subdural hematomas (19)
  4. Normal variant (transient) (157, 158)
  5. Cerebral atrophy (transient) (3)
  6. Acute meningitis (3, 147, 322)
  7. Following subarachnoid hemorrhage, remote (339)
 B. Uncommon
  1. Cerebellar degeneration (186)
  2. Dandy-Walker malformation (associated with cystic fourth ventricle visualization) (124)
  3. Status post brain surgery (89)
  4. Achondroplasia (145)
  5. Associated with porencephaly (106, 149)

      6. Noncommunicating hydrocephalus with patent ventriculocisternal shunt (4)

      7. Communicating hydrocephalus, post shunt (204)

      8. Alzheimer's disease (51)

IV. Entities displaying delayed clearance and/or absent migration over the cerebral convexities plus visualization of the lateral ventricles

    A. Obstructive communicating hydrocephalus, idiopathic normal pressure hydrocephalus (67, 88, 122, 150, 158, 180, 313)

    B. Obstructive communicating hydrocephalus of childhood (8, 95, 148, 201)

      1. Secondary to meningitis

      2. Following head trauma

      3. Secondary to subarachnoid hemorrhage

      4. Post intracranial surgery

    C. Obstructive communicating hydrocephalus following subarachnoid hemorrhage, acute and remote (67, 88, 149, 240, 268, 313, 339, 340)

      1. Ruptured arteriovenous malformation

      2. Ruptured arterial aneurysm

    D. Obstructive communicating hydrocephalus following head trauma (88, 91, 149, 202)

    E. Communicating hydrocephalus associated with cerebral atrophy (149)

    F. Following evacuation of subdural hematoma (19)

    G. Acute and status post meningitis (88, 147, 149, 313, 322)

      1. Tuberculous (311)

      2. Coccidioidal (297)

      3. Cryptococcal (336)

    H. Normal pressure hydrocephalus associated with hypertensive cerebrovascular disease (75, 118)

    I. Obstructive communicating hydrocephalus associated with Alzheimer's disease (51, 292)

    J. Absorptive hydrocephalus secondary to defective pacchionian granulations (107)

    K. Acetazolamide (Diamox) therapy (237)

    L. Cerebral atrophy (transient ventricular filling) (28, 88, 149)

    M. "Compensated" communicating hydrocephalus (8, 107)

    N. Dandy-Walker malformation (122)

    O. Communicating hydrocephalus associated with ectatic basilar artery (28, 313)

    P. Normal pressure hydrocephalus associated with Cockayne's syndrome (40)

    Q. Communicating hydrocephalus associated with arachnoid cysts (92)

V. Conditions causing asymmetric visualization and/or distortion of the subarachnoid spaces and lateral ventricles (see Section VI)

A. Common

    1. "Normal" variant, asymmetric ascent over the cerebral convexities (157)

    2. Status post head trauma and post traumatic adhesive arachnoiditis (67, 86, 91, 149)

    3. Subdural hematoma or hygroma (19, 256, 340)

    4. Following evacuation of subdural hematomas (19)

    5. Tumors

        a. cerebral hemispheres (86, 340)

        b. olfactory groove meningioma (89)

        c. pituitary adenoma (89)

        d. metastases (115A)

    6. Status post brain and skull surgery (88, 89, 122, 148, 149)

    7. Intracerebral hematoma (160)

    8. Acute and status post meningitis and subdural effusions (149, 322)

    9. Status post subarachnoid hemorrhage (149)

    10. Acute cerebrovascular accident (119)

B. Uncommon

    1. Radionuclide cisternography performed immediately after pneumoencephalography with incomplete unilateral ventricular visualization (210)

    2. Leptomeningeal leukemic infiltrates (304)

    3. Basilar invagination in states of skull softening, i.e. Paget's disease (123)

    4. Arnold-Chiari malformation (201, 311)

    5. Dandy-Walker malformation (123)

    6. Achondroplasia, elongated cisterna magna (123, 145)

    7. Sturge-Weber syndrome (48)

    8. Status post hemispherectomy (88)

    9. Leptomeningeal cyst (122)

VI. Conditions causing apparent partial or complete spinal subarachnoid space blocks

    A. Artefactual: subdural or epidural injection of the radionuclide and/or post injection leakage (157, 176, 334)

        1. Subdural injection of radionuclide ("train track" pattern)

        2. Epidural injection of radionuclide ("Christmas tree" pattern)

        3. Spinal ligament or muscle injection

    B. Disc herniation and rupture (21, 73, 139, 246)

    C. Spinal cord tumors

        1. Multiple myeloma (139)

        2. Metastatic carcinoma (21)

        3. Leukemic infiltrates (139)

        4. Epidural lymphosarcoma (139, 246)

    5. Meningioma (234, 246)

    6. Angioma (73)

    7. Dermoid tumor (246)

    8. Neurinoma, single or multiple (70, 73, 234)

    9. Liposarcoma (246)

D. Spinal arachnoiditis (70, 73, 246)

E. Spondyloarthrosis (70)

F. Arachnoid cyst (246)

G. Epidural abscess (246)

H. Post-injection leakage associated with recent lumbar puncture and pneumo-encephalography (176)

I. Spine chondrosarcoma (22)

VII. Conditions causing focal areas of radionuclide concentration or retention

  A. Common

    1. Radionuclide leakage following suboccipital injection or lumbar injection (86, 334)

    2. Anatomical variant, large cisterna magna (123)

    3. Cerebral porencephalic cysts (106, 123, 146)

    4. Post-craniotomy cysts (122, 146, 149)

    5. Cerebrospinal fluid fistula or leaks (3) (Section VIII)

    6. Subdural hematoma (6, 19, 256)

    7. Basilar invagination, i.e. Paget's disease (123)

    8. Basilar impression (123)

    9. Cerebellar degeneration, congenital or acquired (123, 146, 186)

    10. Focal atrophy associated with cerebral embolic or thrombotic disease (198)

    11. Skull fracture (311)

    12. Posterior fossa cysts (123, 146)

    13. Following neurosurgical procedures (88, 89)

  B. Uncommon

    1. Unilateral reflux into a lateral ventricle (65)

    2. Associated with arteriovenous malformation (198)

    3. Meningoceles and myelomeningoceles (9, 146)

    4. Encephalomeningoceles (98, 106, 311)

    5. Acquired leptomeningeal cysts, traumatic (32, 146, 311)

    6. Subdural hygroma

      a. traumatic (291)

      b. following subdural hematoma evacuation (19)

    7. Congenital arachnoid cysts (55, 92, 123)

    8. Sturge-Weber syndrome (48)

    9. Spinal cord cysts (149)

    10. Artefact caused by residual oropharyngeal ^{99m}Tc pertechnetate (59)

    11. Lymphosarcoma, spinal (139)

12. Dandy-Walker cysts (122)
13. Crouzon's disease (148)
14. Artefact from radionuclide retention in hydronephrotic kidney (10)

VIII. Conditions causing cerebrospinal fluid leaks: often associated with other patterns caused by various underlying conditions (3, 67)

A. Common
  1. Traumatic fractures (3, 15, 57, 67) of:
    a. cribriform plate
    b. roof of frontal sinus
    c. anterior wall of sella turcica
    d. posterior fossa
    e. petrous bone
  2. Post craniotomy (3, 15, 122)
    a. transsphenoidal hypophysectomy
    b. tumor resection
    c. paranasal sinus surgery
B. Uncommon
  1. Traumatic cerebrospinal fluid leak (96, 157, 176, 181, 182)
    a. surgical
    b. penetrating wound
    c. following diagnostic and therapeutic lumbar punctures (152)
  2. Leaks associated with encephaloceles (3, 153)
  3. Spontaneous rhinorrhea (153)
  4. Congenital anomaly of the tegmen tympani (318)
  5. Spinal cord leak secondary to dorsal column stimulator implantation (285)
  6. Artefact from residual oropharyngeal pertechnetate (59)
  7. Bronchopleural-subarachnoid fistula (133)

IX. Entities displaying a normal cisternographic pattern in spite of presence of subarachnoid and/or intraventricular space disease (documented false negative results)

A. Status post craniotomy and brain surgery (89)
B. "Compensated" communicating hydrocephalus (107, 201, 204, 311)
C. Communicating hydrocephalus with functioning diversionary shunts and subsequent obstruction of the Sylvian aqueduct (67, 122, 201)
D. Communicating hydrocephalus with functioning shunt (204)
E. Obstructive noncommunicating hydrocephalus (8, 107, 149, 150, 204)
F. Obstructive noncommunicating hydrocephalus plus ventricular decompression (201)
G. Acute meningitis, current or past (3)
H. Obstructive noncommunicating hydrocephalus with patent shunt (149)

I. Communicating hydrocephalus, artefactual absence of intraventricular filling when cisternogram follows pneumoencephalogram on same day (210)

J. Pseudotumor cerebri (62, 88)

K. Obstructive noncommunicating hydrocephalus associated with spina bifida cystica (33)

L. Arnold-Chiari malformation (33)

X. Conditions characterized by accelerated clearance of the radionuclide from subarachnoid spaces

    A. Normal pattern in children (203)

    B. Normal variant (157)

    C. Hypoliquorrhea

        1. Spontaneous essential, low pressure headaches syndrome (172)

        2. Idiopathic, associated with lateral ventricle visualization (16)

References for this chapter may be found at the end of Chapter 15, page 75.

Chapter 14

Shunt Evaluation in Hydrocephalus

MARIANO FERNANDEZ-ULLOA

I. Obstructive noncommunicating hydrocephalus: shunt evaluation by radionuclide injection within the ventricles or into the shunts

    A. Patterns indicating intact and functioning shunt (4, 8, 67, 103, 107, 143, 148, 149, 175, 269)

        1. Lateral ventricle visualization with subsequent rapid clearance

        2. Decreasing of size of ventricles

        3. Radionuclide accumulation at shunt draining sites

            a. superior vena caval and atrial: causes radionuclide accumulation in kidneys and bladder

            b. pleural cavity

            c. peritoneal cavity

The use of an asterisk* in this chapter indicates that this entity has been observed by the author but the case report has not been published.

        d. subarachnoid space (ventriculocisternal shunts)
- **4.** Time-activity curves over the head indicating rapid radionuclide clearance
- **5.** Serial quantitative cisternography indicating adequate drainage
- **6.** Absence of radionuclide extravasation

B. Abnormal patterns
- **1.** Radionuclide accumulation indicating extravasation caused by broken catheter and loose connections (143)
- **2.** Patterns indicating shunt obstruction of proximal (ventricular) or distal limbs (4, 8, 107, 175)
  - **a.** stagnation of the radionuclide within the ventricles as indicated by scintigraphs and time-activity curves
  - **b.** nonvisualization of distal limb of shunt
  - **c.** persistent distal limb visualization may be present if obstruction is distal
  - **d.** radionuclide accumulation at draining sites not present
  - **e.** if obstruction is located at the proximal limb of shunt, ventricular filling is not observed

C. Causes of shunt obstruction (143)
- **1.** Encasement of proximal catheter by the choroid plexus
- **2.** Proximal limb situated within the brain tissue
- **3.** Catheter displacements caused by subdural hematomas
- **4.** Valve blocked by clots, tissue fragments, tumor
- **5.** Valve with improper opening pressure
- **6.** Separated connectors
- **7.** Breaks at motion points

II. Obstructive noncommunicating hydrocephalus: shunt assessment by intrathecal radionuclide administration

A. Patent shunt
- **1.** Normal cisternographic pattern present (203, 204)
- **2.** Pre-shunt pattern of delayed clearance or basilar cistern subarachnoid block may persist (203)
- **3.** Reflux into the ventricles may occur if ventriculocisternal shunting performed (4)

B. Obstructed shunt: cisternography returns to pre-shunt patterns:
- **1.** Normal cisternography*
- **2.** Basilar subarachnoid block (143)
- **3.** Delayed radionuclide clearance*

III. Obstructive communicating hydrocephalus: shunt evaluation by radionuclide administration into the shunt or ventricles (71, 175, 269)

A. Functioning shunt

      1. Patterns are similar to those previously described in Section I

      2. Partial passage of radionuclide into subarachnoid space may be observed

  B. Obstructed shunt, proximal (ventricular) or distal limb

      1. Ventricular shunt filling followed by absent or slow clearance as indicated by serial scintigraphs and clearance curves

      2. Absent visualization of distal shunt limb

      3. Lack of radionuclide accumulation at draining sites

      4. If shunt obstruction is located in the proximal limb, the lateral ventricles fail to visualize; distal limb visualization is possible

  C. "Non-utilized shunt." Radionuclide promptly leaves the ventricles and follows the normal subarachnoid space paths (107)

IV. Obstructive communicating hydrocephalus: shunt evaluation by intrathecal radionuclide administration (9, 67, 103, 107, 143, 148, 149)

  A. Patterns indicating a functioning shunt

      1. Subarachnoid space over the cerebral convexities nonvisualized

      2. Lateral ventricle visualization with subsequent clearing

      3. Normal or slightly delayed overall radionuclide clearance

      4. Visualization of distal shunt and draining sites

      5. Quantitative cisternography reflecting prompt clearance (62, 143, 199)

      6. In children absent ventricular visualization may occur caused by conversion into a noncommunicating hydrocephalus (143)

  B. Obstructed shunt

      1. Pattern returns to one of obstructive communicating hydrocephalus (143)

        a. persistent lateral ventricle visualization

        b. basilar subarachnoid block

        c. delayed radionuclide clearance

      2. Faint visualization of spaces over the convexities may be present (107)

      3. Nonvisualization of distal shunt (143)

      4. Absent radionuclide accumulation at draining sites (143)

      5. Quantitative cisternography: decreased radionuclide clearance (62)

  C. Patterns indicating radionuclide extravasation as previously described (Chapter 13, VI A)

  D. "Non-utilized shunt" pattern

      1. Pattern evolves to a closely normal one with mild delay of radionuclide clearance (107, 203)

References for this chapter may be found at the end of Chapter 15, page 75.

Chapter 15

Ventriculography

MARIANO FERNANDEZ-ULLOA

I. Normal patterns (95)

    A. Temporary filling of injected ventricle (in first 24 hours)
    B. Rapid ventricular clearing by 24 hours
    C. Secondary visualization of subarachnoid space pathways and clearance in a normal fashion

II. Communicating hydrocephalus (93, 236, 313)

    A. Pattern
        1. Enlarged ventricle
        2. Slow radionuclide drainage from lateral ventricle present
        3. Visualization of basal cisterns may be present

III. Noncommunicating hydrocephalus (8, 72, 88, 93, 236, 311)

    A. Pattern
        1. Enlarged ventricular system
        2. Absent or markedly decreased radionuclide clearing from ventricles
    B. Causes
        1. Post meningitis (107)
        2. Aqueduct of Sylvius stenosis associated with occipital encephalocele (106)
        3. Atresia of the aqueduct of Sylvius (8, 88)
        4. Stenosis of foramen of Magendie (4, 88)
        5. Posterior fossa tumor (4)
        6. Tumors of the third ventricle (4)
        7. Aqueduct of Sylvius stenosis secondary to tumors (4)

IV. Evaluation of cerebrospinal fluid shunts (see Chapter 14)

V. Distorted ventricles caused by brain tumors (72)

VI. Evaluation of central nervous system malformations
  A. Arnold-Chiari malformation (47, 106)
    1. With associated obstructive noncommunicating hydrocephalus
      a. visualization of dilated lateral and third ventricles
      b. nonvisualized fourth ventricle
      c. nonvisualized subarachnoid space
    2. Without associated noncommunicating hydrocephalus
      a. slow ventricle clearance
      b. radionuclide passage into and visualization of the subarachnoid space
  B. Dandy-Walker malformation (55, 106, 124)
    1. Dilated ventricular system and stasis
    2. Visualization of cystic fourth ventricle
    3. Subarachnoid spaces usually nonvisualized but seen in rare instances
  C. Hydranencephaly (8, 9, 106)
    1. Radionuclide accumulation and stagnation in single large cavity
  D. Cerebral agenesis (106)
    1. Prompt emptying of normal ventricle
    2. Radionuclide pooling and stagnation in large cerebral cavity
  E. Encephaloceles (106, 311)
    1. Pattern
      a. radionuclide pooling in encephalocele present or absent
      b. features of noncommunicating hydrocephalus may be present

VII. Status post hemispherectomy (88, 106)
  A. Pooling and stagnation of the radionuclide in postoperative cavity
  B. Communication between the subarachnoid space and postoperative cavity may be present

VIII. Focal radionuclide accumulations
  A. Extraventricular
    1. Needle tracks, tissue radionuclide contamination (72)
    2. Radionuclide pooling in encephaloceles (106)
    3. Radionuclide accumulation in post-hemispherectomy cavities (88)
    4. Porencephalic cysts (93)
  B. Intraventricular
    1. Single ventricle, cyclopean ventricle (93)
    2. Unilateral and persistent ventricular filling in asymmetric hydrocephalus secondary to ventriculitis (93)

REFERENCES[1]

1. Addlestone R, Workman JB: Lipoma of the corpus callosum. J Nucl Med 15:714–716, 1974.
2. Aita JF, Keyes JW: Radionuclide studies in vascular infantile hemiplegia. J Nucl Med 15:300–302, 1974.
3. Akerman M, deTovar G, Guiot G: Abnormal CSF circulation and occult hydrocephalus in association with CSF rhinorrhea, in Harbert JC, McCullough DC, Luessenhop AJ, et al (eds): Cisternography and Hydrocephalus: A Symposium. Springfield, IL: Charles C. Thomas, 1972, pp. 293–302.
4. Akerman M, deTovar G, Guiot G: Radionuclide cisternography and ventriculography in noncommunicating hydrocephalus, in Harbert JC, McCullough DC, Luessenhop AJ, et al (eds): Cisternography and Hydrocephalus: A Symposium. Springfield, IL: Charles C. Thomas, 1972, pp. 483–501.
5. Alavi A, Devenney JE, Arendale S, et al: Radionuclide angiography in evaluation of chemodectomas of the jugular glomus. Radiology 121:673–676, 1976.
6. Alazraki NP, Halpern SE, Rosenberg RN, et al: Accumulation of ^{131}I-labelled albumin in a subdural hematoma demonstrated by cisternography. J Nucl Med 12:758–760, 1971.
7. Alderson PO, Gilday DL, Mikhael M, et al: Value of routine cerebral radionuclide angiography in pediatric brain imaging. J Nucl Med 17:780–785, 1976.
8. Alker GJ, Glasauer FE, Leslie EV: Isotope cisternography and ventriculography in hydrocephalus of children, in Harbert JC, McCullough DC, Luessenhop AJ, et al (eds): Cisternography and Hydrocephalus: A Symposium. Springfield, IL: Charles C. Thomas, 1972, pp. 385–396.
9. Alker GJ, Glasauer FE, Leslie EV: Long-term experience with isotope cisternography. JAMA 219:1005–1010, 1972.
10. Alker GJ, Abdel-Dayem, HM, Oh, YS, et al: False positive dynamic imaging of the cerebral circulation due to a congenital anomaly. Clin Nucl Med 6:532–536, 1981.
11. Anderson JM, MacMillan JJ: Intracranial tuberculoma: increasing problem in Britain. J Neurol Neurosurg Psy 38:194–201, 1975.
12. Antunes JL, Schlesinger EB, Michelsen WJ: The abnormal brain scan in demyelinating diseases. Arch Neurol 30:269–271, 1974.
13. Apfelbaum RI, Newman SA, Zingesser LH: Dynamics of technetium scanning of subdural hematomas. Radiology 107:571–576, 1973.
14. Arkies LB, Andrews JT, Steven LW: A reappraisal of the scan diagnosis of subdural hematomas. Am J Roentgenol 115:62–71, 1972.
15. Ashburn WL, Harbert JC, Briner WH, et al: Cerebrospinal fluid rhinorrhea studied with the gamma scintillation camera. J Nucl Med 9:523–529, 1968.
16. Baldwin RD, Gouldin JA, Spencer RP: Hyperdynamic radionuclide cerebrospinal fluid study. Clin Nucl Med 7:82, 1982.
17. Banna M: Craniopharyngioma: Based on 160 cases. Br J Radiol 49:206–233, 1976.
18. Barnes BD, Winestock DP: Dynamic radionuclide scanning in the diagnosis of thrombosis of the superior sagittal sinus. Neurology 27:656–661, 1977.
19. Barnes BD, Hoff JT: Radionuclide cisternography after head injury. Arch Neurol 33:21–25, 1976.

[1]This list contains references for Chapters 11–15.

20. Barrett IR, Mishkin FS: Brain scans in infantile cerebral paralysis. Radiology 112:389–392, 1974.

21. Bauer FK, Yuhl ET: Myelography by means of I-131: The myeloscintigram. Neurology 3:341–346, 1953.

22. Bauer FK, Yuhl ET: Radioisotope myelography. Int J of Appl Rad Isotop 2:52–58, 1957.

23. Baum S, Rothballer AB, Shiffman F, et al: Brain scanning in the diagnosis of acoustic neuromas. J Neurosurg 36:141–147, 1972.

24. Beauchamp JM, Belanger MA, Neitzschman HR: An unusual cause of "doughnut" sign in brain scanning. J Nucl Med 16:432–433, 1975.

25. Bekier A: Displacement of anterior cerebral vessels in cerebral dynamic study in cases of chronic subdural hematomas. J Nucl Med 16:86–88, 1975.

26. Bennahum DA, Messner RP, Shoop JD: Brain scan findings in central nervous system involvement by lupus erythematosus. Ann Int Med 81:763–765, 1974.

27. Benson DF, LeMay M, Patten DH, et al: Diagnosis of normal-pressure hydrocephalus. New England J Med 283:609–615, 1970.

28. Benson DF, Patten DH, LeMay M: Hydrocephalic dementia, in Harbert JC, McCullough DC, Luessenhop AJ, et al (eds): Cisternography and Hydrocephalus: A Symposium. Springfield, IL: Charles C. Thomas, 1972, pp. 343–355.

29. Benua RS: Abnormal brain scan in eosinophilic granuloma of the skull. J Nucl Med 11:89–91, 1970.

30. Bernard JD, McDonald RA, Verdon TA: Brain scanning for subdural hematoma: problems in interpretation (abstract). J Nucl Med 10:322, 1969.

31. Binet EF, Loken MK: Scintiangiography of cerebral arteriovenous malformations and aneurysms. Am J Roentgenol 109:707–713, 1970.

32. Black P, Cooper M: Posterior fossa cyst demonstrated by isotopic cisternography. J Nucl Med 14:944–946, 1973.

33. Bligh AS, Shurtleff DB, Leach KG, et al: Isotope cisternography using ^{99m}Tc labeled human albumin in spina bifida cystica, in Harbert JC, McCullough DC, Luessenhop AJ, et al (eds): Cisternography and Hydrocephalus: A Symposium. Springfield, IL: Charles C. Thomas, 1972, pp. 397–412.

34. Bligh AS, Weaver CM, Wells CEC: Isotope encephalography in the management of acute herpesvirus encephalitis. J Neurol Neurosurg Psy 35:569–581, 1972.

35. Bogdanowicz WM, Wilson DH: Dermoid cyst of fourth ventricle demonstrated on brain scan: case report. J Neurosurg 36:228–230, 1972.

36. Briggs RC, Skor RB: Choroid plexus meningioma of the lateral ventricle: two cases demonstrated by brain scanning. J Nucl Med 9:131–134, 1968.

37. Brill DR, Shoop JD: Sensitivity of radionuclide isotope brain scan in cerebral melioidosis: case report. J Nucl Med 18:987–989, 1977.

38. Brooks WH, Mortara RH, Preston D: The clinical limitations of brain scanning in metastatic disease. J Nucl Med 15:620–621, 1974.

39. Brugge KGT, Meindok H: Rim sign in brain scintigraphy of epidural hematoma. J Nucl Med 14:709–710, 1973.

40. Brumback RA, Yoder FW, Andrews AD, et al: Normal pressure hydrocephalus. Recognition and relationship to neurological abnormalities in Cockayne's Syndrome. Arch Neurol 35:337–345, 1978.

41. Buonanno FS, Moody DM, Ball MR, et al: Radionuclide sinography: Diagnosis of lateral sinus thrombosis by dynamic and static brain imaging. Radiology 130:207–213, 1979.

42. Buozas DJ, Barrett IR, Mishkin FS: Diagnosis of epidural hematoma by brain scan and perfusion study: case report. J Nucl Med 17:975–976, 1976.

43. Burrows EH: Clinical reliability of posterior fossa scintigraphy. Clin Radiol 27:473–481, 1976.

44. Burrows EH: Scintigraphic diagnosis of acoustic neurofibromas. Br J Radiol 48:1000–1006, 1975.

45. Burt RW: Brain scan abnormalities produced by electroencephalographic procedures. J Nucl Med 15:369–370, 1974.

46. Case Records of the Massachusetts General Hospital: Case 40–1977. Scully RE, Galdabini JJ, McNeely BU (eds). N Engl J Med 297:773–780, 1977.

47. Castellino RA, Zatz LM, DeNardo GL: Radioisotope ventriculography in Arnold-Chiari Malformation. Radiology 93:817–821, 1969.

48. Chang JC, Jackson GL, Baltz R: Isotopic cisternography in Sturge-Weber syndrome. J Nucl Med 11:551–553, 1970.

49. Chatterton BE: Progressive abnormalities in the brain scan in adrenal leukodystrophy. Am J Roentgenol 129:939–940, 1977.

50. Ciric IS, Quinn JL, Bucy PC: Mercury-197 and technetium-99m brain scans in the diagnosis of non-neoplastic intracranial lesions. J Neurosurg 27:119–125, 1967.

51. Coblentz JM, Mattis S, Zingesser LH, et al: Presenile dementia: Clinical aspects and evaluation of cerebrospinal fluid dynamics. Arch Neurol 29:299–308, 1973.

52. Cohan SL, Fermaglich J, Auth TL: Abnormal brain scans in multiple sclerosis. J Neurol Neurosurg Psy 38:120–122, 1975.

53. Conway JJ: Radionuclide imaging of the central nervous system in children. Radiol Clin North Am 10:291–312, 1972.

54. Conway JJ, Vollert JM: The accuracy of radionuclide imaging in detecting pediatric dural fluid collections. Radiology 105:77–83, 1972.

55. Conway JJ, Yarzagaray L, Welch D: Radionuclide evaluation of the Dandy-Walker malformation and congenital arachnoid cyst of the posterior fossa. Am J Roent 112:306–314, 1971.

56. Cowan RJ, Maynard CD, Lassiter KR: Technetium-99m pertechnetate brain scans in the detection of subdural hematoma: A study of the age of the lesion as related to the development of positive scan. J Neurosurg 32:30–34, 1976.

57. Cowan J, Maynard CD: Trauma to brain and extracranial structures. Sem Nucl Med 4:319–338, 1974.

58. Cowan RJ, Maynard CD, Meschan I, et al: Value of the routine use of the cerebral dynamic radioisotope study. Radiology 107:111–116, 1973.

59. Cowan RJ, Murphy MP, Maynard CD: Production of cerebrospinal fluid leak artifact by residual ^{99m}Tc-pertechnetate. J Nucl Med 16:434, 1975.

60. Cradduck TD, Duggan HE: Effect of skull plates on postoperative brain scans. J Nucl Med 10:140–142, 1969.

61. Curl FD, Harbert JC, Luessenhop AD, et al: Radionuclide cerebral angiography in a case of bilateral carotid-cavernous fistula. Radiology 102:391–392, 1972.

62. Curl FD, Harbert JC, McCullough DC: Quantitative cisternography: An aid to diagnosis, in Harbert JC, McCullough DC, Luessenhop AJ, et al (eds): Cisternography and Hydrocephalus: A Symposium. Springfield, IL: Charles C. Thomas, 1972, pp. 441–451.

63. Daly MJ, Patton DD: Ventriculitis: Diagnosis with technetium-99m DTPA. J Nucl Med 19:1233–1234, 1978.

64. David RB, Beiler D, Hood H, et al: Scintillation brain scanning in children. Am J Dis Child 112:197–204, 1966.

65. Deisenhammer E, Gund A, Hammer B, et al: Unilateral ventricular reflux: case report. J Nucl Med 16:716–717, 1975.

66. DeLand FH, Garcia F: Perfusion studies in the diagnosis of cerebral aneurysms. J Nucl Med 15:358–360, 1974.

67. DeLand FH, James AE, Wagner HN, et al: Cisternography with [169]Yb-DTPA. J Nucl Med 12:683–689, 1971.

68. DeLand FH, Wagner HN: Tuberculous ventriculitis, in Brain: Atlas of Nuclear Medicine, vol. I. Philadelphia: W.B. Saunders, p. 48, 1969

69. DeLong JF: Subdural empyema associated with an apparent regional hyperperfusion (luxury perfusion). Clin Nucl Med 3:485–486, 1978.

70. De Rossi G, Simone F, Troncone L, et al: La nostra esperienza di mielografia radioisotopica. Sistema Nervoso 22:335–347, 1970.

71. DiChiro G, Grove AS: Evaluation of surgical and spontaneous cerebrospinal fluid shunt by isotope scanning. J Neurosurg 24:743–748, 1966.

72. DiChiro G, Reames PM, Matthews WB: RISA-ventriculography and RISA-cisternography. Neurology 14:185–191, 1964.

73. Dietrich VJ, Lobe J: Erfahrungen mit der Myeloszintigraphie unter verwendung von ^{131}I-human-serum albumin. Zbl Neurochir Band 32:155–166, 1971.

74. Dodson WE, Prensky AL, Siegel BA: Radionuclide imaging in subacute sclerosing panencephalitis. Neurology 29:749–752, 1979.

75. Earnest MP, Fahn S, Karp JH, et al: Normal pressure hydrocephalus and hypertensive cerebrovascular disease. Arch Neurol 31:262–266, 1974.

76. Fagan JA, Cowan RJ: The effect of potassium perchlorate on the uptake of ^{99m}Tc-pertechnetate in choroid plexus papillomas: A report of two cases. J Nucl Med 12:312–314, 1971.

77. Farkas R, Binet E, McAfee JG, et al: Scintigraphy of meningiomas: Radiologic-pathologic correlations in 32 cases. Int J Nucl Med and Biol 4:1–12, 1977.

78. Feigin DS, Welsh DM, Siegel BA, et al: The efficacy of the brain scan in diagnosis of brain stem gliomas. Radiology 116:117–120, 1975.

79. Ferry DJ, Mylander K, Hardman J: Radiographic identification and surgical removal of teratoid tumor of roof of third ventricle: case report. J Neurosurg 36:231–234, 1972.

80. Fischer RJ, Miale A: Evaluation of cerebral vascular disease with radionuclide angiography. Stroke 3:1–9, 1972.

81. Fish MB, Barnes B, Pollycove M: Cranial scintiphotographic blood flow defects in arteriographically proven cerebral vascular disease. J Nucl Med 14:558–564, 1973.

82. Fish MB, Pollycove M, O'Reilly S, et al: Vascular characterization of brain lesions by rapid sequential cranial scintiphotography. J Nucl Med 9:249–259, 1968.

83. Fitzer PM: Radionuclide angiography—brain and bone imaging in craniofacial fibrous dysplasia (CFD): case report. J Nucl Med 18:709–712, 1977.

84. Fitzer PM: Nuclide angiography in Paget's disease of the skull: case report. J Nucl Med 16:619–621, 1975.

85. Fitzer PM, Rinaldi I: Abnormal radionuclide angiogram in proven intracranial fibromuscular dysplasia: case report. J Nucl Med 15:190–192, 1976.

86. Fleming JFR, Sheppard RH, Turner VM: CSF scanning in the evaluation of hydrocephalus: A clinical review of 100 patients, in Harbert JC, McCullough DC, Luessenhop AJ, et al (eds): Cisternography and Hydrocephalus: A Symposium. Springfield, IL: Charles C. Thomas, 1972, pp. 261–284.

87. Fowler GW, Williams JP: Technetium brain scans in tuberous sclerosis. J Nucl Med 14:215–218, 1973.

88. Frigeni G, Gaini SM, Paoletti P, et al: Isotope cisternography. Considerations on abnormal pictures. Acta Neurochirurgica 25:145–163, 1971.

89. Frigeni G, Gaini SM, Paoletti P, et al: Study of possible postsurgical complications in neurosurgery using radioisotope cisternography, in Harbert JC, McCullough DC, Luessenhop AJ, et al (eds): Cisternography and Hydrocephalus: A Symposium. Springfield, IL: Charles C Thomas, 1972, pp. 303–316.

90. Front D: Distinctive imaging characteristics of different types of brain tumors. Clin Nucl Med 4:211–218, 1979.

91. Front D, Beks JWF, Giorganas CL, et al: Abnormal patterns of cerebrospinal fluid flow and absorption after head injuries. Diagnosis by isotope cisternography. Neuroradiology 4:6–13, 1972.

92. Front D, Minderhoud JM, Beks WF, et al: Leptomeningeal cysts diagnosed by isotope cisternography. J Neurol Neurosurg Psy 36:1018–1023, 1973.

93. Front D, Overbeek WJ, Penning L: The study of infantile hydrocephalus with combined air and isotope ventriculography. J Neurol Neurosurg Psy 35:456–462, 1972.

94. Fulmer LR, Sfakianakis GN: Cerebral ventricle visualization during brain scanning with ^{99m}Tc-pertechnetate. J Nucl Med 15:202–204, 1974.

95. Gaini SM, Paoletti P, Villani R, et al: High specific activity ^{131}I and ^{99m}Tc albumin for studying the cerebrospinal fluid circulation in infantile and childhood hydrocephalus. Acta Neurochirurgica 23:31–46, 1970.

96. Gass H, Goldstein AS, Ruskin R, et al: Chronic postmyelogram headache. Isotopic demonstration of dural leak and surgical cure. Arch Neurol 25:168–170, 1971.

97. Gates GF, Dore EK, Taplin GV: Interval brain scanning with sodium pertechnetate Tc-99m for tumor detectability. JAMA 215:85–88, 1971.

98. Gelfand MJ, Walus M, Tomsick T, et al: Nasoethmoidal encephalomeningocele demonstrated by cisternography: case report. J Nucl Med 18:706–708, 1977.

99. Gilday DL: Various radionuclide patterns of cerebral inflammation in infants and children. Am J Roentgenol 120:247–253, 1974.

100. Gilday DL, Coates G, Goldenberg D: Subdural hematoma—what is the role of brain scanning in its diagnosis? J Nucl Med 14:283–287, 1973.

101. Gilday DL, Eng B, Ash J: Accuracy of brain scanning in pediatric craniocerebral neoplasms. Radiology 117:93–97, 1975.

102. Gilday DL, Eng B, Ash J, et al: Dural fluid collections in infants and children. A successful nuclear medicine approach. Radiology 114:367–372, 1975.

103. Gilday DL, Kellam J: ^{111}In-DTPA evaluation of CSF diversionary shunts in children. J Nucl Med 14:920–923, 1973.

104. Gilday DL, Reba RC, Longo R: Comparison of techniques for obtaining the vertex view in brain scanning. J Nucl Med 11:503–507, 1970.

105. Gize RW, Mishkin FS: Brain scans in multiple sclerosis. Radiology 97:297–300, 1970.

106. Glasauer FE: Isotope cisternography and ventriculography in congenital abnormalities of the central nervous system. J Neurosurg 43:18–26, 1975.

107. Glasauer FE, Alker GJ, Leslie EV: Isotope cisternography and ventriculography. Evaluation of hydrocephalus in children. Am J Dis Child 120:109–114, 1970.

108. Glass ED, Stadalnik RC, Barnett CA: Ventricular visualization on brain scan with intracranial hemorrhage in disseminated phycomycosis. Clin Nucl Med 3:429–431, 1978.

109. Go RT, Chiu CL, Neuman LA: Diagnosis of superior sagittal sinus thrombosis by dynamic and sequential brain scanning. Neurology 23:1199–1204, 1973.

110. Go RT, Ptacek JJ: Localization of ^{99m}Tc in the choroid plexus. J Nucl Med 14:352–353, 1973.

111. Go RT, Suzuki Y, Schapiro RL, et al: The scintigraphic features of the occipital sinus. Radiology 112:635–638, 1974.

111A. Goldfarb CR, Daiz AS: Trauma in the Pagetoid: Beware the non-specific scintigram. Clin Nucl Med 3:404–405, 1978.

112. Goodman JM, Heck LL: Confirmation of brain death at bedside by isotope angiography. JAMA 238:966–968, 1977.

113. Goodman JM, Mishkin FS, Dyken M: Determination of brain death by isotope angiography. JAMA 209:1869–1872, 1969.

114. Goodman SJ, Hayes M: Value of cerebral isotope flow studies in timing of surgery for ruptured aneurysms when there is vasospasm and neurologic deficit. J Nucl Med 15:1113–1116, 1974.

115. Goodrich JK, Tutor FT: The isotope encephalogram in brain tumor diagnosis. J Nucl Med 6:541–548, 1965.

115A. Grossman SA, Trump DL, Chen DCP, et al: Cerebrospinal fluid flow abnormalities in patients with neoplastic meningitis: An evaluation using [111]indium-DTPA ventriculography. Am J Med 73:641–647, 1982.

116. Hahn FJY, Rice AC, Christie JH: Occlusion of the posterior cerebral artery: scintiscan and angiographic findings. Radiology 112:131–133, 1974.

117. Hahn FJY, Schapiro RL: Brain image manifestation in the patient with cavernous sinus occlusion. Radiology 118:113–114, 1976.

118. Haidri NH, Modi SM: Normal pressure hydrocephalus and hypertensive cerebrovascular disease. Dis Nervous Systems 38:918–921, 1977.

119. Halpern SE, Alazraki N, Hurwitz S, et al: Changes in the radioisotope cisternogram in cerebrovascular-occlusive disease. J Nucl Med 13:493–497, 1972.

120. Halpern SE, Smith CW, Ficken V: [99m]Tc brain scanning in herpes virus type I encephalitis. J Nucl Med 11:548–550, 1970.

121. Handa J, Janda H, Hamamoto K, et al: Sequential brain imaging as an aid in understanding disease etiology. Sem Nucl Med 1:56–59, 1971.

122. Harbert JC: Radionuclide cisternography. Sem Nucl Med 1:90–106, 1971.

123. Harbert JC, James AE: Posterior fossa abnormalities demonstrated by cisternography. J Nucl Med 13:73–80, 1972.

124. Harbert JC, McCullough DC: Radionuclide studies in an unusual case of Dandy-Walker cyst. Radiology 101:363–366, 1971.

125. Hattner RS: Posterior fossa scintiangiography: Documentation of genetic penetrance of Von Hippel-Lindau syndrome in a clinically unaffected girl and her father. J Nucl Med 16:828–830, 1975.

126. Hattner RS, Putman C, Shames DM: Decompression hyperostosis: Cranial hyperostosis mimicking bilateral subdural hematoma on brain scintigraphy. Radiology 115:673–674, 1975.

127. Hawes DR, Mishkin FS: Brain scans in watershed infarction and laminar cortical necrosis. Radiology 103:131–134, 1972.

128. Hayt DB, Blatt CJ, Goldman SM, et al: Hypervascular presentation of multiple myeloma involving the skull, demonstrated on encephaloscintigraphy. J Nucl Med 20:125–126, 1979.

129. Hayt DB, Perez LA: Cervical venous reflux in dynamic brain scintigraphy. J Nucl Med 16:9–12, 1975.

130. Heiser WJ, Quinn JL, Mollihan WV: The crescent pattern of increased radioactivity in brain scanning. Radiology 87:483–488, 1966.

131. Higgins CB, Taketa RM, Halpern SE: Abnormal brain scans in adrenal leukodystrophy.

Radiology 114:667–669, 1975.

132. Hill TC, Hoffer PB, Levin VA: A comparison of 1- and 2-hr delayed brain scans in patients undergoing chemotherapy for primary brain tumors. J Nucl Med 18:877–880, 1977.

133. Hofstetter KR, Bjelland JC, Patton DD, et al: Detection of bronchopleural-subarachnoid fistula by radionuclide myelography: case report. J Nucl Med 18:981–983, 1977.

134. Hofstetter KR, Patton DD, Henry RE: Cerebral perfusion deficit masked by Paget's disease of the skull. J Nucl Med 19:197–199, 1978.

135. Holloway W, Gammal TE, Pool WH: Doughnut sign in subdural hematomas. J Nucl Med 13:630–632, 1972.

136. Holmes RA, Golle R: Appearance of the transverse sinuses by brain scanning. Am J Roentgenol 106:340–343, 1969.

137. Holmquest DL, Launey WS: Abnormal scintiangiographic findings associated with seizure activity. Radiology 111:147–150, 1974.

138. Hopkins GB, Kristensen KAB: Rapid sequential scintiphotography in the radionuclide detection of subdural hematomas. J Nucl Med 14:288–290, 1973.

139. Hubner KF, Brown DW: Scanning of the spinal subarachnoid space after intrathecal injection of ^{131}I labeled human serum albumin. J Nucl Med 6:465–472, 1965.

140. Hulvat GF, Batnitzky S, Wellman HN: Epidural hematoma of the posterior fossa: Radionuclide features. Radiology 127:194, 1978.

141. Hurley PJ: Effect of craniotomy on the brain scan related to time elapsed after surgery. J Nucl Med 13:156–158, 1972.

142. Jain KK, Schober B: Diagnosis of extradural hematoma by brain scan. Can Med Assoc J 107:218–219, 1972.

143. James AE, DeBlanc HJ, DeLand FH, et al: Refinements in cerebrospinal fluid diversionary shunt evaluation by cisternography. Am J Roentgenol 115:766–773, 1972.

144. James AE, DeLand FH, Hodges FJ, et al: Radionuclide imaging in detection and differential diagnosis of craniopharyngiomas. Am J Roentgenol 109:692–700, 1970.

145. James AE, Dorst JP, Mathews ES, et al: Hydrocephalus in achondroplasia studied by cisternography. Pediatrics 49:46–49, 1972.

146. James AE, Harbert JC, DeLand FH, et al: Localized enlargement of the cerebrospinal fluid space demonstrated by cisternography. Neuroradiology 2:184–190, 1971.

147. James AE, Hodges FJ, Jordan CE, et al: Angiography and cisternography in acute meningitis due to *Hemophilus influenzae*. Radiology 103:601–606, 1972.

148. James AE, Hurley PJ, Heller RM, et al: CSF imaging (cisternography) in pediatric patients. Ann Radiol 14:591–600, 1971.

149. James AE, Mathews ES, DeBlanc HJ, et al: Cerebrospinal fluid imaging: Its current status. J Can Assoc Radiol 23:157–167, 1972.

150. James AE, New PFJ, Heinz ER, et al: A cisternographic classification of hydrocephalus. Am J Roentgenol 115:39–49, 1972.

151. Jayaraman A, Garofalo M, Donnenfeld H, et al: Huntington's chorea and normal pressure hydrocephalus. New York State J Med 78:1465–1468, 1978.

152. Kadrie H, Driedger AA, McInnis W: Persistent dural cerebrospinal fluid leak shown by retrograde radionuclide myelography: case report. J Nucl Med 17:797–799, 1976.

153. Kan MK, Hopkins GB: Spontaneous rhinorrhea in a 52-year-old woman. JAMA 239:2375–2376, 1978.

154. Kapp JP, Alfred HC, Jones T: Isotope sinograms. Technical note. J Neurosurg 44:393–394, 1976.

155. Karlin CA, Robinson RG, Hinthorn DR, et al: Radionuclide imaging in herpes simplex

encephalitis. Radiology 126:181–184, 1978.
156. Kieffer SA, Loken MK: Positive "brain" scans in fibrous dysplasia and other lesions of the skull. Am J Roentgenol 106:731–738, 1969.
157. Kieffer SA, Wolff JM, Prentice WB, et al: Scinticisternography in individuals without known neurological disease. Am J Roentgenol 112:225–236, 1971.
158. Kieffer SA, Wolff JM, Westreich G: The borderline scinticisternogram. Radiology 106:133–140, 1973.
159. Kilgore BB, Bonte FJ: Scintigraphic demonstration of cerebral infarction in a "watershed" distribution. J Nucl Med 12:756–757, 1971.
160. Kim EE: Ipsilateral cessation of CSF flow in a patient with cerebral hematoma. Clin Nucl Med 3:64, 1978.
161. Kim EE, DeLand FH, Maruyama Y: Brain and lung involvement of mycosis fungoides demonstrated by radionuclide imaging. J Nucl Med 20:240–242, 1979.
162. Kim EE, DeLand FH, Montebello J: Sensitivity of radionuclide brain scan and computed tomography in early detection of viral meningoencephalitis. Radiology 132:425–429, 1979.
163. Kirchner P, McKusick KA: Serendipity in cisternography. J Nucl Med 14:59–60, 1973.
164. Kirsh J, Rosenthal L, Finlayson MH, et al: Progressive multifocal leukoencephalopathy. Radiology 119:399–400, 1976.
165. Kitching GB, Hasso AN, Hieshima GB: Interhemispheric infarction. Radiology 120:111–115, 1976.
166. Klingensmith WC, Datu J: Tuberculous meningitis of the Sylvian fissure. Clin Nucl Med 3:315–317, 1978.
167. Koulouris S, Lang ER, Fox JL: Intracranial Hodgkin's disease simulating pterional meningioma. Med Ann District of Columbia 38:86–97, 1969.
168. Krishnamurthy GT, Methat A, Tomiyasu AN, et al: Clinical value and limitation of ^{99m}Tc brain scan: an autopsy correlation. J Nucl Med 13:373–378, 1972.
169. Krishnamurthy M, Nusbacher N, Elguezaba A, et al: Granulocytic sarcoma of the brain. Cancer 39:1542–1546, 1977.
170. Kryst-Widzgowska T, Kozlowski P, Binkiewicz M, et al: The angiographic and scintigraphic picture of dolichoectasia of the anterior cerebral artery. Eur J Nuc Med 5:387–389, 1980.
171. Kuhl DE, Bevilacqua JE, Mishkin MM, et al: The brain scan in Sturge-Weber syndrome. Radiology 103:621–626, 1972.
172. Labadi EL, Van Antwerp J, Bamford CR: Abnormal lumbar isotope cisternography in an unusual case of spontaneous hypoliquorrheic headache. Neurology 26:136–139, 1976.
173. Lake P, Friedenberg MJ, McCammon CJ: Diagnosis of basal meningeal gliomatosis by brain scan: significance of basal cistern sign. J Neurosurg 37:100–102, 1972.
174. Landman S, Ross P: Radionuclides in the diagnosis of arteriovenous malformations of the brain. Radiology 108:635–639, 1973.
175. Larson SM, Johnston GS, Ommaya AK, et al: The radionuclide ventriculogram. JAMA 224:853–857, 1973.
176. Larson SM, Schall GL, DiChiro G: The influence of previous lumbar puncture and pneumoencephalography on the incidence of unsuccessful radioisotope cisternography. J Nucl Med 12:555–557, 1971.
177. Larson SM, Schall GL, DiChiro G: The unsuccessful injection in cisternography: Incidence, cause and appearance (abstract). J Nucl Med 12:375, 1971.
178. Lee HK: Brain scanning in a case of through and through gunshot head wound. Clin Nucl Med 4:306, 1979.

179. Lee HK: Unilateral pyogenic ventriculitis. J Nucl Med 18:403, 1977.
180. LeMay M, New PFJ: Radiologic diagnosis of occult normal pressure hydrocephalus. Radiology 96:347–358, 1970.
181. Lieberman LM, Tourtellotte WW, Newkirk TA: Prolonged post-lumbar puncture cerebrospinal fluid leakage from lumbar subarachnoid space demonstrated by radioisotope myelography. Neurology 21:925–929, 1971.
182. Liebeskid AL, Herz DA, Rosenthal AD, et al: Radionuclide demonstration of spinal dural leaks. J Nucl Med 14:356–358, 1973.
183. Lin MS: Diagnostic scintigraphic sign in epidural hematoma at the vertex: case report. J Nucl Med 17:972–974, 1976.
184. Lisbona R, Lacourciere Y, Rosenthall L: Aspergillomatous abscesses of the brain and thyroid. J Nucl Med 14:541–542, 1973.
185. Lusins J: Delayed appearance of ''doughnut'' uptake demonstrated by sequential brain scanning. Clin Nucl Med 2:166–168, 1977.
186. Lusins J: Status of ^{111}In-DTPA in the posterior fossa in patients with cerebellar degeneration. J Nucl Med 17:349–351, 1976.
187. Maeda T, Mori H, Hisada K, et al: Radionuclide cerebral angiography in moyamoya disease. Clin Nucl Med 4:513–515, 1979.
188. Makhija MC, Vincent NR: Scintigraphy in epidermoid tumor of the skull. Clin Nucl Med 5:122–124, 1980.
189. Maki Y, Nakada Y, Nose T, et al: Clinical and radioisotopic follow-up study of ''moyamoya.'' Childs Brain 2:257, 1976
190. Makler PT, Gutowicz MF, Kuhl DE: Methotrexate-induced ventriculitis: Appearance on routine radionuclide scan and emission computer tomography. Clin Nucl Med 3:22–23, 1980.
191. Maroon JC, Jones R, Mishkin FS: Tuberculous meningitis diagnosed by brain scan. Radiology 104:333–335, 1972.
192. Martin TR, Moore JS, Shafer RB: Evaluation of the posterior flow study in brain scintigraphy. J Nucl Med 17:13–16, 1976.
192A. Martins AN, Johnston JS, Henry JM et al: Delayed radiation necrosis of the brain. J Neurosurg 47:336–345, 1977.
193. Marty R, Cain ML: Effects of corticosteroid (Dexamethasone) administration on the brain scan. Radiology 107:117–121, 1973.
194. Matin P, Goodwin DA, Nayyar SN: Radionuclide cerebral angiography in diagnosis and evaluation of carotid-cavernous fistula. J Nucl Med 15:1105–1109, 1974.
195. Maynard CD, Hanner TG, Witcofski RL: Positive brain scans due to lesions of the skull. Arch Neurol 18:93–97, 1968.
196. Maynard CD, Witcofski RL, Janeway R, et al: ''Radioisotope arteriography'' as an adjunct to the brain scan. Radiology 92:908–912, 1969.
197. McAllister JD, Marasco JA: Correlation of brain scans with radiographic findings (abstract). J Nucl Med 10:419–420, 1969.
198. McClelland RR: Focally increased activity on scinticisternography: Report of two cases. J Nucl Med 17:626–629, 1976.
199. McCullough DC, Fox JL, Curl FD, et al: Effects of CSF shunts on intracranial pressure and CSF dynamics, in Harbert JC, McCullough DC, Luessenhop AJ, et al (eds): Cisternography and Hydrocephalus: A Symposium. Springfield, IL: Charles C. Thomas, 1972, pp. 335–342.
200. McCullough DC, Harbert JC: Isotope demonstration of CSF pathways: Guide to antifungal therapy in coccidioidal meningitis. JAMA 209:558–560, 1969.

201. McCullough DC, Harbert JC: Pediatric radionuclide cisternography. Sem Nucl Med 2:343–352, 1972.

202. McCullough DC, Harbert JC, DiChiro G, et al: Prognostic criteria for cerebrospinal fluid shunting from isotope cisternography in communicating hydrocephalus. Neurology 20:594–598, 1970.

203. McCullough DC, Luessenhop AJ: Evaluation of photoscanning of the diffusion of intra-thecal RISA in infantile and childhood hydrocephalus. J Neurosurg 30:673–678, 1969.

204. McCullough DC, Harbert JC, Luessenhop AJ: Pediatric hydrocephalus: Contributions of radioisotope in cisternography to diagnosis and management, in Harbert JC, McCullough DC, Luessenhop AJ, et al (eds): Cisternography and Hydrocephalus: A Symposium. Springfield, IL: Charles C. Thomas, 1972, pp. 375–383.

205. McDaniel MM, Zobell RL, Morton ME: Periventricular spread of tumor shown on 67-Ga-citrate scan. Clin Nucl Med 3:231, 1978.

206. McLaughlin AF, Crocker EF, Morris JC: Brain scanning in intracranial infection (abstract). J Nucl Med 13:451, 1972.

207. Meschan I, Lytle WP, Maynard CD, et al: Statistical relationship of brain scans, cervicocranial dynamic studies, and cerebral arteriograms. Radiology 100:623–629, 1971.

208. Messert B, Miley C: Isotope cisternography in the diagnosis of chronic subdural hematoma. Neurology 24:828–833, 1974.

209. Messert B, Tyson IB, Barron SA: Limitations of radionuclide flow studies in bilateral carotid thrombosis. Stroke 6:67–71, 1975.

210. Milhorat TH, Chien T, Majd M, et al: Unreliability of combined pneumoencephalography and scinticisternography. J Nucl Med 17:54–56, 1976.

211. Miller JH, Pena AM, Segal HD: Radiological investigation of sellar region masses in children. Radiology 134:81–87, 1980.

212. Miller MS, Simmon GH: Optimization of timing and positioning of the technetium brain scan. J Nucl Med 9:429–435, 1968.

213. Miller SW, Potsaid MS: Focal brain scan abnormalities in multiple sclerosis. J Nucl Med 15:131–133, 1974.

214. Mishkin F: Brain scanning in children. Sem Nucl Med 2:328–342, 1972.

215. Mishkin F: Determination of cerebral death by radionuclide angiography. Radiology 115:135–137, 1975.

216. Mishkin F, Dyken M: Increased early radionuclide activity in the nasopharyngeal area in patients with internal carotid artery obstruction: "Hot Nose." Radiology 96:77–80, 1970.

217. Mishkin F, Truksa J: The diagnosis of intracranial cyst by means of the brain scan. Radiology 90:740–746, 1968.

218. Mishkin F, Weber K: Brain scan in hyperparathyroidism. J Nucl Med 12:763–764, 1971.

219. Mishkin FS: Radionuclide angiogram and scan findings in a case of herpes simplex encephalitis. J Nucl Med 11:608–609, 1970.

220. Molinari GF, Pircher F, Heyman A: Serial brain scanning using technetium-99m in patients with cerebral infarction. Neurology 17:627–636, 1967.

221. Moody RA, Olsen JO, Gottschalk A, et al: Brain scans of the posterior fossa. J Neurosurg 36:148–152, 1972.

222. Moore J, Goldberg ME, Kieffer SA: Positive dynamic radionuclide flow studies in intracranial tumors: Correlation with angiographic studies. J Nucl Med 14:430–431, 1973.

223. Moreno JB, DeLand FH: Brain scanning in the diagnosis of astrocytomas of the brain. J Nucl Med 12:107–111, 1971.

224. Morley JB, Langford KH: Abnormal brain scan with subacute extradural hematoma. J Neurol Neurosurg Psy 33:679–686, 1970.

225. Moses DC, Davis LE, Wagner HN: Brain scanning with ^{99m}TcO$_4$ in multiple sclerosis: J Nucl Med 13:847–848, 1972.

226. Moses DC, James AE, Strauss HW, et al: Regional cerebral blood flow estimation in the diagnosis of cerebrovascular disease. J Nucl Med 13:135–141, 1972.

227. Mosher MB, Schall GL, Wilson J: Progressive multifocal leukoencephalopathy. Positive brain scan. JAMA 218:226–228, 1971.

228. Nordlander S, Wiklund PE, Asard PE: Cerebral angioscintigraphy in brain death and in coma due to drug intoxication: J Nucl Med 14:856–857, 1973.

229. Norwood CW, Kelly DL: Intracerebral sarcoidosis acting as a mass lesion. Surg Neurol 2:367–372, 1974.

230. Nusynowitz ML, Clark RW: False positive brain scan associated with febrile convulsions. Am J Roentgenol 110:71–73, 1970.

231. Ogawa TK, So SK, Gerberg E, et al: Jugular-dural sinuses-jugular reflux in dynamic brain-flow imaging as a sign of unilateral innominate vein obstruction: case report. J Nucl Med 18:39–41, 1976.

232. O'Mara RE, Subramanian G, McAfee JG, et al: Comparison of ^{113}In and other short-lived agents for cerebral scanning. J Nucl Med 10:18–27, 1969.

233. Ostertag C, Mundinger F, McDonnell D, et al: Detection of 247 midline and posterior fossa tumors by combined scintigraphic and digital gammaencephalography. J Neurosurg 39:224–229, 1974.

234. Otto H, Saver J, Fieback O, et al: Die Myeloszintigraphie als praoperative Untersuchungsmethode bei raumfordernden Prozessen des Spinalkanals. Fortschr Rontgenstr 116:766–772, 1972.

235. Palacios E, Lawson RC: Choroid plexus papillomas of the lateral ventricles. Am J Roentgenol 115:113–119, 1972.

236. Paoletti P, Villani R: Radioactive isotopes as a diagnostic aid in pediatric neurosurgery. Progr Neurol Surg 4:54–101, 1971.

237. Papanicolaou N, McNeil BJ, Funkenstein HH, et al: Abnormal cisternogram associated with Diamox therapy. J Nucl Med 19:501–503, 1978.

238. Park HM: Inflamed pierced ear on brain scan. J Nucl Med 17:1108–1109, 1976.

239. Partain CL, Guinto FC, Scatliff JH, et al: Cerebral venous angioma: Correlation of radionuclide brain scan, transmission computed tomography, and angiography. J Nucl Med 20:1166–1169, 1979.

240. Patten DH, Benson DF: Diagnosis of normal-pressure hydrocephalus by RISA cisternography. J Nucl Med 9:457–461, 1968.

241. Patton DD, Brasfield DL: "Ear" artifact in brain scans. J Nucl Med 17:305–306, 1976.

242. Patton DD, Hertsgaard DB, Staab EV: Frontal lucency sign on brain scans. Radiology 106:353–356, 1973.

243. Peart RA, Driedger AA: Effect of obstructed mediastinal venous return on dynamic brain blood flow studies: case report. J Nucl Med 16:622–625, 1975.

244. Penning L, Front D: Scintigraphic demonstration of a bullet track in the brain. J Nucl Med 15:140–141, 1974.

245. Perkerson RB, Smith CS, Weller WF: The rim sign of subdural hematoma. J Nucl Med 13:637–639, 1972.

246. Perryman CR, Noble PR, Bragdon FH: Myeloscintigraphy: A useful procedure for localization of spinal block lesions. Am J Roentgenol 80:104–111, 1958.

247. Pexman JHW: The angiographic and brain scan features of acute herpes simplex encephalitis. Br J Radiol 47:179–184, 1974.

248. Planiol TL, Degiovanni E, Groussin P, et al: Les hematomes intracerebraux en gamma-angio-encephalographie. Rev Neurol (Paris) 131:301–318, 1975.

249. Polga JP, Dann RH: Sebaceous cysts of the scalp presenting as doughnut lesions on radionuclide brain imaging. Clin Nucl Med 3:300, 1978.

250. Prather JL, Long JM, van Heertum R, et al: Multicentric and isolated multifocal glioblastoma multiforme simulating metastatic disease. Br J Radiol 48:10–15, 1975.

251. Preimesberger KF, Loken MK, Shafer RB: Abnormal brain scan in Paget's disease of bone—confusion with subdural hematoma. J Nucl Med 15:880–883, 1974.

252. Prensky AL, Swisher CN, DeVivo DC: Positive brain scans in children with idiopathic focal epileptic seizures. Neurology 23:798–807, 1973.

252A. Preston, DF: Personal communication, 24 March 1976.

253. Puri S, Spencer RP, Gordon ME: Positive brain scan in toxoplasmosis. J Nucl Med 15:641–642, 1974.

254. Ramsey RG, Quinn JL: Comparison of accuracy between initial and delayed ^{99m}Tc-pertechnetate brain scans. J Nucl Med 13:131–134, 1972.

255. Reinke DB, Shafer RB, Wolff JM, et al: Radionuclide angiography in the diagnosis of traumatic middle meningeal artery to meningeal vein fistula. Clin Nucl Med 2:239–242, 1977.

256. Rinaldi I, Harris WO, DiChiro G: Radionuclide cisternography in subdural hematoma. Radiology 105:597–602, 1972.

257. Rockett J, Hamilton F, Robertson J, et al: Scintigraphic appearance of bifrontal epidural hematoma: case report. J Nucl Med 16:908–909, 1975.

258. Rockett JF, Kaplan ES, Hudson JS, et al: Intracerebral hemorrhage demonstrated by nuclear cerebral angiogram: case report. J Nucl Med 16:459–461, 1975.

259. Rockett JF, Kaplan ES, Moinuddin M: Scintiangiographic visualization of an occipitoparietal, extradural hematoma. J Nucl Med 18:496–497, 1977.

260. Rockett JF, Kaplan ES, Ray M, et al: Scintiphotographic demonstration of bilateral infarction in the distribution of the anterior cerebral arteries. Radiology 112:135–137, 1974.

261. Rockett JF, Ray M, Moinuddin M, et al: A brain tumor detected by the nuclear cerebral angiogram. J Nucl Med 15:1050–1051, 1974.

262. Rockett JF, Moinuddin M, Robertson JT, et al: Vertebral artery fistula detected by radionuclide angiography: case report. J Nucl Med 16:24–25, 1975.

263. Rockett JF, Moinuddin M, Tyson JW: Bilateral middle cerebral artery occlusions. Clin Nucl Med 3:415, 1978.

264. Rosenthall L: Intravenous and intracarotid radionuclide cerebral angiography. Sem Nucl Med 1:70–84, 1971.

265. Rosenthall L: Detection of altered cerebral arterial blood flow using ^{99m}Tc and the gamma-ray scintillation camera. Radiology 88:713–718, 1967.

266. Rosenthall L, Chan J, Stratford J: Intraarterial radionuclide cerebral angiography. Radiology 95:325–332, 1970.

267. Rosler H, Huber P: Serial cerebral scanning: Results in 208 patients. Fortschr Geb Rontgenstrachlen 111:467–480, 1969.

268. Rudd TG, O'Neal JT, Nelp WB: Cerebrospinal fluid circulation following subarachnoid hemorrhage: J Nucl Med 12:61–63, 1971.

269. Rudd TG, Shurtleff DB, Loeser JD, et al: Radionuclide assessment of cerebrospinal fluid shunt function in children. J Nucl Med 14:683–686, 1973.

270. Rujanavech N, Mattar AG, Coleman RE: Abnormal rapid-sequence imaging in a patient with subdural empyema: case report. J Nucl Med 17:980–981, 1976.

271. Ryo UY, Siddiqui A, Pinsky S: Visualization of nonvascular cranial tumor in cerebral flow study: case report. J Nucl Med 16:462–464, 1975.

272. Samuels LD: Scan visualization of mycotic aneurysm of a branch of right middle cerebral artery. J Nucl Med 13:695–696, 1972.
273. Savage JP, Gilday DL, Eng B, et al: Cerebrovascular disease in childhood. Radiology 123:385–391, 1977.
274. Schall GL, Heffner RR, Handmaker H: Brain scanning in oligodendrogliomas. Radiology 116:367–372, 1975.
275. Schleif A, Alazraki N, Halpern S, et al: A vertex view artifact on 99mTc-pertechnetate brain scan in a child. J Nucl Med 13:393–394, 1972.
276. Schrumpf J, Hoffer PB: Cerebral echinococcal cyst demonstrated on radionuclide angiogram: case report. Radiology 125:170, 1977.
277. Schulhof LA, Heimburger RF: Frontal lobe epidermoid tumor with positive brain scan. Surg Neurol 1:265–266, 1973.
278. Serafini AN, Weinstein MB: Radionuclide evaluation of a carotid body tumor. J Nucl Med 13:640–642, 1972.
279. Shafer RB, Wolff JM: Fenestrated sagittal sinus mimicking posterior cerebral infarction. Clin Nucl Med 3:425–428, 1978.
280. Shapiro K, Tabaddor K: Cerebral aspergillosis. Surg Neurol 4:465–471, 1975.
281. Sharma SM, Quinn JL: Brain scans in autopsy proved cases of intracerebral hemorrhage. Arch Neurol 28:270–271, 1973.
282. Sheldon JJ, Smoak WM, Gargano FP, et al: Dynamic scintigraphy in intracranial meningiomas. Radiology 109:109–115, 1973.
283. Shishikura A, DeLand FH, Gilday D: Sensitivity of brain scanning in the detection of arteriovenous malformations. Radiology 97:95–98, 1970.
284. Shivers JA, Adcock DF, Guinto FC, et al: Radionuclide imaging in primary intracerebral hemorrhage. Radiology 111:211–212, 1974.
285. Short DB, Kirchner PT: Radioisotope myelography in detection of spinal fluid leaks due to dorsal column stimulator implantation: case report. J Nucl Med 16:616–618, 1975.
286. Silberstein EB: Epidural hematoma with decreased radionuclide uptake: case report. J Nucl Med 15:712–713, 1974.
287. Silver L, Sham R, Klein HA: Cerebral hematoma with intraventricular bleeding. J Nucl Med 15:639–640, 1974.
288. Smoak WM, Gilson AJ: Scintillation visualization of a vascular rim in subdural hematoma. J Nucl Med 11:695–697, 1970.
289. Smoak WM, Sheldon J: Intracranial meningiomas: Dynamic and static scintigraphic characteristics. Clin Nucl Med 1:41–44, 1976.
290. Snow RM, Keyes JW: The "luxury-perfusion syndrome" following a cerebrovascular accident demonstrated by radionuclide angiography. J Nucl Med 15:907–909, 1974.
291. So SK, Ogawa T, Gerberg E, et al: Tracer accumulation in a subdural hygroma: case report. J Nucl Med 17:119–121, 1976.
292. Sohn RS, Siegel BA, Gado M, et al: Alzheimer's disease with abnormal cerebrospinal fluid flow. Neurology 23:1058–1065, 1973.
293. Soin JS, Burdine JA: Acute cerebral vascular accident associated with hyperperfusion. Radiology 118:109–112, 1976.
294. Soin JS, Holmes RA: An unusual cause of apparent regional hyperperfusion on radionuclide cerebral angiography study: case report. J Nucl Med 17:1057–1059, 1976.
295. Sostre S: Vein of Galen malformation. Clin Nucl Med 1:211–212, 1976.
296. Soucek CD: Sinusitis demonstrated by brain scanning. J Nucl Med 16:89–91, 1975.
297. Stadalnik RC, Goldstein E, Hoeprich PD, et al: Use of radiologic modalities in coccidioidal meningitis. Arch Int Med 141:75–81, 1981.

298. Stebner FC: Steroid effect on the brain scan in a patient with cerebral metastases. J Nucl Med 16:320–321, 1975.

299. Stein MA, Winter J: Delayed appearance of anterior cerebral arteries on isotopic cerebral flow study: a sign of bleeding anterior communicating artery aneurysm. J Nucl Med 15:1217–1219, 1974.

300. Steinbach JJ, Mattar AG, Mahin DT: Alteration of the cerebral bloodflow study due to reflux in internal jugular veins. J Nucl Med 17:61–64, 1976.

301. Stevens JS, Mishkin FS: Abnormal radionuclide angiogram in cervical lymphadenitis: case report. J Nucl Med 17:26, 1976.

302. Stevens JS, Mishkin FS: Abnormal radionuclide cerebral angiograms and scans due to seizures. Radiology 117:113–115, 1975.

303. Strauss HW, James AE, Hurley PJ, et al: Nuclear cerebral angiography. Usefulness in the differential diagnosis of cerebrovascular disease and tumor. Arch Intern Med 131:211–216, 1973.

304. Sty J, Kun L, Thorp S: Scintigraphy in acute lymphocytic cell leukemia. J Nucl Med 20:1101–1102, 1979.

304A. Sty JR, Murphy J, Thorp S: Brain scintigraphy: sinus pericranii. Clin Nucl Med 6:184–185, 1981

305. Sty JR, Starshak RJ, Boedecker R: "Doughnut" sign due to metastatic Wilm's tumor. Clin Nucl Med 3:33–34, 1978.

306. Sty JR, Swick H: "Doughnut" sign in adrenoleukodystrophy. Clin Nucl Med 3:158, 1978.

307. Suwanwela C, Poshyachinda V, Poshyachinda M: Isotope cisternography and ventriculography in frontoethmoidal encephalomeningocele. Acta Radiol 14:5–8, 1972.

308. Sy WM, Khatib R, Bay R: Rim and "doughnut" signs, and variants: review and reappraisal. Clin Nucl Med 1:186–189, 1976.

309. Sy WM, Weinberg G, Ngo N, et al: Imaging patterns of subdural hematoma—a proposed classification. J Nucl Med 15:693–698, 1974.

310. Tanasescu DE, Wolfstein RS, Brachman MB, et al: Early and delayed Tc-99m glucoheptonate brain scintigraphy: are routine early images indicated? J Nucl Med 20:287–290, 1979.

311. Tandon PN, Rao MAP, Basu AK, et al: ^{131}I-RIHSA CSF scanning in pediatric neurosurgical practice. Neuroradiology 7:119–123, 1974.

312. Tarcan YA, Fajman W, Marc J, et al: "Doughnut" sign in brain scanning. Am J Roentgenol 126:842–852, 1976.

313. Tator CH, Fleming JFR, Sheppard RH, et al: A radioisotopic test for communicating hydrocephalus. J Neurosurg 28:327–340, 1968.

314. Tauxe WN, Thorsen HC: Cerebrovascular permeability studies in cerebral neoplasms and vascular lesions: optimal dose-to-scan interval for pertechnetate brain scanning. J Nucl Med 10:34–39, 1969.

315. Teates CD, Allen DM: Superficial cortical atrophy simulating bilateral subdural hematomas. Clin Nucl Med 1:156–158, 1976.

316. Teplic SK, VanHeertum RL, Clark RE, et al: Pseudoparasagittal masses caused by displacement of the falx and superior sagittal sinus. J Nucl Med 15:1047–1049, 1974.

317. Thompson RW, DeNardo GL, Kottra JJ: The diagnostic value of brain scanning in intracranial lymphomas. Radiology 102:111–116, 1972.

318. Touya E, Osorio A, Touya JJ, et al: Bilateral cerebrospinal fluid otorrhea due to congenital malformation—a cisternoscintillography diagnosis (abstract). J Nucl Med 11:369, 1970.

319. Tow DE, Wagner HN: Scanning for tumors of the brain or bone. Comparison of sodium pertechnetate Tc-99m and ionic strontium-87m. JAMA 199:104–108, 1967.

320. Trackler RT, Mikulicich AG: Diminished cerebral perfusion resulting from kinking of the internal carotid artery. J Nucl Med 15:634–635, 1974.

321. Tulley TE, Shafer RB, Reinke DB, et al: Radionuclide angiography in the diagnosis of carotid cavernous sinus fistula. J Nucl Med 15:797–800, 1974.

322. Tyson JE, Gilmartin RC, Friedman BI, et al: ^{131}I-HSA cisternography in children with meningitis, in Harbert JC, McCullough DC, Luessenhop AJ, et al (eds): Cisternography and Hydrocephalus: A Symposium. Springfield, IL: Charles C. Thomas, 1972, pp. 413–432.

323. Tyson JW, Witherspoon LR, Wilkinson RH, et al: Accuracy of radionuclide cerebral angiograms in the detection of cerebral arteriovenous malformations. J Nucl Med 15:953–958, 1974.

324. Ucmakli A: The pathological significance of corpus callosum involvement in brain scans. J Nucl Med 13:510–516, 1972.

325. VanHouten FX, Holman BL, Treves S: Negative defect in an intracranial teratoma. J Nucl Med 13:122–124, 1972.

326. Vityé B, Ostiguy G, LeBel E: Abnormal ^{99m}Tc brain scan in cerebral sarcoidosis. Canad Med Assoc J 101:169–170, 1969.

327. Wallace JC: Radionuclide brain scanning in investigation of late-onset seizures. Lancet 2:1467–1470, 1974.

328. Waltino O, Eistola P, Vuolio M: Brain scanning in detection of intracranial arteriovenous malformations. Acta Neurol Scandinav 49:434–442, 1973.

329. Watson DD, Nelson JP, Gottlieb S: Rapid bolus injection of radioisotopes. Radiology 106:347–352, 1973.

330. Watts G, Mena I, Joe SH: Cerebral radioisotope angiogram: The significance of increased external carotid circulation (abstract). J Nucl Med 17:527, 1976.

331. Wechsler AF, Tomiyasu AN: Unusual radiographic-brain scan dissociation pattern with reticulum cell sarcoma (microglioma) of the brain. Bull Los Angeles Neurol Soc 39:1–8, 1974.

332. Weisbaum SD, Garnett ES: Brain scan in Schilder's disease. J Nucl Med 14:291–292, 1975.

333. Weiss S, Conway JJ: The hole in the head: An artifact of immediate brain imaging. J Nucl Med Tech 6:145–148, 1978.

334. Welch DM, Coleman E, Siegel BA: Cisternographic imaging patterns: Effects of partial extra-arachnoid radiopharmaceutical injection and post-injection CSF leakage. J Nucl Med 16:267–269, 1975.

335. Welch DM, Siegel BA: Posterior fossa infarction: results of brain scanning. Radiology 110:403–406, 1974.

336. Wilhelm JP, Siegel BA, James AE: Brain scanning and cisternography in cryptococcosis. Radiology 109:121–124, 1973.

337. Wilkins RH, Wilkinson RH, Odom GL: Abnormal brain scans in patients with cerebral arterial spasm. J Neurosurg 36:133–140, 1972.

338. Willemse JL, van Dorssen JG, de Haas G, et al: Computerized axial tomography and cerebral scintigraphy in leukodystrophy. Arch Neurol 35:603–607, 1978.

339. William JP, Lynde RH, Pribram HFW: Cisternographic changes following subarachnoid hemorrhage, in Harbert JC, McCullough DC, Luessenhop AJ, et al (eds): Cisternography and Hydrocephalus: A Symposium. Springfield, IL: Charles C. Thomas, 1972, pp. 285–291.

340. Williams JP, Pribram HFW, Lynde RH, et al: Isotope cisternography in the evaluation of patients with subarachnoid hemorrhage. J Nucl Med 11:592–596, 1970.
341. Williamson BRJ, Teates CD: Value of routine flow studies in nuclide brain scanning. South Med J 71:1082–1086, 1978.
342. Williamson BRJ, Teates CD, Bray ST, et al: Radionuclide brain scan findings in superior sagittal sinus thrombosis. Clin Nucl Med 3:184–187, 1978.
343. Witcofski RL, Janeway R, Maynard CD, et al: Visualization of the choroid plexus on the technetium-99m brain scan. Arch Neurol 16:286–289, 1967.
344. Witcofski RL, Maynard D, Meschan I: The utilization of ^{99m}technetium in brain scanning. J Nucl Med 6:121–130, 1965.
345. Witcofski RL, Maynard CD, Roper TJ: A comparative analysis of the technetium-99m pertechnetate brain scan: followup of 1000 patients. J Nucl Med 8:187–196, 1967.
346. Witcofski RL, Roper TJ, Maynard CD: False positive brain scans from extracranial contamination with 99m technetium. J Nucl Med 6:524–527, 1965.
347. Witherspoon LR, Tyson JW, Goodrich JK: The appearance of peripheral postsurgical activity on cerebral dynamic studies. J Nucl Med 15:709–711, 1974.
348. Wolfstein RS, Tanasescu D, Sakimura IT, et al: Brain imaging with ^{99m}Tc-DTPA: A clinical comparison of early and delayed studies. J Nucl Med 15:1135–1137, 1974.
349. Wolpert SM, Carter BL, Ferris EJ: Lipomas of the corpus callosum, an angiographic analysis. Am J Roentgenol 115:92–99, 1972.
350. Yarnell PR, Burdick D, Sanders B, et al: Focal seizures, early veins, and increased flow: A clinical, angiographic, and radioisotopic correlation. Neurology 24:512–516, 1974.
351. Yarnell PR, Burdick D, Sanders B: The "Hot Stroke." Arch Neurol 30:65–69, 1974.
352. Yeh EL, Meade RC: Quantitative analysis of brain scans. J Nucl Med 14:176–178, 1973.
353. Yeh EL, Pohlman GP, Ruetz PP, et al: Jugular venous reflux in cerebral radionuclide angiography. Radiology 118:730–732, 1976.
354. Zilkha A, Irwin GAL: The rim sign in epidural hematoma: case report. J Nucl Med 17:977–979, 1976.
355. Zwas ST, Czerniak P: Head and brain scan findings in rhinocerebral mucormycosis: case report. J Nucl Med 16:925–927, 1975.

Part III

Endocrine System

Chapter 16

Thyroid

HARRY R. MAXON III

D. G. VARMA

I. Asymmetrical size of thyroid lobes (on images with Tc-99m pertechnetate or radioiodide I-123 or I-131)

  A. Common

     1. Normal variation (50, 145, 198)

        a. right lobe larger than left about 48% (220, 234, 245)

        b. left lobe larger than right about 15% (245)

     2. Post partial thyroidectomy

  B. Uncommon

     1. Intrathyroidal lesions (see Sections VII & VIII)

  C. Rare

     1. Unilateral congenital hypoplasia (8)

     2. Congenital absence, portion of a lobe (181, 207), usually upper left

II. Nonvisualization of one thyroid lobe

  A. Common

     1. Hemithyroidectomy

  B. Uncommon

     1. Total replacement of lobe by intrathyroidal lesions (100) (see Section VII)

The use of an asterisk * in this chapter indicates that this entity has been observed by one of the authors but the case report has not been published.

C. Rare
  1. Thyroid hemiagenesis (90–95% left lobe) (8, 17, 100, 207)
    a. occasionally right lobe (207)

III. Pyramidal lobe

  A. Common
    1. Normal variation
      a. anatomical incidence 43–48% (45, 106, 113, 145, 151)
      b. visualization on images 35% (113)
    2. Post-thyroidectomy
    3. Associated with hyperthyroidism
    4. Associated with goiter

IV. Absent isthmus

  A. Common
    1. Normal variation (85, 145)
    2. Replacement by intrathyroidal lesions (see Section VII)

V. Focal concentration of radioiodide or Tc-99m pertechnetate outside of usual site of thyroid gland due to ectopic thyroid tissue (see also Section XIV, Metastatic thyroid carcinoma)

  A. Uncommon
    1. Mediastinal goiter (best demonstrated with radioiodide) (29)
      a. downward extension from cervical thyroid (75, 226)
    2. Esophageal retention of swallowed radioactivity in saliva (192)
    3. Lingual thyroid
      a. anatomical incidence 10%, much lower incidence by imaging (196)
      b. 85–90% symptomatic patients are females (104, 169)
      c. equal distribution in males and females at autopsy (209)
  B. Rare
    1. Mediastinal goiter without apparent connection to cervical thyroid (61, 75, 120)
    2. Lingual thyroid with hyperthyroidism (163) or malignant transformation (5, 196, 236)
    3. Midline cervical ectopic thyroid tissue (foramen cecum to lower neck)
      a. subhyoid median (105, 152, 205)
      b. thyroid malignancy in thyroglossal duct remnants (19, 44, 66, 137, 166)
      c. carcinoma in median ectopic thyroid (117, 137)
      d. with lingual thyroid (4, 140)
    4. Lateral rests of embryonic thyroid tissue (23, 66)

    5. Accessory thyroid tissue in mediastinum (24, 33, 75, 111, 120, 208, 214, 244)

        a. esophagus (187, 253)

        b. heart, aorta and pericardium (204)

    6. Struma ovarii (26, 257, 259) makes up 1% of ovarian tumors (257)

        a. teratomatous tumor with "true" thyroid tissue (144, 185, 186)

        b. with hyperthyroidism (26, 122)

        c. with malignant transformation (81, 122, 257)

        d. with metastases (122, 257)

        e. pseudostruma ovarii (radioiodide in hemorrhagic ovarian cyst with no thyroid tissue) (172)

VI. Goiter (thyroid gland over normal mass of 15–20 grams in adults) [methods of estimating mass on images (6, 30, 82, 235) in combination with palpation (141, 230, 235)]

  A. Common

    1. Iodine deficiency (endemic goiter in certain geographic areas) (167, 168)

    2. Non-toxic nodular goiter (42)

    3. Toxic nodular goiter (157)

    4. Diffuse toxic goiter (Graves' disease) (42)

    5. Post-surgical hypertrophy (143)

    6. Thyroiditis (99, 179, 227) (suppurative, lymphocytic, or subacute)

    7. Misdiagnosis of normal larger glands, especially in females and children (85)

  B. Less common

    1. Congenital goiter from maternal ingestion of iodide (109)

    2. Congenital goiter from maternal ingestion of anti-thyroid drugs (49, 62)

    3. Familial goiter due to dyshormonogenesis

        a. sporadic goitrous cretins (11)

        b. sporadic non-toxic familial goiters (3, 11, 46)

        c. Pendred's syndrome (3, 11, 80, 164)

        d. "peroxidase" defect (170, 221)

        e. "coupling" defect (3)

    4. Iodide-induced goiter (15, 237) in children or adults

    5. Artefact from excessive overlying soft tissue or an unusually high location of the thyroid (91)

VII. The "cool," "cold," or non-functional nodule

  A. Due to extrinsic non-thyroidal disease impinging on the thyroid

    1. Large parathyroid cysts (243)

    2. Parathyroid adenomas (147, 161, 243)

    3. Tortuous innominate artery (186)

    4. Any extrinsic neck mass in the vicinity of the thyroid may simulate a "cold" nodule

B. Due to intrathyroidal disease

    1. Diseases of thyroid parenchyma

        a. adenoma (65, 86, 124, 150, 176, 232, 241, 246, 258)

        b. Hashimoto's thyroiditis and chronic lymphocytic thyroiditis (179)

            (1) irregular, patchy bilateral uptake (32, 108, 179)

            (2) focal disease may occur (179)

        c. subacute thyroiditis

            (1) focal (101, 133)

            (2) diffuse (87, 99, 101)

        d. acute suppurative thyroiditis (53, 93, 129, 227, 247)

        e. papillary carcinoma (9, 104, 176, 195, 232, 246)

        f. follicular carcinoma (232, 246)

        g. undifferentiated anaplastic carcinoma (232)

        h. medullary carcinoma (7)

        i. cysts (47, 150, 153, 158, 246)

    2. Diseases of other intrathyroidal tissue

        a. lymphoma (212, 232, 246)

        b. teratoma (130)

        c. hemangioma (182)

        d. nonchromaffin paraganglioma (92)

    3. Neoplasms metastatic to thyroid (60, 72, 104, 211, 246)

        a. malignant melanoma

        b. breast tumors

        c. lung tumors

        d. gastrointestinal tumors

        e. pancreatic tumors

        f. genitourinary tumors

            (1) kidney

            (2) prostate

        g. head and neck tumors

        h. lymphomas

        i. rhabdosarcoma

        j. liposarcoma

        k. bile duct tumors

        l. adrenal tumors

        m. parotid tumors

        n. central nervous system tumors

    4. Miscellaneous causes

        a. abscess (including tuberculosis and acute suppurative thyroiditis) (53, 79, 93, 107, 124, 129, 135, 142, 227, 247)

        b. post-surgical changes (143, 203, 260)

        c. Riedel's struma (232)

      d. pseudosarcomatous nodular fasciitis (246)
      e. hematoma*
      f. amyloid*
      g. hemochromatosis*

VIII. A focus of markedly increased radioisotope concentration relative to the rest of the gland ("hot nodule")

  A. The autonomous hyperfunctioning nodule (31, 34, 57, 97, 121, 148, 156, 160, 194, 213, 262)
    1. TSH independent or dependent (156)
    2. No definite correlation between nodule size and degree of function (34, 160, 194)
    3. Autonomous nodules due to adenomas, adenomatous hypertrophy, or nodular goiter (34, 154, 160)
  B. Acquired (surgical) absence of one lobe (203, 260)
  C. Tissue of relatively normal function with surrounding poorly functional areas of degeneration or thyroiditis (156)
  D. Asymmetric lobulated gland with greater concentration of radioiodine in one portion of the gland than the other (156)
  E. Carcinoma in an autonomously functioning nodule (1, 22, 67, 77, 126, 150, 225)
    1. Uncertainty whether reported carcinomas in "hot nodules" have been precisely related to the "hyperfunctioning" areas noted on scan (13, 188, 256)
  F. Congenital absence of one lobe (207) (cf. thyroid hemiagenesis)

IX. The multinodular gland

  A. Toxic multinodular goiter (42, 155, 157, 185)
    1. The Marine-Lenhart syndrome (cold nodules in a toxic diffuse goiter) may have the appearance of a multinodular gland (40)
  B. Non-toxic multinodular goiter (41, 42, 157, 191)
  C. Lymphocytic thyroiditis (179)
  D. Compensatory hyperplasia in hemiagenesis (42) or post-surgical glands (203)
  E. Malignancy in multinodular glands (71)
    1. Primary (71)
    2. Metastatic (123)

  X. The radioactive iodine uptake test (35, 37, 74, 84, 96, 98, 103, 131, 173, 174, 190, 199, 202, 206, 215, 251)

A. With increasing dietary intake of iodides, the current normal radioiodine uptake values appear lower than those previously reported (76, 139, 183, 201)

B. Elevated radioactive iodine uptake test

   1. Common

      a. hyperthyroidism (2, 69, 206)

         (1) Graves' disease

         (2) toxic adenoma

         (3) multinodular toxic goiter

         (4) secondary to pituitary overactivity

            (a) adenoma

            (b) non-adenomatous hyperfunctional pituitary thyrotrophic cells

      b. Hashimoto's disease (27)

      c. sub-acute thyroiditis (in the "recovery" phase) (48, 240)

      d. following cessation of thyroid hormone therapy (88, 200)

   2. Less common

      a. following anti-thyroid drug therapy (drugs inhibiting organification) (20, 58, 215)

      b. iodine deficiency (58, 215) (more common outside United States)

      c. following cessation of iodine therapy (228)

      d. following recovery after exposure to iodinated contrast media (219)

      e. iodotyrosyl coupling defect (221)

      f. pregnancy (70, 95)

      g. euthyroid Graves' disease (endocrine ophthalmopathy) (90, 248, 249)

   3. Rare

      a. hydatiform mole from extremely high levels of HCG (56)

      b. choriocarcinoma from extremely high levels of HCG (56, 175)

      c. embryonal carcinoma of the testis from high levels of a TSH-like activity, probably HCG (222)

      d. liver dysfunction, especially cirrhosis (165)

      e. nephrotic syndrome with prolonged iodide clearance related to renal failure; in nephrotic syndrome protein bound iodine may be lost in the urine and the thyroid gland may compensate for this (197)

C. Low radioactive iodine uptake test

   1. Common

      a. hypothyroidism (58, 69)

         (1) congenital

         (2) spontaneous acquired

         (3) post thyroidectomy

         (4) post radiation (external or I-131 iodide)

      b. Hashimoto's thyroiditis (27, 54, 73, 78, 217)

     c. sub-acute thyroiditis ("early" phase) (48, 112, 177, 240)
     d. anti-thyroid (sulfonylurea) drug administration (20, 58)
     e. thyroid hormone administration (58, 88)
     f. iodide administration (58, 64, 219, 228)
        (1) Lugol's solution or SSKI
        (2) kelp
        (3) mineral supplements
        (4) radiographic contrast media
        (5) eye drops (39)
  2. Uncommon
     a. iodide trapping defect (221)
     b. TSH deficiency, pituitary or hypothalamic (138, 159)
     c. adrenal corticosteroid administration (18)
     d. phenylbutazone administration (134)
     e. goitrogenic foods in excess
        (1) kale
        (2) turnips
     f. toxic struma ovarii (122)
     g. thyrotoxicosis factitia (55, 102)
     h. metastatic well-differentiated thyroid carcinoma (with hyperthyroidism) (55, 102)
     i. severe hepatitis (51)
     j. gram-negative septicemia (rats) (119)

XI. Abnormal perchlorate discharge test (indicates an organification defect)

  A. Hashimoto's thyroiditis (11, 25, 83, 163, 178, 223, 229)
  B. Thiouracil or methimazole administration (10)
  C. Sporadic goitrous cretinism (11)
  D. Sporadic non-toxic familial goiters (3, 11, 46)
  E. Pendred's syndrome (11, 80, 164)
  F. Peroxidase defect (171, 221)
  G. "Coupling defect" (3)

XII. The T_3 suppression uptake test (positive test indicates autonomy of some or all of the thyroid gland) (43, 89, 215, 242, 252, 254)

  A. Conditions associated with iodine uptake not adequately suppressible by T_3 or T_4 (autonomy)
    1. Graves' disease (110, 149, 250)
    2. Autonomous adenoma (148, 154, 157, 160)
    3. Autonomy in a multinodular goiter
      a. with thyrotoxicosis (155)
      b. without thyrotoxicosis (180)
    4. Euthyroid Graves' disease (90, 248, 249)

5. Post-therapy for hyperthyroidism (36, 38, 94, 249)

XIII. The TSH stimulation uptake test (21, 28, 68, 115, 116, 127, 132, 189, 210, 215, 218, 231, 255)

  A. Untoward reactions may occur following injection of TSH (261)
  B. TSH responsivity of the thyroid uptake and scan
    1. Normal thyroid gland (normal patient) (59)
    2. Patient taking thyroid hormone who does not have primary hypothyroidism (21)
    3. Secondary or tertiary hypothyroidism (138, 159)
    4. In infants with marasmus (12)
    5. Suppressed normal thyroid tissue (154)
  C. Absent or impaired response
    1. Hashimoto's thyroiditis (218)
    2. Sub-acute thyroiditis (118, 218)
    3. Primary hypothyroidism (68, 231)
    4. Post-therapy for Graves' disease (115, 146)
    5. After the ingestion of large amounts of iodine compounds or iodides (21, 32)
    6. In pituitary or hypothalamic insufficiency (including Sheehan's syndrome) (231)
    7. In patients with Turner's syndrome with positive thyroid antibodies (261)

XIV. The ^{131}I total body scan for metastatic thyroid carcinoma[1] (14, 125, 233)

  A. Non-thyroidal ^{131}I concentration (false positive)
    1. Common
      a. due to saliva and nasal secretions containing [131]I
        (1) in dental cavities (216)
        (2) in tracheotomy tubes (216)
        (3) in the esophagus, linear (216) or localized (238)
      b. physiologic uptake
        (1) stomach
        (2) bowel
        (3) bladder
        (4) salivary glands
    2. Rare
      a. due to normal concentration in the thymus (114)
      b. due to concentration by primary lung carcinoma (239)

---

[1] Not all papillary or follicular carcinomas have a sufficient iodine concentrating mechanism to permit detection by ^{131}I scanning (128).

B. Visualization of metastatic well-differentiated adenocarcinomas of the thyroid with ^{131}I (14, 16, 125, 233)

REFERENCES

1. Abdel-Razzak M, Christie J: Thyroid carcinoma in an autonomously functioning nodule. J Nucl Med 20(9):1001, 1979.
2. Adams D, Purves H: The change in thyroidal ^{131}I content between 8 and 48 hours as an index of thyroid activity. J Clin Endocr 17:126, 1957.
3. Agerback H: Non-toxic goiter: dyshormogenesis. Acta Endocrinologica 72:671, 1973.
4. Alexandre J, Allen W: Co-existent lingual and median-cervical ectopic thyroid. Surgical Management. JAMA 195(2):133, 1966.
5. Al-Hindawi A, et al: The clinical presentation of ectopic thyroid gland with results of radioiodine studies. Br J Clin Pract 23:372, 1969.
6. Allen H Jr, Goodwin W: The scintillation counter as an instrument for *in vivo* determination of thyroid weight. Radiology 58:68, 1952.
7. Anderson R, Sizemore G, Wahner H, Carney A: Thyroid scintigram in familial medullary carcinoma of the thyroid gland. Clin Nucl Med 3:147, 1978.
8. Andrew I: On the incidence and functional condition of congenital thyroid gland anomalies especially in partial aplasia and hypoplasia. Deutsch Gesundh 23:1297, 1968.
9. Ashkar F, Smoak W: "Owl eye" sign of benign autonomous thyroid nodule. JAMA 214:1563, 1970.
10. Astwood E: Chemotherapy of hyperthyroidism. Harvey Lectures, 1944–45, Series XL 195, 1945.
11. Baschieri L, Benedetti G, et al: Evaluation and limitations of the perchlorate test in the study of thyroid function. J Clin Endocr 23:786, 1963.
12. Beas F, Monckeberg F, Horwitz I: The response of the thyroid gland to thyroid stimulation hormone (TSH) in infants with malnutrition. Pediatrics 38(6) Part 1:1003, 1966.
13. Becker F, Economou P, Schwartz T: The occurrence of carcinoma in "hot" nodules. Ann Int Med 58:877, 1963.
14. Beckerman C, Gottschalk A, Hoffer P: Optimal time for ^{131}I total body imaging to detect metastatic thyroid carcinoma (abstract). J Nucl Med 15:477, 1974.
15. Begg T, Hall R: Iodide goiter and hypothyroidism. Q.J. Med 32:351, 1963.
16. Beierwaltes W: Radioiodine in the therapy for thyroid carcinoma, in Spencer RP (ed): Therapy in Nuclear Medicine, New York: Grune and Stratton, 1978 p. 101.
17. Bell R, Wolfe L: Lateral unilobular thyroid gland: a report of two cases. Journal of the Tennessee Medical Association 66(12):1149, 1973.
18. Berson S, Yalow R: The effect of cortisone on the iodine accumulating function of the thyroid gland in euthyroid subjects. J Clin Endocr 12:407, 1952.
19. Bhagvan Belur S, Govindaro D, Weinberg T: Carcinoma of thyroglossal duct cyst: case report and review of the literature. Surgery 67(2):281, 1970.
20. Beierwaltes W, Johnson P, Solari A: Clinical Use of Radioisotopes. Philadelphia: W.B. Saunders, 1957, p. 69.
21. Bishopric G, Garrett N, Nicholson W: Clinical value of the TSH test in the diagnosis of thyroid diseases. Am J Med 18:15, 1955.
22. Black B, Woolner L, Blackburn C: The uptake of radioactive iodine by carcinoma of the thyroid gland. A study of 128 cases. J Clin Endocr Metab 13:1378, 1953.
23. Block M, Wylie J, Patton R, et al: Does benign thyroid tissue occur in the lateral part of the neck? Am J Surg 112:476, 1966.

24. Boardman P (for Bayliss R): An unusual mediastinal tumor defined with radioiodine. Proceedings of the Royal Society of Med 60:651, 1967.
25. Boyle J, Thompson J, Murray I, et al: Phenomenon of iodide inhibition in various states of thyroid function with observations on one mechanism of its occurrence. J Clin Endocr 25:1255,1965.
26. Brown Q, Shetty K, Rosenfeld P: Hyperthyroidism due to struma ovarii. Demonstration by radioiodine scan. Acta Endocrinologica 73:266, 1973.
27. Buchanan W, Koutras D, Alexander W, et al: Iodine metabolism in Hashimoto's thyroiditis. J Clin Endocr 21:806, 1961.
28. Burke G: The thyrotropin stimulation test. Ann Int Med 69:(6)1127, 1968.
29. Burkell C, Cross J, Kent H, Nanson E: Mass lesions of the mediastinum. Curr Probl Surg 2:57, 1969.
30. Burkinshaw L: A method of measuring the mass of the thyroid gland *in vivo*. Acta Radiol (Stockh) 49:308, 1958.
31. Burman K, Earll J, et al: Clinical observations on the solitary autonomous thyroid nodule. Arch Intern Med 134:915, 1974.
32. Burns W, Thomas C: Radioisotope scanning in the diagnosis of lymphoproliferative disorders of the thyroid. Am Surg 38:35, 1972.
33. Caballero C, Perez D: Retrosternal goiter. Bol Asoc Med PR 68(2):41, 1976.
34. Campbell W, Santiago H, et al: The autonomous thyroid nodule: correlation of scan appearance and histopathology. Radiology 107:133, 1973.
35. Caplan R, Kujak R: Thyroid uptake of radioactive iodine: a reevaluation. JAMA 215:916, 1971.
36. Cassidy C: Use of thyroid suppression test as a guide to prognosis of hyperthyroidism treated with anti-thyroid drugs. J Clin Endocr 25:155, 1965.
37. Cassidy C, Vanderlaan W: Laboratory aids to diagnosis in thyroid disease. N Eng J Med 258:828, 1958.
38. Cassidy C, Vanderlaan W: Thyroid-suppression test in the prognosis of hyperthyroidism treated by anti-drugs. N Eng J Med 262:1228, 1960.
39. Ceccarelli C, Grasso L, Martion E, et al: Reduction of thyroid uptake by iodine absorbed with eye-drop therapy. J Nuc Med 23:364,1982.
40. Charkes D: Graves' disease with functioning nodules (Marine-Lenhart syndrome). J Nucl Med 13:(12):885, 1972.
41. Charkes D: Radioisotope scanning in the management of benign thyroid disease. Delaware Medical Journal 42(9):227,1970.
42. Charkes D: Scintigraphic evaluation of nodular goiter. Sem Nucl Med 1(3):326, 1971.
43. Charkes D, Cantor R, Goluboff B: A three day double isotope l-triiodothyronine suppression test of thyroid autonomy. J Nucl Med 8:627,1967.
44. Choy F, Ward R, Richardson R: Carcinoma of the thyroglossal duct. Am J Surg 108:361, 1964
45. Christopher F: A Textbook of Surgery, 4th Edition. Philadelphia: W.B. Saunders, 1945, p. 274.
46. Clayton G, Smith J, Leiser A: Familial goiter with defect in intrinsic metabolism of thyroxine without hyperthyroidism. J Pediatrics 52:129, 1958.
47. Crile G: Treatment of thyroid cysts by aspiration. Surgery 59:210, 1966.
48. Czerniak P, Harell-Steinberg A: The chronology of events in the development of subacute thyroiditis, studied by radioactive iodine. J Clin Endocr 17:1448, 1957.
49. David L, Forbes W: Thiouracil in pregnancy, effect on foetal thyroid. Lancet 2:740, 1945.

50. Deland F, Wagner H Jr: Atlas of Nuclear Medicine, Vol. 3. Reticuloendothelial System, Liver, Spleen and Thyroid. Philadelphia: W.B. Saunders, 1972.
51. Desai KB, Ganatra RD, Sharma SM, et al: Thyroid uptake in infectious hepatitis. J Nucl Med 12:828–830, 1971.
52. Dische S, Berg P: An investigation of the thyroglossal tract using the radioisotope scan. Clin Rad 14:298,1963.
53. Donato J: Acute suppurative thyroiditis: report of two cases. Int Surg 57:750, 1972.
54. Doniach D, Hudson R, Roit I: Human auto-immune thyroiditis. Clinical Studies. Br Med J 1:365, 1960.
55. Dorfman S: Hyperthyroidism: usual and unusual causes. Arch Int Med 137:995, 1977.
56. Dowling T, Ingbar S, Freinkel N: Iodine metabolism in hydatiform mole and choriocarcinoma. J Clin Endocr Metab 20(1):1, 1960.
57. Drexler A: In CPC: A functioning thyroid nodule in a patient previously tested with irradiation for Hodgkins disease. Am J Med 68:432, 1980.
58. Drummy W: The use of radioactive iodine in the detection of thyroid dysfunction. N Eng J Med 249:970, 1953.
59. Einhorn J, Larsson L: Studies on the effect of thyrotropin on human thyroid function. J Clin Endocr 19:28, 959.
60. Elliott R, Frantz-Kneeland V: Metastatic carcinoma masquerading as primary thyroid cancer. Ann Surg 151(4):551, 1960.
61. Ellis F, Good C, Seybold W: Intrathoracic goiter. Ann Surg 135:79, 1952.
62. Elphinstone N: Thiouracil in pregnancy: its effect on the foetus. Lancet 1:1281, 1953.
63. Endo Y: Subacute thyroiditis of aberrant thyroid gland. JAMA 245:1632, 1981.
64. Feinberg W, Hoffman D, Owen C: The effects of varying amounts of stable iodide on the function of the human thyroid. J Clin Endocr 19:567, 1959.
65. Ferriman D, Hennebry T, Tassopoulos C: True thyroid adenoma. Quarterly J of Med, New Series XLI 162:127, 1972.
66. Fish J, Moore R: Ectopic thyroid tissue and ectopic thyroid carcinoma: a review of the literature and report of a case. Ann Surg 157(2):221, 1963.
67. Fitzgerald P, Foote F: Function of various types of thyroid carcinoma as revealed by the radioautographic demonstration of radioactive iodine (^{131}I). J Clin Endocr 9:1153, 1949.
68. Fletcher R, Besford H: A test of thyroid and pituitary function using thyrotropin. Clin Sci 17:113, 1958.
69. Freedberg A, Chamovitz D, Kurland G: Thyroid function in normal and pathologic states as revealed by radioactive iodine studies. 1. Thyroid ^{131}I uptake and turnover in euthyroid, hyperthyroid and hypothyroid subjects. Metabolism 1:26, 1952.
70. Freedberg I, Hamolsky M, Freedberg S: The thyroid gland in pregnancy. N Eng J Med 256(11):505, 1957.
71. Freeman L, Johnson P: Nodular goiter, in Clinical Scintillation Imaging. New York: Grune and Stratton, 1975, p. 684,.
72. Friberg S, Kinnman J: Renal adenocarcinoma with metastases to the thyroid gland. Acta Oto-laryngologica 67:552, 1969.
73. Furr W, Crile G, McCullagh E, et al: Struma lymphomatosa: Clinical manifestations and response to therapy. J Clin Endocr Metab 14:79, 1954.
74. Gaffney G, Gregerman R, Shock N: Relationship of age to the thyroidal accumulation, renal excretion and distribution of radioiodide in euthyroid man. J Clin Endocr 22:784, 1962.
75. Georgiadis N, Katsas A, Leoutsakes B: Substernal goiter. Int Surg 54:(2):116, 1970.
76. Ghahreman G, Hoffer P, Oppenheim B, et al: New normal values for thyroid uptake of radioactive iodine. JAMA 217(3):337, 1971.

77. Ghose M, Genuth S, Abellera R, et al: Functioning primary thyroid carcinoma and metastases producing hyperthyroidism. J Clin Endocr Metab 33:639, 1971.
78. Gluck F, Nusynowitz M, Plymate S: Chronic lymphocytic thyroiditis, thyrotoxicosis and low radioactive iodine uptake. N Eng J Med 293(13):624, 1975.
79. Goldfarb H, Schifrin D, Craig F: Thyroiditis caused by tuberculous abscess of the thyroid gland. Am J Med 38:825, 1965.
80. Gomez-Pan A, Evered D, Hall R: Pituitary-thyroid function in Pendred's syndrome. Br Med J 911(2):152, 1974.
81. Gonzalez A, Kaufman R, Braungardt C, et al: Adenocarcinomas of thyroid arising in struma ovarii (malignant struma ovarii): report of 2 cases and review of the literature. Obstet Gynec 21:567, 1963.
82. Goodwin W, Cassen B, Bauer F: Thyroid gland weight determination from thyroid scintigrams with post-mortem verification. Radiology 61:88, 1953.
83. Gray H, Greig W, Thompson J, et al: Intravenous perchlorate test in the diagnosis of Hashimoto's disease. Lancet 1:853, 1974.
84. Grayson R: Factors which influence the radioactive iodine thyroidal uptake test. Am J Med 28:397, 1960.
85. Gray's Anatomy: 26th Edition. Philadelphia: Lea and Febiger, 1956.
86. Greenberg H: Low radioiodine uptake and high serum PBI levels from hemorrhage into thyroid adenoma. J Nuc Med 7:787, 1966.
87. Greene J: Subacute thyroiditis. Am J Med 51:97, 1971.
88. Greer M: The effect of endogenous thyroid activity of feeding dessicated thyroid to normal human subjects. N Eng J Med 244:385, 1951.
89. Greer M, Smith G: Method for increasing the accuracy of radioiodine uptake as a test for thyroid function by the use of dessicated thyroid. J Clin Endocr 14:1374, 1954.
90. Guinet P, Descour C: Etude critique du test de Werner. Rev. Lyon Med 11, 501, 1962.
91. Gwinup G, Mortin M: The high lying thyroid: a cause of pseudogoiter. J Clin Endocr Metab 40:37, 1975.
92. Haegert D, Wang N, Farrer P, et al: Non-chromaffin paragangliomatosis manifesting as a cold thyroid nodule. Am J Clin Path 61:561, 1974.
93. Hajjar E, Salti I: Tuberculosis of the thyroid. Leb Med J 26:272, 1973.
94. Hales L, Myhill J, et al: Thyroid suppressibility after therapy for thyrotoxicosis. J Clin Endocr 21:569, 1961.
95. Halman K: The radioiodine uptake of the human thyroid in pregnancy. Clin Sci 17:281, 1958.
96. Halpern S, Alazrake N, Littenberg R, et al: [131]I thyroid uptakes: capsule versus liquid. J Nucl Med 14:507, 1973.
97. Hamburger J: Solitary autonomously functioning thyroid lesions. Am J Med 58:740, 1975.
98. Hamburger J: Application of the radioiodine uptake to the clinical evaluation of thyroid disease. Sem Nucl Med 1:287, 1971.
99. Hamburger J: Sub-acute thyroiditis: Diagnostic difficulties and simple treatment. J Nucl Med 15:81, 1974.
100. Hamburger J, Hamburger S: Thyroidal hemiagenesis: report of a case and comments on clinical ramifications. Arch Surg 100:319, 1970.
101. Hamburger J, Kadian G, Rossin H: Sub-acute thyroiditis—evolution depicted by serial ^{131}I scintigram. J Nuc Med 6:560, 1965.
102. Hamilton C, Maloof F: Unusual types of hyperthyroidism. Medicine 52:195, 1973.
103. Harvey R: Influence of body weight on thyroidal uptake of radioiodine. J Clin Endocr Metab 28:912, 1968.

104. Heidendal G, Roos P, Thijs L, et al: Evaluation of cold areas on the thyroid scan with ^{67}Ga-citrate. J Nuc Med 16:793, 1975.

105. Heilman J, Huey K: The subhyoid median ectopic thyroid. Arizona Medicine 29:855, 1972.

106. Hollingshead W: Anatomy for Surgeons, Vol. 1. New York: Paul B. Hoeber, 1954, p. 519.

107. Howbaker E: Thyroid abscess. Am Surg 37:290, 1971.

108. Hung W, LoPresti J: Thyroid scintiscans in children and adolescents with chronic lymphocytic thyroiditis. J Ped 77:302, 1970.

109. Iancu T, Bodyanower Y, Laurian N: Congenital goiter due to maternal ingestion of iodide. Am J Dis Child 128:528, 1974.

110. Ingbar S: Physiological considerations in treatment of diffuse toxic goiter. Arch Int Med 107:932, 1961.

111. Irwin R, Braman S, Arvanitidi S, et al: [131]I thyroid scanning in the preoperative diagnosis of mediastinal goiter. Ann Int Med 89:73, 1978.

112. Ivy H: Permanent myxedema: An unusual complication of granulomatous thyroiditis. J Clin Endocr 21:1384, 1961.

113. Izenstark J, Forsaith A, Horwitz N: The pyramidal lobe in thyroid imaging. J Nuc Med 10:519, 1969.

114. Jackson G, Graham W, Flickinger F, et al: Thymus accumulation of radioactive iodine. Pennsylvania Medicine 82:37, 1979.

115. Jeffries W, Kelley L, et al: The significance of low thyroid reserve. J Clin Endocr 16:1438, 1956.

116. Jeffries W, Levy R, Storassli J: Use of the TSH test in the diagnosis of thyroid disorders. Radiology 73:341, 1959.

117. Judd E: Thyroglossal duct cysts and sinuses. Surgical Clinics of North America 43:1023, 1963.

118. Kamio N, Kobayashi I, et al: Permissive role of thyrotropin on thyroid radioiodine uptake during the recovery phase of subacute thyroiditis. Metabolism 26:295, 1977.

119. Kan MK, Garcia JF, McRae J, et al: Marked suppression of thyroid function in rats with gram-negative septicemia. J Nucl Med 17:104–107, 1976.

120. Kaplan W, Watnick M, Holman L: Scintigraphic identification of complete thoracic goiter with normal appearing cervical thyroid: a case report. J Can Assoc of Radiologists 25:193, 1974.

121. Karlberg B: Thyroid nodule autonomy: its demonstration by the thyrotropin releasing hormone (TRH) stimulation test. Acta Endocr 73:689, 1973.

122. Kempers R, Dockerty M, Hoffman D, et al: Struma ovarii—ascitic, hyperthyroid, and asymptomatic syndromes. Ann Int Med 72:883, 1970.

123. Kim E, Mattar A: Primary and secondary carcinomata with focal nodular hyperplasia in a multinodular thyroid: case report. J Nucl Med 17:983, 1976.

124. Kirkland R, Kirkland J, et al: Solitary thyroid nodules in 30 children and report of a child with a thyroid abscess. Pediatrics 51:85, 1973.

125. Krishnamurthy G, Bland W: Diagnostic and therapeutic implications of long-term radioisotope scanning in the management of thyroid cancer. J Nuc Med 13:924, 1972.

126. Lamberg B, Makinen J, Murtomaa M: Papillary thyroid carcinoma in a toxic adenoma. Nuklearmedizin 15:138, 1976.

127. Lashmet M, Gurney C, Beierwaltes W: Thyroid response to TSH in normal subjects. Univ Mich Med Bull 23:161, 1957.

128. Leeper J: The effects of [131]therapy on survival of patients with metastatic papillary or

follicular thyroid carcinoma. J Clin Endocr Metab 36:1143, 1973.

129. Leers W, Dussault J, Mullen J, et al: Suppurative thyroiditis: an unusual case caused by *Actinomyces naeslundi*. Can Med Assoc J 101:714, 1969.
130. Levey M: An unusual thyroid tumor in a child. Laryngoscope 12:1864, 1976.
131. Levy R, Caughey P, Turell D. Daily variation in the thyroidal uptake of ^{131}I in human subjects. J Clin Endocr 19:632, 1959.
132. Levy R, Kelly L, Jeffries W: The study of thyroid function by means of a single injection of thyrotropin. J Clin Invest 32:583, 1953.
133. Lewitusz R, Lubin E: Sequential scanning of the thyroid as an aid in the diagnosis of subacute thyroiditis. Israel J Med Sci 3:847, 1967.
134. Linsk J, Paton B, Persky M, et al: The effect of phenylbutazone and a related analogue (G25671) upon thyroid function. J Clin Endocr 17:416, 1957.
135. Lisbona R, Lacourciere Y, Rosenthal L: Aspergillomatous abscesses of the brain and thyroid. J Nuc Med 14:541, 1973.
136. Little G, et al: "Cryptothyroidism," the major cause of sporadic "athyreotic" cretinism. J Clin Endocr 25:1529, 1965.
137. Livolsi V, Perzin K, Svetsky L: Carcinoma arising in median ectopic thyroid (including thyroglossal duct tissue). Cancer 34:1303, 1974.
138. Lohrenz F, Fernandez R, Doe R: Isolated thyrotropin deficiency. Review and report of three cases. Ann Int Med 60:990, 1964.
139. London W, Wought R, Brown F: Bread-dietary source of large quantities of iodine. N Eng J Med 273:381, 1965.
140. Long R, Evans A, Beggs J: Surgical management of ectopic thyroid: report of a case with simultaneous lingual and subhyoid median ectopic thyroid. Ann Surg 160:824, 1964.
141. Malamos B, Vagenakis A, Pandos P, et al: Comparison of scanning and palpation in the assessment of the weight of the thyroid gland. Endocrinologie 56:232, 1970.
142. Mann C: Thyroid abscess in a 3½ year old child. Arch Otolarygol 103:299, 1977.
143. Marchetta F, Krause L, Sako K: Interpretation of scintigrams obtained after thyroidectomy. Surg Gynec Obstet 116:647, 1963.
144. Marcus C, Marcus S: Struma ovarii: a report of 7 cases and a review of the subject. Amer J Obstet Gynec 81:752, 1961.
145. Marshall C: Variations in the form of the thyroid gland in man. J Anat and Physiology 29:235, 1895.
146. Martin J, Stanbury J: The response of the ^{131}I-treated thyroid gland to thyrotropic hormone. J Clin Endocr 15:811, 1955.
147. McCormack K: An unusual "thyroid" nodule "cold" to scintiscan. California Medicine 103:282, 1965.
148. McCormack K, Sheline G: Long term studies of solitary autonomous thyroid nodules. J Nuc Med 8:701, 1967.
149. McKenzie J: Neonatal Grave's disease. J Clin Endocr 24:660, 1964.
150. Meadows P: Scintillation scanning in the management of the clinically single thyroid nodule. J Amer Med Assoc 277:229, 1961.
151. Means J, DeGroot L, Stanbury J: The Thyroid and Its Diseases, 3rd Edition. New York: McGraw-Hill, 1963, p. 7.
152. Meyerowitz B, Bucholz R: Midline cervical ectopic thyroid tissue. Surg 65:358, 1969.
153. Michael K, Ong G: Cystic thyroid nodules. Br J Surg 62:205, 1975.
154. Miller J, Horn R, Block M: The evaluation of toxic nodular goiter. Arch Intern Med 113:72, 1964.
155. Miller M, Block M: Functional autonomy in multinodular goiter. JAMA 214:535, 1970.

156. Miller M, Hamburger J: The thyroid scintigram: the hot nodule. Radiology 84:66, 1965.
157. Miller M, Horn R, Block M: The evolution of toxic nodular goiter. Arch Int Med 113:72, 1964.
158. Mishkin M, Rosen I, Walfish P: B-mode ultrasonography in assessment of thyroid gland lesions. Ann Int Med 75:505,1973.
159. Miyai K, Azukizawa M, Kumahara Y: Familial isolated thyrotropin deficiency with cretinism. N Eng J Med 285:1043, 1971.
160. Molnar G, Wilber R, Lee R, et al: On the hyperfunctioning solitary thyroid nodule. Mayo Clin Proc 40:665, 1965.
161. Montero J, Pascual V, et al: Extrathyroidal parathyroid adenoma presenting as a cold nodule on ^{131}I thyroid scan. VA Med Mon 100:643, 1973.
162. Montgomery M: Lingual thyroid—a comprehensive review. West J Surg 43:661, 1935, and 44:54,122,189,237,303,378,442, 1936.
163. Morgans M, Trotter W: Defective organic binding of iodine by the thyroid in Hashimoto's thyroiditis. Lancet 1:553, 1957.
164. Morgans M, Trotter W: Association of congenital deafness with goiter: the nature of the thyroid defect. Lancet 1:607, 1958.
165. Mueller R, Bruasch C, Hirsch E, et al: Uptake of radioactive iodine in the thyroid of patients with impaired liver function. J Clin Endocr and Metab 14:1287, 1954.
166. Nachlas N: Thyroglossal duct cysts. Ann Otol, Rhin & Laryng 59:381, 1950.
167. Najjar S: Hypothyroidism in children from an endemic goiter area. J of Ped 64:372, 1964.
168. Najjar S, Woodruff C: Some observations on goiter in Lebanon. Am J Clin Nutrition 13:46, 1963.
169. Neinas F, Gorman C, Devine K, et al: Lingual thyroid, clinical characteristics of 15 cases. Ann Int Med 79:205, 1973.
170. Neinas FW, Gorman CA, Devine KD, et al: Lingual thyroid. Ann Int Med 79:205–211, 1973.
171. Niepominiszce H, DeGroot L, Hagen G: Abnormal thyroid peroxidase causing iodide organification defect. J Clin Endocr 34:607, 1972.
172. Nodine J, Maldia G: Pseudostruma ovarii. Obstet Gynec 17:460, 1961.
173. Oddie T, Myhill J, Pirnique F, et al: Effect of age and sex on the radioiodine uptake in euthyroid subjects. J Clin Endocr 28:766, 1968.
174. Oddie T, Pirnique F, et al: Geographic variation of radioiodine uptake in euthyroid subjects. J Clin Endocr 28:761, 1968.
175. Odell W, Bates R, Rivlin R, et al: Increased thyroid function without clinical hyperthyroidism in patients with choriocarcinoma. J Clin Endocr Metab 23:658, 1963.
176. Oyamada H, Tabei T: Scintigraphic evaluation of cold thyroid nodules. Tohoku J Exp Med 123:315, 1977.
177. Papapetrou P, Jackson I. Thyrotoxicosis due to "silent" thyroiditis. Lancet 1:363, 1975.
178. Paris J, McConahey W, Tauxe W, et al: The effect of iodides on Hashimoto's thyroiditis. J Clin Endocr 21:1037, 1961.
179. Paull B, Alderson P, Siegel B: Thyroid imaging in lymphocytic thyroiditis. Radiology 115:129, 1975.
180. Pedras W, et al: Our experience with the suppression test in the diagnosis of thyroid dysfunction. Nuklearmedizin 3:263, 1963.
181. Pellegrini A, Cenni L, Po V: An unusual finding—congenital absence of the upper pole of the lobe of thyroid gland and radioactive scanning. J Kansas Med Soc 67:491,500, 1966.

182. Pickelman J, Lee J, Straus F II, et al: Thyroid hemangioma. Amer J of Surg 129:331, 1975.
183. Pittman J, Dailey G, Geschi R: Changing normal values for thyroidal radioiodine uptake. N Eng J Med 280:1431, 1979.
184. Plaut A: Ovarian struma: a morphologic, pharmacologic and biologic examination. Amer J of Obstet Gynec 25:351, 1933.
185. Plummer H: Clinical and pathological relationship of simple and exophthalmic goiter. Amer J Med Sci 146:790, 1913.
186. Polacheck A: Tortuous innominate artery simulating thyroid nodule. New York State J of Med 75:1276, 1975.
187. Porto G: Esophageal nodule of thyroid tissue. Laryngoscope 70:1336, 1960.
188. Psarras A, Papadoupoulos S, Livadas D, et al: The single thyroid nodule. Brit J Surg 59:545, 1972.
189. Querido A, Stanbury J: The response of the thyroid gland to thyrotropic hormone as an aid in the differential diagnosis of primary and secondary hypothyroidism. J Clin Endocr 10:1192, 1950.
190. Quimby E, Werner S, Schmidt C: Influence of age, sex, and season upon the radioiodine uptake by the human thyroid. Proc Soc Exp Biol Med 75:537, 1950.
191. Quinn J, Brand W: Pertechnetate-99m thyroid scans obtained incidental to brain scans. J Nuc Med 8:481, 1967.
192. Rajguru H, Poulose K, Reba R: Esophageal tracer retention simulating substernal goiter. J Nuc Med 18:404, 1977.
193. Ramgopal E, Stanbury J: Studies of distribution of iodine and protein in a struma ovarii. J Clin Endocr 25:526, 1965.
194. Ramsay I, Richardson P, Marsden P, et al: Thyroid "hot" nodules. Post-Graduate Med J 48:577, 1972.
195. Ravel R: "Owl eye" sign in thyroid nodule of papillary carcinoma: Case report. J Nuc Med 17:985, 1976.
196. Reaume C, Sofie V: Lingual thyroid. Review of the literature and report of a case. Oral Surgery 45:841, 1978.
197. Recan T, Riggs D: Thyroid function in nephrosis. J Clin Invest 31:789, 1952.
198. Renda F, Holmes R, North W, et al: Characteristics of thyroid scans in normal persons, hyperthyroidism and nodular goiter. J Nuc Med 9:156, 1968.
199. Report of an International Atomic Energy Agency panel: Thyroid radionuclide uptake measurements. Int Journal Appl Rad and Isotopes 23:305, 1972.
200. Rich C: Thyroid function of euthyroid patients during and after treatment with triiodothyronine. J Clin Endocr 18:1024, 1958.
201. Robertson J, Nolan N, Wagner H, et al: Thyroid radioiodine uptakes and scans in euthyroid patients. Mayo Cl Proc 50:79, 1975.
202. Robertson J, Verhasselt M, Wahner H: Use of ^{123}I for thyroid uptake measurements and depression of ^{131}I thyroid uptakes by incomplete dissolution of capsule filler. J Nuc Med 15:770, 1974.
203. Robinson E, Horn Y: The scanogram of the thyroid following partial sub-total or total thyroidectomy. Oncology 24:81, 1970.
204. Rogers W, Kesten H: Case report: a thyroid mass in the ventricular septum obstructing the right ventricular outflow tract and producing a murmur. J Cardiovascular Surg 4:175, 1963.
205. Rosen I, Walfish P: Case report: the subhyoid ectopic median thyroid. Canad Med Assoc J 96:544, 1967.

206. Rosenberg I: Evaluation of thyroid function. N Eng J Med 286:924, 1972.
207. Russotto J, Boyar R: Thyroid hemiagenesis. J Nuc Med 12:186, 1971.
208. Salvatore M, Gallo A: Accessory thyroid tissue in the anterior mediastinum: Case report. J Nuc Med 16:1135, 1975.
209. Sauk J Jr: Ectopic lingual thyroid. J Pathol 102:239, 1970.
210. Schneeberg N, Perloff W, Levy L: Diagnosis of equivocal hypothyroidism using thyrotropin hormone (TSH). J Clin Endocr 14:223, 1954.
211. Shimaoka K, Sokal J, Pickren J: Metastatic neoplasms in the thyroid gland. Cancer 15:557, 1962.
212. Shimkin P, Sagerman R: Lymphoma of the thyroid gland. Radiology 92:812, 1969.
213. Silverstein G, Burke G, Cogan R: The natural history of the autonomous hyperfunctioning thyroid nodule. Ann Internal Med 67:539, 1967.
214. Silverstein G, Burke G, Goldberg D, et al: Superior vena caval system obstruction caused by benign endothoracic goiter. Dis Chest 56:519, 1969.
215. Sisson J: Principles of, and pitfalls in, thyroid function tests. J Nuc Med 6:853, 1965.
216. Sitterson B, Andrews G: Introduction to thyroid scanning. Progress in Medical Radioisotope Scanning. Oak Ridge, Tenn.: Oak Ridge Inst of Nuc Studies, p. 279, 1963.
217. Skillern P, Crile G, McCullagh E, et al: Struma lymphomatosa: primary thyroid failure with compensatory thyroid enlargement. J Clin Endocr and Metab 16:35, 1956.
218. Skillern P, Evans B: The thyroid stimulating hormone (TSH) test: An aid to the differential diagnosis of non-toxic disease of the thyroid. Arch Int Med 99:234, 1957.
219. Slingerland D: Effects of an organic iodine compound (Priodax) on tests of thyroid function. J Clin Endocr 17:82, 1957.
220. Spencer R, Benever C: Human thyroid growth: a scan study (preliminary report). Investigative Radiology 5:111, 1970.
221. Stanbury J: The metabolic basis for certain disorders of the thyroid gland. Amer J Clin Nutr 9:669, 1961.
222. Steigbigel N, Oppenheim J, Fishman L, et al: Metastatic embryonal carcinoma of the testis associated with elevated plasma TSH-like activity and hyperthyroidism. New Eng J Med 271:345, 1964.
223. Stewart R, Murray I: An evaluation of the perchlorate discharge test. J Clin Endocr 26:1050, 1966.
224. Strickland A, MacAfie J, Van Wyk J, et al: Ectopic thyroid glands simulating thyroglossal duct cysts: hypothyroidism following surgical excision. JAMA 208:307, 1969.
225. Sussman L, Librink L, Clayton G: Hyperthyroidism attributable to a hyperfunctional thyroid carcinoma. J Pediatr 72:208, 1968.
226. Sweet R: Intrathoracic goiter located in the posterior mediastinum. Surg Gynecol Obstet 89:57, 1949.
227. Szego P, Levy J: Recurrent acute suppurative thyroiditis. Can Med Assoc J 103:631, 1970.
228. Taguchi J, Powell C, Nickerson N: Thyroidal ^{131}I uptake patterns following iodides. Arch Intern Med 112:569, 1963.
229. Takeuchi K, Suzuki H, Horiuchi Y, et al: Significance of iodide perchlorate discharge test for detection of iodine organification defect of the thyroid. J Clin Endocr 31:144, 1970.
230. Tannahil A, Hooper M, England M, et al: Measurement of thyroid size by ultrasound, palpation and scintiscan. Clin Endocr 8:483, 1978.
231. Taunton O, McDaniel H, Pittman J: Standardization of TSH testing. J Clin Endocr 25:266, 1965.

232. Thomas C, Pepper F, Owen J: Differentiation of malignant from benign lesion of the thyroid gland using complementary scanning with [75]selenomethionine and radioiodide. Ann Surg 170:396, 1969.

233. Thomas S, Maxon H, Kereiakes J, et al: Quantitative external counting techniques enabling improved diagnostic and therapeutic decisions in patients with well-differentiated thyroid cancer. Radiology 122:731, 1977.

234. Thompson J: The normal thyroid scan. Lancet 2:308, 1966.

235. Tong E, Rubenfeld S: Scan mesurements of normal and enlarged thyroid glands. Am J Roentgenol 115:706, 1972.

236. Turcot J: Lingual and hyoid thyroid. Am J Surg 104:667, 1962.

237. Turner H, Howard R: Goiter from prolonged ingestion of iodide. J Clin Endocr 16:141, 1956.

238. Tysow W, Wilkinson R, Witherspoon L, et al: False positive ^{131}I total body scans. J Nuc Med 15:1052, 1974.

239. Ulloa-Fernandez M, Maxon H, Mehta S, et al: [131]I uptake by primary lung adenocarcinoma. JAMA 236:857, 1976.

240. Volpe R, Johnston M, Huber N: Thyroid function in subacute thyroiditis. J Clin Endocr 18:65, 1958.

241. Wade H: Solitary thyroid nodule. Ann Royal College of Surgeons of England 55:13, 1974.

242. Wallack M, Adelberg H, Nicoloff J: A thyroid suppression test using a single dose of ℓ-thyroxine. N Eng J Med 283: 402, 1970.

243. Wang C, Vickery A, Maloof F: Large parathyroid cysts mimicking thyroid nodules. Ann Surg 175:448, 1972.

244. Wang Y: Radioisotope scanning of superior mediastinal masses. Am J Roentgenol 103:766, 1968.

245. Weiner J, Roos P: Thyroid asymmetry. Bri Med J 3:312, 1968.

246. Weinstein M, Ashkar F, Caron C: [75]Se selenomethionine as a scanning agent for the differential diagnosis of the cold thyroid nodule. Sem Nuc Med 1:390, 1971.

247. Weissel M, Wolf A, Linkesch W: Acute suppurative thyroiditis caused by *Escherichia coli*. Br Med J 2:23, 1977.

248. Werner S: Euthyroid patients with early eye signs of Graves' disease: their responses to ℓ-triiodothyronine and thyrotropin. Am J Med 18:608, 1955.

249. Werner S: Response to triiodothyronine as index of persistence of disease in the thyroid remnant of patients in remission from hyperthyroidism. J Clin Invest 35:57, 1958.

250. Werner S, Hamilton H: Pituitary thyroid relations. Lancet 1:796, 1953.

251. Werner S, Spooner M: Some clinical aspects of thyroid physiology. Med Clin N Amer 39:799, 1955.

252. Werner S, Spooner M: A new and simple test for hyperthyroidism employing ℓ-triiodothyronine and the twenty-four hour I-131 uptake method. Bull NY Acad Med 31:137, 1955.

253. Whale H: Esophageal tumor of thyroid tissue. Bri Med J 2:987, 1921.

254. Williams E, Ekins R, Ellis S: Thyroid suppression test with serum thyroxine concentration as index of suppression. Bri Med J 4:338, 1969.

255. Williams E, Ekins R, Ellis S: Thyroid stimulation test with serum thyroxine concentration as index of thyroid response. Bri Med J 4:336, 1969.

256. Wolfstein R: Enigma of the "hyperfunctioning" carcinoma resolved? J Nuc Med 19:441, 1978.

257. Woodruff J, Rauh J, Markley R: Ovarian struma. Obstet Gynec 27:194, 1966.

258. Yao Y: Thyroid nodules—benign or malignant? Diagnosis. Post-graduate Med 61:76, 1977.

259. Yeh E, Meade R, Ruetz P: Radionuclide study of struma ovarii. J Nuc Med 14:118, 1973.

260. Young H, MacLeod N: The fate and function of the thyroid remnant. A surgical and radioactive iodine study. Bri J Surg 59:726, 1972.

261. Young-McHardy S, Doniach D, Polani P: Thyroid function in Turner's syndrome and allied conditions. Lancet 2:1161, 1970.

Chapter 17

Parathyroid

AMOLAK SINGH

EDWARD B. SILBERSTEIN

I. Parathyroid uptake of ^{75}Se-selenomethionine

   A. Common

      1. Parathyroid adenoma (2, 4, 6)

         a. clear cell (2)

         b. chief cell (4)

         c. oxyphil cell (2)

      2. Parathyroid hyperplasia (6)

         a. clear cell (6)

   B. Uncommon

      1. Carcinoma (6)

      2. Ectopic parathyroid (1)

II. Non-parathyroid uptake of ^{75}Se-selenomethionine in the neck

   A. Thyroid (10)

      1. Common

         a. thyroid adenoma

      b. papillary carcinoma
      c. follicular carcinoma
  2. Uncommon
      a. Hürthle cell carcinoma
      b. substernal thyroid (1)
B. Thymus
  1. Uncommon
      a. thymoma (9)
        (1) with red cell aplasia (5)
        (2) with myasthenia gravis (8)
C. Other neoplastic disease
  1. Common
      a. lung cancer (all cell types) (3)
      b. metastatic squamous cell carcinoma (10)
        (1) laryngeal
        (2) oropharyngeal
      c. metastatic adenocarcinoma (10)
        (1) ovary
      d. lymphoma, non-Hodgkin's (7, 10)
        (1) histiocytic
        (2) non-histiocytic
  2. Uncommon
      a. sarcoma (10)
      b. teratoma (1)
      c. metastatic breast cancer (1)
      d. mesothelioma (1)
      e. esophageal carcinoma (1)
      f. carcinoid tumors (1)
D. Granuloma
  1. Common
      a. tuberculosis (1)
      b. sarcoidosis (1)

REFERENCES

1. Bose A, Tanaka T, Mishkin FS: Selenomethionine uptake in the thorax. Sem Nucl Med 12:220–221, 1982.
2. Colella AC, Pigorini F: Experience with parathyroid scintigraphy. Am J Roentgenol 109:714–723, 1970.
3. Critchley M, Testa HJ, Stretton TB: Combined use of ^{99m}Tc labelled macroaggregates of albumin and 75-selenium selenomethionine in the diagnosis of lung cancer. Thorax 29:421–424, 1974.
4. DiGiulio W, Morales JO: The value of selenomethionine Se-75 scan in pre-operative localization of parathyroid adenomas. JAMA 209:1873–1880, 1969.
5. Min KW, Waddel CC, Pircher FJ, et al: Selective uptake of 75-Se selenomethionine by thymoma with pure red cell aplasia. Cancer 41:1323–1328, 1978.

6. Potchen EJ, Watts HG, Awwad HK: Parathyroid scintiscanning. Radiol Clin North Am 5:267–275, 1967.

7. Spencer RP, Montana G, Scanlon GT, et al: Uptake of selenomethionine by mouse and in human lymphomas, with observations on selenite and selenate. J Nucl Med 8:197–208, 1967.

8. Toole JF, Cowan R, Maynard D, et al: Selenomethionine Se-75 thymus scans in myasthenia gravis. Trans Am Neurol Assoc 100:248–249, 1975.

9. Toole JF, Witcofski R: Selenomethionine Se-75 scan for thymoma. JAMA 198:197–198, 1966.

10. Weinstein MB, Ashkar FS, Caron CD: [75]Se selenomethionine as a scanning agent for the differential diagnosis of the cold thyroid nodule. Sem Nucl Med 1:390–396, 1971.

Chapter 18

Adrenal Medulla[†]

JOHN G. McAFEE

I. Nonvisualization of adrenal areas (at 1–3 days after administration)

  A. Normal adrenal glands (1)

  B. Abnormal adrenergic uptake suppressed by reserpine or tricyclic antidepressant drugs (1)

  C. Small pheochromocytomas, obscured by liver or spleen (about 10% of total tumors) (1, 2)

II. Visualization of one adrenal area (at 1–3 days and beyond)

  A. Pheochromocytoma (1, 2, 3)

III. Visualization of both adrenal areas (at 1–3 days)

  A. Normal adrenal glands (after 1 day) (1)

† Adrenal medullary imaging with I-131 m-iodobenzylguanidine.

B. Bilateral pheochromocytoma (2)

C. Bilateral pheochromocytoma associated with neurofibromatosis (2)

D. Bilateral pheochromocytoma in multiple endocrine neoplasia (3)

E. Adrenal medullary hyperplasia in multiple endocrine neoplasia (3)

IV. Extra-adrenal concentrations

A. Extra-adrenal pheochromocytoma (2)

B. Metastases from malignant pheochromocytoma (2)

C. Normal myocardium (1)

D. Colonic activity (1)

E. Pelvocalyceal renal activity (radioiodide) (1)

REFERENCES

1. Nakajo M, Shapiro B, Copp J, et al: The normal and abnormal distribution of the adreno-medullary imaging agent m-(I-131) iodobenzylguanidine (I-131 MIBG) in man: evaluation by scintigraphy. J Nucl Med 24:672–682, 1983.
2. Sisson JC, Frager MS, Valk TW, et al: Scintigraphic localization of pheochromocytoma. New Engl J Med 305:12–17, 1981.
3. Valk TW, Frager MS, Gross MD, et al: Spectrum of pheochromocytoma in multiple endocrine neoplasia: a scintigraphic portrayal using ^{131}I-metaiodobenzylguanidine. Ann Int Med 94:762–767, 1981.

Chapter 19

Adrenal Cortex[†]

JOHN G. McAFEE

EDWARD B. SILBERSTEIN

I. Symmetrical adrenal uptake without dexamethasone suppression

A. Common

The use of an asterisk * in this chapter indicates that this entity has been observed by one of the authors but the case report has not been published.

[†] Adrenal cortex imaging with ^{131}I-19-iodocholesterol or ^{131}I-6β-iodomethyl-19-norcholesterol.

    1. Normal

    2. Cushing's syndrome with adrenal hyperplasia due to excess ACTH (1, 14)

    3. Low renin, normal aldosterone hypertension (16, 20)

  B. Uncommon

    1. Idiopathic aldosteronism with bilateral hyperplasia (21)

    2. False negative studies

      a. adenoma secreting aldosterone (21)

      b. adrenal carcinoma (21)

II. Symmetrical uptake with increased intensity, without dexamethasone

  A. Common

    1. Idiopathic aldosteronism with bilateral adrenal cortical hyperplasia (21)

    2. Cushing's syndrome with bilateral hyperplasia (1)

III. Symmetrical uptake following dexamethasone suppression, i.e., failure to suppress (usually 0.5 to 2 mg every 6 hours beginning 72–120 hours prior to radiopharmaceutical)

  A. Common

    1. Certain normals (especially with norcholesterol agent and short periods of dexamethasone suppression) (11)

    2. Idiopathic hyperaldosteronism with bilateral hyperplasia (21)

    3. Cushing's syndrome with adrenal hyperplasia due to ACTH excess (20)

    4. Low renin, normal aldosterone, hypertension (16, 17, 20)

    5. Secondary hyperaldosteronism (11A)

      a. oral contraceptives

      b. diuretic therapy

      c. renal artery stenosis

  B. Uncommon

    1. Aldosteronoma (21)

    2. Hyperandrogenism (10)

    3. Bilateral adrenocortical adenoma (2)

    4. Congenital adrenal hyperplasia (e.g. 17- or 21-hydroxylase deficiency) (14A)

    5. Exogenous ACTH (3A)

    6. Aminoglutethimide (18)

    7. Visualization of left adrenal with gallbladder activity simulating right adrenal (11A)

IV. Asymmetrical uptake without dexamethasone suppression

A. Common
　　1. Aldosteronoma (21)
　　2. Idiopathic aldosteronism with bilateral hyperplasia, macronodular or micronodular (23)
　　3. Cushing's syndrome with adrenal hyperplasia (21)
　　4. Pheochromocytoma (on side of decreased uptake) (1)
B. Uncommon
　　1. Normal variation, due to differences in adrenal depth or superimposition of right gland on liver (7)
　　2. Adrenal virilizing adenoma (7)
　　3. Low renin, normal aldosterone, hypertension (16)
C. Rare
　　1. Adrenal medullary hyperplasia (on side of decreased uptake) (20)
　　2. "Functioning" adenoma without overt endocrine abnormality (3, 18)

V. Unilateral uptake without dexamethasone suppression

A. Common
　　1. Unilateral adrenalectomy
　　2. Adrenal adenoma suppressing contralateral gland
　　　　a. with Cushing's syndrome (1)
　　　　b. with hyperaldosteronism (19)
　　3. Metastatic carcinoma to nonvisualized side (19)
B. Uncommon
　　1. Adrenal infarction post-venography (1)
　　2. Adrenal remnant post-total adrenalectomy causing Cushing's syndrome (14)
　　3. Adenoma without overt endocrine abnormality (3, 18)
C. Rare
　　1. Tumors
　　　　a. adrenal cortical carcinoma in nonfunctioning side (13)
　　　　b. pheochromocytoma in nonfunctioning side (1)
　　　　c. neuroblastoma in nonfunctioning side (14)
　　　　d. ganglioneuroma in nonfunctioning side (24)
　　　　e. chemodectoma in nonfunctioning side (24)
　　　　f. sarcoma in nonfunctioning side (24)
　　2. Congenital cyst*
　　3. Congenital unilateral agenesis, more often right sided (19)
　　4. Unilateral calcified adrenal, unknown cause (possibly remote tuberculosis or infarction)*

VI. Focal decreased uptake or defect in one adrenal

A. Common
　　1. Metastatic tumor (15)

B. Uncommon
  1. Pheochromocytoma (4, 22)
  2. Simple cyst (9)
  3. Hematoma (12)

VII. Asymmetrical or unilateral uptake with dexamethasone suppression

  A. Common
    1. Aldosteronoma (21)
  B. Uncommon
    1. Idiopathic aldosteronism with macronodular cortical hyperplasia (21)
    2. Adrenocortical adenoma causing hyperandrogenism (4, 10)
    3. Adenoma in low renin, essential hypertension (17)
    4. Adrenal carcinoma with late increased uptake (4)

VIII. Bilaterally absent or decreased uptake without dexamethasone suppression

  A. Common
    1. Cushing's syndrome due to adrenocortical adenoma or carcinoma (unilateral tumor with functional suppression of opposite gland)(1)
    2. Previous prednisone therapy (1)
  B. Uncommon
    1. Hypopituitarism treated with hydrocortisone (1)
    2. Functioning remnants after bilateral adrenalectomy (1)
    3. Addison's disease (1)
  C. Rare
    1. Histiocytosis X (1)
    2. Elevated serum cholesterol (8, 25)
    3. Adrenal carcinoma, on early scans (4)

IX. Bilaterally absent or decreased uptake with dexamethasone suppression

  A. Common
    1. Normal
    2. Micronodular hyperplasia associated with hyperaldosteronism (6, 21)
    3. Macronodular hyperplasia associated with hyperaldosteronism (1, 6)
  B. Uncommon
    1. Hyperandrogenism (10)
    2. Low renin, essential hypertension (17)

X. Uptake of adrenal agents focally within the liver
  A. Rare
    1. Hepatic metastases from adrenal cortical carcinoma (5, 26)

REFERENCES

1. Anderson BG, Beierwaltes WH: Adrenal radiocholesterol in the diagnosis of adrenal disorders. Adv Intern Med 19:327–343, 1974.
2. Barliev GB: Adrenal scintigraphy with [131]I-19-iodocholesterol. Eur J Nucl Med 4:449–451, 1979.
3. Beierwaltes WH, Sturman MF, Ryo U, et al: Imaging functional nodules of the adrenal glands with [131]I-19-iodocholesterol. J Nucl Med 15:246–251, 1974.
3A. Blair RJ, Beierwaltes WH, Liebermann LM, et al: Radiolabeled cholesterol as an adrenal scanning agent. J Nucl Med 12:176–182, 1971.
4. Chatal JF, Charbonnel B, Guihard D: Radionuclide imaging of the adrenal glands. Clin Nucl Med 3:71–76, 1978.
5. Chatal JF, Charbonnel B, LeMevel BP, et al: Uptake of [131]I-19-iodocholesterol by an adrenal cortical carcinoma and its metastases. J Clin Endocrinol Metab 43:248–251, 1976.
6. Conn JW, Cohen EL, Herwig KR: The dexamethasone modified adrenal scintiscan in hyporeninemic aldosteronism (tumor versus hyperplasia) with adrenal venography and adrenal venous aldosterone. J Lab Clin Med 88:841–855, 1976.
7. Freitas JE, Thrall JH, Swanson DP, et al: Normal adrenal imaging (abstract). J Nucl Med 18:599, 1977.
8. Gordon L, Mayfield RK, Levine JH, et al: Failure to visualize adrenal glands in a patient with bilateral adrenal hyperplasia. J Nucl Med 21:49–51, 1980.
9. Gross MD, Freitas JE, Silver TM: Documentation of adrenal cyst by adrenal scanning techniques. J Nucl Med 19:1092, 1978.
10. Gross MD, Freitas JE, Swanson DP, et al: Dexamethasone-suppression adrenal scintigraphy in hyperandrogenism. J Nucl Med 22:12–17, 1981.
11. Gross MD, Freitas JE, Swanson DP, et al: Dexamethasone suppression (DS) adrenal scans in normal controls (abstract). J Nucl Med 19:677, 1978.
11A. Gross MD, Valk TW, Swanson DP: The role of pharmacologic manipulation in adrenal cortical scintigraphy. Sem Nucl Med 11:128–148, 1981.
12. Heyman S, Treves S: Adrenal hemorrhage in the newborn: scintigraphic diagnosis. J Nucl Med 20:521–523, 1979.
13. Hogan MJ, McRae J, Schambelan M, et al: Location of aldosterone-producing adenomas with [131]I-19-iodocholesterol. N Engl J Med 294:410–414, 1976.
14. Lieberman LM, Beierwaltes WH, Conn JW, et al: Diagnosis of adrenal disease by visualization of human adrenal glands with [131]I-19-iodocholesterol. N Engl J Med 285:1387–1393, 1971.
14A. Moses DC, Beierwaltes WH: Adrenal imaging in children, in James AE, Wagner HH, Cooke RE (eds): Pediatric Nuclear Medicine. Philadelphia: W.B. Saunders, 1974, pp. 399–409.
15. Parthasarathy KL, Bakshi S, Ackerhalt RE, et al: Adrenal scintigraphy utilizing [131]I-19-iodocholesterol. Clin Nucl Med 1:150–155, 1976.
16. Rifai A, Beierwaltes WH, Freitas JE, et al: Adrenal scintigraphy in low renin essential hypertension. J Nucl Med 18:599, 1977.
17. Rifai A, Beierwaltes WH, Freitas JE, et al: Adrenal scintigraphy in low renin essential hypertension. Clin Nucl Med 3:282–286, 1978.
18. Rizza RA, Wahner HW, Spelsberg TC, et al: Visualization of nonfunctioning adrenal adenomas with iodocholesterol: possible relationship to subcellular distribution of tumor. J Nucl Med 18:600, 1977.

19. Ryo UY: Unilateral visualization of the adrenal gland. Sem Nucl Med 11:224–225, 1981.
20. Sarkar SD, Cohen EL, Beierwaltes WH, et al: A new and superior adrenal imaging agent, [131]I-6β-iodomethyl-19-norcholesterol. J Clin Endocrinol Metab 45:353–362, 1977.
21. Seabold JE, Cohen EL, Beierwaltes WH, et al: Adrenal imaging with [131]I-19-iodocholesterol in the diagnostic evaluation of patients with aldosteronism. J Clin Endocrinol Metab 42:41–51, 1976.
22. Sturman MF, Moses DC, Beierwaltes WH, et al: Radiocholesterol adrenal images for the localization of pheochromocytoma. Surg Gyn Obstet 135:177–180, 1974.
23. Thrall JH, Gross MD, Freitas JE, et al: Clinical applications of adrenal scintigraphy. Applied Radiol 9:115–124, 1980.
24. Troncose L, Falappa PG, Focacci C, et al: [131]I-19-iodocholesterol scintigraphy for the localization of medullary tumors. J Nucl Med Allied Sci 21:159–164, 1977.
25. Valk TW, Gross MD, Freitas JE, et al: The relationship of serum lipids to adrenal gland uptake of 6β-(^{131}I) iodomethyl-19-norcholesterol in Cushing's syndrome. J Nucl Med 21:1069–1072, 1980.
26. Watanabe K, Kamoi I, Nakaymam C, et al: Scintigraphic detection of hepatic metastases with ^{131}I-labeled steroid in recurrent adrenal carcinoma. J Nucl Med 17:904–906, 1076.

Part IV

The Eye

Chapter 20

Dacryoscintigraphy

MARIANO FERNANDEZ-ULLOA

I. Normal pattern (2, 4)

    A. Consecutive visualization of all portions of lacrimal drainage apparatus
        1. Canaliculi
        2. Lacrimal sac
        3. Nasolacrimal duct
        4. Nasal cavity
    B. Prompt and symmetric drainage into the nasal cavity
    C. Rapid tear drainage as assessed by quantitative scintigraphy (6)

II. Obstruction

    A. Patterns (2)
        1. Delayed or nonvisualized lacrimal drainage apparatus with duct ectasia
        2. Decreased or lack of nasal radioactivity
        3. Occasional duct distortion
    B. Causes
        1. Common
            a. stone (dacryolith) (2, 14)
            b. lid injury; enucleation, orbital fracture (2, 14)
            c. radiation stricture (1, 14)
            d. chronic dacryocystitis (2)
                (1) mycotic canaliculitis (12A)
            e. obstruction post-dacryocystorhinostomy (3)
            f. mucus plug (5); mucocele (9)

      g. idiopathic stenosis (5)
  2. Uncommon
      a. anomalous valve of Krause or of Taillefer (5)
      b. basal cell carcinoma (1)
      c. surgically occluded puncta (9)
      d. absent puncta (9)

III. Delayed clearance without obstruction

  A. Common
    1. Lax lids and poor orbicularis palpebrarum tone; ectropion (2, 9)
      a. acquired
      b. congenital
    2. Spasmodic blinking (14)
    3. Reduced tear secretion after skull fracture (14)
    4. Facial nerve palsy (9, 14)
    5. Functional blocks (4)
  B. Uncommon
    1. Thyroid ophthalmopathy with decreased lacrimation and slow clearance (9)
    2. Diverticulum of lacrimal sac (9)

IV. Focal retention

  A. Uncommon
    1. Diverticula (9)
    2. Focal retention in ectropion (1)
    3. Fistula (12A)

V. Assessment of dacryocystorhinostomy and lid surgery for epiphora (3, 9)

  A. Restored patency (normal)
  B. Residual obstruction; functional blocks as above

References for this chapter may be found at the end of Chapter 21, page 123.

Radioactive Phosphorus (^{32}P-Phosphorus) for the Detection of Ocular Malignancy

MARIANO FERNANDEZ-ULLOA

I. Abnormal uptake in suspected lesion in excess of 65% over average of uninvolved quadrants (11)

  A. Common
1. Malignant melanoma of the choroid and ciliary body (spindle cell, epithelioid cell or mixed) (7, 11)
2. Posterior uveal melanoma (7, 10)
3. Metastases (11)
   a. lung cancer (7)
   b. breast carcinoma (13)

  B. Uncommon (false positive)
1. Adenoma of retinal pigment epithelium (11)
2. Choroidal hemangioma (10)
3. Chorioretinal granuloma, tuberculous (9)
4. Choroidal nerves (9)
5. Technical factors (9)

II. No increased uptake

  A. Common
1. Choroidal hemangioma (7)
2. Benign nevus (8)

  B. Uncommon
1. Choroidal hematoma (7)
2. Melanoma (7, 11)
3. Ciliary body cysts (8)
   a. with retinal detachment (8)
4. Coats' disease (8)
5. Choroiditis (8)
6. Technical error (8)
7. Hyperplasia of the retinal pigment epithelium (7)
8. Choroidal effusions (13)
9. Nerve fibers (8)

REFERENCES[1]

1. Brizel HE, Sheils WC, Brown M: The effect of radiotherapy on the nasolacrimal system as evaluated by dacryoscintigraphy. Radiology 116:373–381, 1975.
2. Brown M, El Gammel TAM, Luxenberg NM, et al: The value, limitations, and applications of nuclear dacryocystography. Sem Nucl Med 11:250–257, 1981.
3. Carlton WH, Trueblood JH, Rossomondo RM: Clinical evaluation of micro cintigraphy of the lacrimal drainage apparatus. J Nucl Med 14:89–92, 1973.
4. Chaudhuri TK: Clinical evaluation of nuclear dacryocystography. Clin Nucl Med 1:83–89, 1976.
5. Chaudhuri TK, Saparoff GR, Dolan KD, et al: A comparative study of contrast dacryocystogram and nuclear dacryocystogram. J Nucl Med 16:605–608, 1975.
6. Chavis RM, Welham RAN, Maisey MN: Quantitative lacrimal scintillography. Arch Ophthal 96:2066–2068, 1978.
7. Hagler WS, Jarrett WH, Humphrey WT: The radioactive phosphorus uptake test in diagnosis of uveal melanoma. Arch Ophthal 83:548–557, 1970.
8. Hagler WS, Jarrett WH, Schnauss RH, et al: The diagnosis of malignant melanoma of the ciliary body or choroid. So Med J 65:49–54, 1972.
9. Hurwitz JJ, Maisey MN, Welham RAN: Quantitative lacrimal scintillography. Br J Ophthal 59:312–313, 1975.
10. Lanning R, Shields JA: Comparison of radioactive phosphorus (^{32}P) uptake test in comparable sized choroidal melanomas and hemangiomas. Am J Ophthal 87:769–772, 1979.
11. Larose JH, Hagler WS, Jarrett WH: Phosphorus-32 eye tumor identification test. JAMA 236:1617–1618, 1976.
12. McLean IW, Shields JA: Prognostic value of ^{32}P uptake in posterior uveal melanomas. Ophthalmol 87:543–548, 1980.
12A. Pettie TH, Coin CG: Anatomy and physiology of the lacrimal drainage systems. Radiol Clin North Am 10:129–138, 1972.
13. Ruiz RS, Howerton EE: ^{32}P testing for posterior segment lesions. Trans Am Acad Ophthal Otolaryngal 79:287–296, 1975.
14. Søensen T, Jensen FT: Lacrimal pathology evaluated by dynamic lacrimal scintigraphy. Acta Ophthalmologica 58:597–607, 1980.

[1] This list contains references for Chapters 20 and 21.

Part V

Gallium Imaging

Chapter 22

Gallium-67

EDWARD B. SILBERSTEIN

I. Patterns of normal uptake for gallium-67

    A. Commonly seen organs

        1. Liver (71, 96)

        2. Bone and marrow cavities, especially epiphyseal regions (71, 96)

            a. sternum and spine uptake may hide mediastinal lesions on anterior and posterior views

        3. Spleen (96)

        4. Colon (96, 151)

        5. Salivary glands (71, 72, 96)

        6. Nasopharynx–minor salivary glands (71, 72, 96)

        7. Kidneys up to 24 hours (96)

    B. Less commonly seen

        1. Female breast and milk, non-lactating or lactating (75, 96)

        2. Male pubertal gynecomastia, occasionally unilateral (199)

        3. Lacrimal glands (72, 96, 125)

        4. Placenta (135)

        5. Spleen (71, 72, 96)

    C. Common with pediatric imaging

        1. Thymus (51, 69)

        2. Growth plate areas (51, 71)

        3. Spleen (51)

II. Abnormal causes of uptake in the head and neck (percentage is reported sensitivity for lesion)

A. Neoplastic
  1. Brain tumors: 90–91% (71, 178, 193)
    a. meningioma (6, 73, 117, 205, 206)
    b. glioma, grades I–IV (73, 117, 207, 208)
    c. metastases: 85% (73, 117, 207, 208)
    d. retinoblastoma (32, 33, 218)
    e. medulloblastoma (32, 33, 218)
    f. ependymoma (33)
    g. pinealoma (198)
    h. neuroblastoma (33, 218)
  2. Epidermoid and miscellaneous tumors of the head and neck: 50–85%
    a. sinuses (15, 57, 58, 117, 179, 194)
    b. pharynx (57, 63, 143, 179, 182, 194)
    c. larynx (57, 143, 179, 194)
    d. tongue (63, 117)
    e. tonsil (63)
    f. parotid cylindroma (117)
    g. floor of mouth (117)
    h. lacrimal gland adenoid cystic carcinoma (51)
    i. ameloblastoma (142)
    j. thyroid carcinoma (94, 178, 193)
    k. lymphoma (see Section III)
B. Non-neoplastic
  1. Head
    a. brain abscess (117, 210)
    b. meningitis/cerebritis (210)
    c. tuberculoma (218)
    d. osteomyelitis (210)
    e. mastoiditis (210)
    f. sinusitis (56, 108, 208)
    g. cerebral infarction (161, 206)
    h. craniotomy site (14)
    i. retro-orbital abscess (180)
    j. arterio-venous malformation (117)
    k. lacrimal gland inflammation
      (1) sarcoid (55, 144, 177, 211)
      (2) actinomycosis (111)
    l. salivary glands
      (1) sarcoid (55, 144, 177, 211)
      (2) radiation sialadenitis (100, 168)
      (3) sialadenitis from lupus erythematosus, renal failure, Sjögren's syndrome, etc. (54, 58)
      (4) actinomycosis (111)
  2. Neck
    a. thyroid gland
      (1) subacute thyroiditis (47)

    (2) Hashimoto's thyroiditis (35)
    (3) nontoxic nodular goiter (167)
  b. thymus gland
    (1) benign cyst (68)

III. Abnormal uptake in lymph nodes of neck, mediastinum, abdomen, including spleen

  A. Lymphoproliferative diseases
    1. Hodgkin's disease: 85–90% (2, 70, 71, 94, 117, 178)
    2. Non-Hodgkin's lymphoma: 33–75% (2, 7, 22, 71, 94, 117, 178)
    3. Angioimmunoblastic lymphadenopathy (45)
    4. Thymoma: 82% (150, 189, 193)
    5. Mycosis fungoides (84)
    6. Burkitt's lymphoma (32, 33, 162)
    7. Lymphoepithelioma (143)
  B. Metastatic carcinoma (72)
  C. Non-neoplastic
    1. *Yersinia pestis* (184)
    2. Mesenteric adenitis (213)
    3. Giant lymph node hyperplasia (204)
    4. After Lipiodol (102)
    5. Candidiasis (146)
    6. Actinomycosis (111)

IV. Abnormal thoracic uptake

  A. Neoplastic
    1. Breast: 65–70%
      a. adenocarcinoma (58, 85, 94, 97, 117, 163, 201)
      b. anaplastic carcinoma (94)
      c. malignant cystic mesodermal breast tumor (38)
      d. fibroadenoma (38)
      e. Burkitt's lymphoma (101)
    2. Thymoma (149, 189, 193)
    3. Thyroid cancer substernal, metastatic (94, 178, 193)
      a. adenocarcinoma: 27–40% (35, 53, 58, 77, 90, 94)
      b. anaplastic: 56–60% (35, 53, 94, 117)
      c. adenoma (35, 53)
      d. medullary carcinoma (35)
    4. Parathyroid substernal adenoma (oxyphilic) (12)
    5. Lung
      a. bronchogenic carcinoma: 86–95% (28, 29, 58, 71, 86, 94, 177, 178, 193)
        (1) adenocarcinoma (86, 94, 178)
        (2) squamous cell carcinoma (86, 94, 178)

         (3) oat cell carcinoma (86, 94, 178)

         (4) anaplastic carcinoma (86, 94, 178)

     b. carcinoid (117)

     c. lymphoma (115)

     d. mesothelioma (26, 107, 205)

  6. Cardiac metastases (219)

  7. Mediastinal seminoma (10)

  8. Leukemia (82)

B. Non-neoplastic

  1. Breast

     a. abscess (38)

     b. granuloma (38)

     c. hematoma (38)

     d. adjacent to breast prosthesis (102)

     e. secondary to phenothiazine-induced galactorrhea (157)

     f. estrogen (4, 85)

  2. Pulmonary

     a. sarcoid (55, 144, 177)

     b. infectious pneumonitis

         (1) bacterial (pneumococcus, *Legionella*, etc.) (58, 137, 214)

         (2) tuberculosis: 95% (58)

         (3) viral (58, 180)

             (a) cytomegalovirus (49)

             (b) Korean hemorrhagic fever (174)

             (c) psittacosis (8)

         (4) *pneumocystis carinii* (181, 200)

         (5) *coccidioides* (9)

         (6) paragonimiasis (94)

         (7) aspergilloma (159)

         (8) hydatid cyst (116)

     c. drug-induced pneumonitis (112)

         (1) bleomycin (164)

         (2) cyclophosphamide (116)

         (3) busulfan (118)

         (4) drug abuse (?talc) (115)

         (5) lipiodal lymphangiography (94, 98)

     d. radiation pneumonitis: 50% (177, 202)

     e. abscess: > 90% (48, 58, 97, 177, 180)

         (1) septic emboli (82)

     f. pneumoconiosis: > 90% (136)

         (1) silicosis: > 90% (58, 177)

         (2) asbestosis: > 90% (177)

     g. lupus erythematosus (136, 195)

     h. rheumatoid pleuritis (48)

     i. idiopathic pulmonary pneumonitis (136, 177) and fibrosis (54, 105)

        j. eosinophilic granuloma (67)

        k. uremic pneumonitis (82)

        l. bronchitis (82)

  3. Heart

        a. endocarditis, bacterial (48, 92, 215)

        b. cardiomyopathy (165)

        c. myocardial abscess (183)

        d. myocardial infarction (91, 172)

        e. phlebothrombosis (147)

        f. mycotic aneurysm (48, 121)

        g. pericarditis

            (1) tuberculosis (128, 190A)

            (2) histoplasmosis (190A)

            (3) viral (139)

            (4) rheumatoid arthritis (139)

            (5) post-pericardiotomy syndrome (165)

        h. luetic myocarditis (60)

        i. infection of synthetic vascular graft (23)

        j. sarcoidosis (191)

        k. Kawasaki disease myocarditis (186)

        l. amyloidosis (21)

        m. hypersensitivity angiitis (174AA)

  4. Esophagus

        a. esophagitis (187)

V. Abnormal abdominal uptake

  A. Neoplastic

    1. Gastrointestinal tract

        a. liver

            (1) hepatoblastosarcoma (32, 33, 51, 104, 218)

            (2) hepatoma: 86–90% (58, 94, 109, 117, 178, 188, 193)

            (3) cholangioma (188)

            (4) metastases (109, 188)

            (5) angiomyolipoma (160)

            (6) hepatocholangiocarcinoma (93A)

        b. pancreatic adenocarcinoma: 10–14% (83, 99, 178, 193)

        c. gastric

            (1) adenocarcinoma: 36–38% (31, 94, 97, 117, 178, 193)

            (2) lymphoma (156)

        d. esophageal adenocarcinoma: 47–50% (58, 89, 94, 117)

        e. ileal carcinoid (117)

        f. colonic adenocarcinoma: 30–38% (58, 94, 97, 117, 134, 201)

    2. Genitourinary

        a. renal: 59–74% (178, 193)

            (1) Wilms tumor (51, 104, 218)

        (2) nephroblastoma (32, 33, 104)
        (3) hypernephroma: 57–80% (117, 126, 171, 201)
        (4) lipoma (117)
        (5) metastases (41)
    b. testicular: 57–80% (178, 193)
        (1) teratocarcinoma (33, 51)
        (2) anaplastic teratoma (33)
        (3) chorionepithelioma (33)
        (4) seminoma (65, 153)
        (5) embryonal cell carcinoma (152)
        (6) choriocarcinoma (153)
    c. uterus: 50%
        (1) adenocarcinoma (212)
        (2) leiomyosarcoma (190)
        (3) rhabdomyosarcoma (190)
    d. ovary: 36–54% (71, 191)
        (1) adenocarcinoma: 60–75% (97, 190, 212)
        (2) mesonephric carcinoma (188)
    e. prostate: 55–60% (94, 117, 178, 193, 201)
    f. cervix: 28–36% (178, 193)
        (1) adenocarcinoma (190)
        (2) squamous carcinoma (117, 190)
    g. vaginal adenocarcinoma (117)
    h. bladder: 33–41% (117, 171)
  3. Endocrine system
    a. adrenal carcinoma (149)
    b. neuroblastoma: 85% (16, 32, 104, 218)
    c. sympathicoblastoma (33)
B. Non-neoplastic
  1. Gastrointestinal tract
    a. gastritis (34)
    b. stomach after cis-dichlorodiamine platinum (102)
    c. delayed gastric retention of parenterally administered gallium (203)
    d. infarction (170)
    e. Crohn's disease (46, 113) and regional enteritis (52, 74)
    f. ulcerative colitis (76)
    g. pseudomembranous colitis (196)
    h. hernias
        (1) incarcerated inguinal hernia (20, 173)
        (2) Petit's hernia with bowel protruding through lateral abdominal wall (155)
    i. pancreas
        (1) pseudocyst, infected (80)
        (2) pancreatitis, acute: > 80% (130, 132, 192)

       (3) pancreatitis, chronic: 25% (129, 192)

       (4) abscess (54)

    j. gallbladder

       (1) cholecystitis, acute: > 90% (108, 209)

         (a) *Salmonella* (155)

       (2) cholecystitis, chronic: 25% (209)

       (3) empyema: > 90% (48, 54, 110)

       (4) cholangitis (54)

    k. appendiceal mucocele (5)

2. Genitourinary

    a. renal

       (1) pyelonephritis (81, 92, 93, 109)

       (2) vasculitis (93)

       (3) acute tubular necrosis (93)

       (4) cortical necrosis (93)

       (5) hydronephrosis (93)

       (6) transplant rejection (43)

       (7) kidney post-transplant with normal function (36)

       (8) abscess (39, 93, 149)

       (9) medullary necrosis (3)

       (10) Wegener's granulomatosis (92)

       (11) renal vein thrombosis (92)

       (12) interstitial nephritis (217)

       (13) perinephric abscess (59)

       (14) after cis-dichlorodiamine platinum (102)

       (15) amyloidosis (13)

       (16) with severe hepatocellular disease (4A)

    b. testicles—scrotal area

       (1) epididymo-orchitis (14)

       (2) Petit's hernia (155)

    c. bladder—ureter

       (1) cystitis (109)

       (2) urinoma (37)

3. Peritonitis or diffuse peritoneal exudation

    a. local (130)

    b. diffuse

       (1) vasculitis (130)

       (2) bacterial, gram-positive or negative (130, 152)

       (3) tuberculous (11, 152, 185)

    c. hypoproteinemia (84A)

4. Intra-abdominal abscess: 90%

    a. perirenal (133)

    b. psoas (42, 145)

    c. paravertebral (92)

    d. perihepatic (27, 39, 92)

      e. intrarenal abscess (30)

      f. intrahepatic abscess, bacterial, mycotic, amebic (30, 44, 54, 61, 109, 114, 127)

      g. intrasplenic abscess (30)

      h. pericecal abscess (175)

      i. subphrenic (27, 30, 54, 61)

      j. pelvic (48, 192)

      k. colon (39)

      l. appendicitis (58)

      m. retroperitoneal (54)

      n. starch granuloma (1)

  5. Vascular

      a. aortic graft abscess (23)

  6. Retroperitoneal fibrosis (120)

VI. Abnormal skeletal and/or marrow uptake

  A. Neoplastic

    1. Any metastasis (94)

    2. Myeloma (includes plasmacytoma): 17–31% (62, 71, 117, 201)

    3. Myeloblastoma (95)

    4. Leukemia, acute lymphocytic: 57% (71, 123)

    5. Leukemia, acute myelogenous: 59% (71, 123)

    6. Leukemia, chronic myelogenous (71, 94)

    7. Myelofibrosis with myeloid metaplasia (18)

    8. Osseous tumors (58, 94, 97, 117, 134, 201)

      a. Ewing's sarcoma: 95–100% (17, 40, 71)

      b. osteogenic sarcoma (33, 58, 141)

      c. histiocytosis X (141)

      d. enchondromatosis (141)

      e. giant cell tumor (141)

      f. chondrosarcoma: 95–100% (79)

      g. eosinophilic granuloma (33)

      h. fibrous dysplasia (33)

      i. ameloblastoma (58, 142)

      j. osteoblastoma (173)

      k. osteoid osteoma (169)

  B. Non-neoplastic

    1. Osteomyelitis (88, 106, 117)—rarely photon deficient

      a. fungal

        (1) coccidioidomycosis (9)

      b. pyogenic (88)

      c. *Salmonella* (154)

    2. Sinusitis—mastoiditis (56, 210)

    3. Disk-space infection (138)

4. Septic arthritis (54, 88, 106)
5. Pseudarthrosis—diminished or increased uptake (64)
6. Paget's disease (141)
7. Rheumatoid arthritis (107)
8. Healing fracture or osteotomy (119, 169)
9. Reiter's syndrome (195)
10. Diffuse bone uptake after dialysis or chronic renal disease (102)
11. Gout (117)
12. Eosinophilic granuloma (33)
13. Rheumatic fever, acute (216)
14. Bone infarcts in sickle cell disease (25)
15. Costochondritis (124)
16. Synovitis (169)
17. Septic ischemic bone-decreased uptake (169)
18. Around orthopedic prosthesis and orthopedic stabilizing devices (169)
    a. sterile inflammation as in a reactive bursa (169)
    b. loosening (169)
    c. with osteomyelitis (169)
    d. in area of heterotopic bone (169)

VII. Soft tissue—(muscle, skin, connective tissue)

  A. Neoplastic
    1. Sarcomas
      a. rhabdomyosarcoma: 50–86% (15, 17, 32, 79)
      b. leiomyosarcoma: gastric, thyroidal, arterial (17, 79, 131)
      c. fibrous histiocytoma, malignant (17, 79, 143)
      d. liposarcoma (17, 79)
      e. synovial cell sarcoma (17, 79)
      f. neurofibrosarcoma (50, 79)
      g. fibrosarcoma (17, 79)
      h. lymphangiosarcoma (79)
      i. chondrosarcoma (79)
      j. undifferentiated (79)
      k. malignant schwannoma (17)
      l. myxoliposarcoma (72)
    2. Melanoma: 55–70% (66, 71, 94, 122)
    3. Kaposi's sarcoma (117)
    4. Squamous cell carcinoma (117)
    5. Mycosis fungoides (174A)
  B. Non-neoplastic
    1. In any incision for up to 4 weeks (14)
    2. Abscess
      a. injection site of *Cornynebacterium parvum*; other infected injection sites (97, 103, 117)

      b. at site of peritoneal dialysis (78)

  3. Intramuscular antibiotic injection site (102)

  4. Cellulitis (106)

  5. Pressure lesions (102)

  6. Purpura fulminans (180)

  7. Sarcoidosis (166)

  8. Pseudohypertrophic muscular dystrophy (19)

  9. Muscle hypertrophy (140)

10. Panniculitis (24)

11. Rhabdomyolysis (197)

12. Pyomyositis (158)

13. Acne vulgaris (201)

14. Polymyositis (199)

15. Calcium gluconate extravasation (186A)

REFERENCES

1. Abrenio JK, Jhingran SG, Johnson PC: Abnormal gallium-67 image of the abdomen in starch granulomatous disease. J Nucl Med 20:902–903, 1979.
2. Adler S, Parthasarathy KL, Bakshi SP: Gallium-67-citrate scanning for the localization and staging of lymphoma. J Nucl Med 16:255–260, 1975.
3. Adler SN: Nonobstructive pyelonephritis initially seen as acute renal failure. Arch Int Med 138:816–817, 1978.
4. Ajmani SK, Pircher FJ: Ga-67 citrate in gynecomastia. J Nucl Med 19:560–561, 1978.
4A. Alazraki N, Sterkel B, Taylor A: Renal gallium accumulation in the absence of renal pathology in patients with severe hepatocellular disease. J Nucl Med 8:200–204, 1983.
5. Alpert L, Friedman R: Gallium scintigraphy demonstration of an appendiceal mucocele. Clin Nucl Med 6:378–379, 1981.
6. Amici F, Salvolini U: Results of brain scanning with different radioisotopes. Neuroradiology 9:157-161, 1975.
7. Andrews GA, Hubner KF, Greenlaw RH: ^{67}Ga-citrate imaging in malignant lymphoma: final report of Cooperative Group. J Nucl Med 19:1013–1019, 1978.
8. Andrews JT, Fraser JRE: [67]Gallium uptake in psittacosis infection. Aust NZ J Med 9:437–439, 1979.
9. Armbruster TG, Goergen TG, Resnick D, et al: Utility of bone scanning in disseminated coccidioidomycosis. J Nucl Med 18:450–454, 1977.
10. Ayulo MA, Dibos PE, Aisner A, et al: Gallium-67 citrate scanning in primary mediastinal seminoma. J Nucl Med 22:796–797, 1981.
11. Baron RJ, Fratkin MJ: Gallium-67 scanning of tuberculous peritonitis. J Nucl Med 17:1020–1021, 1976.
12. Bekerman C, Schulak JA, Kaplan EL, et al: Parathyroid adenoma imaged by Ga-67 scintigraphy. J Nucl Med 18:1096–1098, 1977.
13. Bekerman C, Vyas MI: Renal localization of ^{67}Ga-citrate in renal amyloidosis. J Nucl Med 17:899–901, 1976.
14. Bell EG, O'Mara RE, Henry CA, et al: Non-neoplastic localization of ^{67}Ga citrate (abstract). J Nucl Med 12:338–339, 1971.
15. Berelowitz M, Blake BCH: [67]Gallium in the detection and localization of tumours. S African Med J 45:1351-1359, 1971.

16. Bidani N, Moohr JW, Kirchner P, et al: Gallium scanning as prognostic indicator in neuroblastoma (abstract). J Nucl Med 19:692, 1978.

17. Bitran JD, Bekerman C, Golomb HM, et al: Scintigraphic evaluation of sarcomata in children and adults by ^{67}Ga citrate. Cancer 42:1760–1765, 1978.

18. Blei CL, Born ML, Rollo FD: Gallium bone scan in myelofibrosis. J Nucl Med 18:445–447, 1977.

19. Bowen P, Lentle BC, Jackson FI, et al: Abnormal localization of gallium-67 citrate in pseudohypertrophic muscular dystrophy. Lancet 2:1072–1073, 1977.

20. Boxen I, Lamki L: Gallium in the sac. Clin Nucl Med 6:495, 1981.

21. Braun SD, Lisbona R, Novales-Diaz JA, et al: Myocardial uptake of ^{99m}Tc-phosphate tracer in amyloidosis. Clin Nucl Med 4:244, 1979.

22. Brown ML, O'Donnell JB, Thrall JH, et al: Gallium-67 scintigraphy in untreated and treated non-Hodgkin's lymphoma. J Nucl Med 19:875–879, 1978.

23. Causey DA, Fajman WA, Perdue GD, et al: [67]Ga scintigraphy in post-operative synthetic graft infection. Am J Roentgenol 134:1041–1045, 1980.

24. Choy D, Murray IPC, Ford JC: Gallium scintigraphy in acute panniculitis. J Nucl Med 22:973–974, 1981.

25. Cox F, Hughes WT: Gallium-67 scanning for the diagnosis of infection in children. Am J Dis Child 133:1171–1173, 1979.

26. Dach J, Patel N, Patel S, et al: Peritoneal mesothelioma: CT, sonography, and gallium-67 scan. Am J. Roentgenol 135:614–616, 1980.

27. Damron JR, Beihn RM, DeLand FH: Detection of upper abdominal abscesses by radionuclide imaging. Radiology 120:131–134, 1976.

28. DeLand FH, Sauerbrunn BJL, Boyd C, et al: ^{67}Ga-citrate imaging in untreated primary lung cancer: preliminary report of Cooperative Group. J Nucl Med 15:408–411, 1974.

29. DeMeester TR, Bekerman C, Joseph JG, et al: Gallium-67 scanning for carcinoma of the lung. J Thor Cardiovasc Surg 72:699–708, 1976.

30. Dhawan VM, Sziklar JJ, Spencer RP, et al: Computerized double-tracer subtraction scanning with gallium-67 citrate in inflammatory disease. J Nucl Med 19:1297–1300, 1978.

31. Douds HN, Berens SV, Long RF, et al: ^{67}Ga-citrate scanning in gastrointestinal malignancies. Clin Nucl Med 3:179–183, 1978.

32. Edeling CJ: Tumor imaging in children. Cancer 38:921–930, 1976.

33. Edeling CJ: Tumor visualization using [67]gallium scintigraphy in children. Radiology 127:727–731, 1978.

34. Eikman EA, Tenorio LE, Frank BA, et al: Gallium-67 accumulation in the stomach in patients with post-operative gastritis. J Nucl Med 21:706–707, 1980.

35. Erjavec M, Auersperg M, Golouh R, et al: Computer-assisted scanning in evaluation of ^{67}Ga-citrate uptake in thyroid disease. J Nucl Med 25:810–813, 1974.

36. Fawwaz RA, Johnson PM: Localization of gallium-67 in the normally functioning allografted kidney. J Nucl Med 20:207–209, 1979.

37. Fishman EK, Moses D: Gallium accumulation in a urinoma secondary to ureteral trauma. Clin Nucl Med 6:175–176, 1981.

38. Fogh J: [67]Ga accumulation in malignant tumors and in the prelactating or lactating breast. Proc Soc Exp Biol Med 138:1086–1090, 1971.

39. Forgacs P, Wahner HW, Keys TF, et al: Gallium scanning for the detection of abdominal abscesses. Am J Med 65:949–954, 1978.

40. Frankel RS, Jones AE, Cohen JA, et al: Clinical correlations of ^{67}Ga and skeletal whole-body radionuclide studies with radiography in Ewing's sarcoma. Radiology

110:597–603, 1974.

41. Frankel RS, Richman SD, Levenson SM, et al: Renal localization of gallium-67 citrate. Radiology 114:393–397, 1975.

42. Fratkin MJ, Sharpe AR: Nontuberculous psoas abscess: localization using [67]Ga. J Nucl Med 14:499–501, 1973.

43. George EA, Codd JE, Newton WT, et al: Ga-67 citrate in renal allograft rejection. Radiology 117:731–733, 1975.

44. Geslien GE, Thrall JH, Johnson MC: Gallium scanning in acute hepatic amebic abscess. J Nucl Med 15:561–563, 1974.

45. Gill SP, Thrall JH, Beauchamp ML, et al: Gallium-67 citrate concentration in angioimmunoblastic lymphadenopathy with dysproteinemia. J Nucl Med 18:312–313, 1977.

46. Goldenberg DJ, Russell CD, Mihas AA, et al: Value of gallium-67 citrate scanning in Crohn's disease. J Nucl Med 20:215–218, 1979.

47. Grove RB, Pinsky SM, Brown TL, et al: Uptake of ^{67}Ga-citrate in subacute thyroiditis. J Nucl Med 14:403, 1973.

48. Habibian MR, Staab EV, Matthews HA: Gallium citrate Ga-67 in febrile patients. JAMA 233:1073–1076, 1975.

49. Hamed IA, Wenzel JE, Leonard JC, et al: Pulmonary cytomegalovirus infection. Arch Int Med 139:286–288, 1979.

50. Hammond JA, Driedger AA: Detection of malignant change in neurofibromatosis (von Recklinghausen's disease) by gallium-67 scanning. Canad Med Assoc J 119:352–353, 1978.

51. Handmaker H, O'Mara RE: Gallium imaging in pediatrics. J Nucl Med 18:1057–1063, 1977.

52. Harvey WC, Podoloff DA, Kopp DT: [67]Gallium in 68 consecutive infection searches. J Nucl Med 16:2–4, 1974.

53. Heidendal GAK, Roos P, Thijs LG, et al: Evaluation of cold areas on the thyroid scan with ^{67}Ga-citrate. J Nucl Med 16:793–794, 1975.

54. Henkin RE: Gallium-67 in the diagnosis of inflammatory disease, in Hoffer PB, Becker C, Henkin R. (eds): Gallium-67 Imaging New York: John Wiley & Sons, 1978, pp. 65–92.

55. Heshiki A, Schatz SL, McKusick KA, et al: Gallium-67 citrate scanning in patients with pulmonary sarcoidosis. Am J Roentgenol 127:744–749, 1974.

56. Higashi T, Aoyama W, Mori Y, et al: Gallium-67 scanning in the differentiation of maxillary sinus carcinoma from chronic maxillary sinusitis. Radiology 123:117–122, 1977.

57. Higashi T, Kashima I, Shimura K, et al: Gallium-67 scanning in the evaluation of therapy of malignant tumors of the head and neck. J Nucl Med 18:243–249, 1977.

58. Higashi T, Nakayama Y, Murata A, et al: Clinical evaluation of ^{67}Ga-citrate scanning. J Nucl Med 13:196–201, 1972.

59. Hopkins GB, Hall RL, Mende CW: Gallium-67 scintigraphy for the diagnosis and localization of perinephric abscess. J Urol 115:126–128, 1976.

60. Hopkins GB, Kan M, Schwartz LJ: Myocardial involvement in secondary syphilis detected by [67]Gallium scintigraphy. Clin Nucl Med 2:208,1977.

61. Hopkins GB, Menke CW: Gallium-67 and subphrenic abscesses—is delayed scintigraphy necessary? J Nucl Med 16:609–611, 1975.

62. Hubner KF, Andrews GA, Hayes RL: The use of rare-earth radionuclides and other bone-seekers in the evaluation of bone lesions in patients with multiple myeloma and plasmacytoma. Radiology 125:171–176, 1977.

63. Hurst WB, Andrews JT, Chmiel RL, et al: The use of [67]gallium citrate scanning to stage malignancies of the head and neck. Australas Radiol 18:19–26, 1974.

64. Hurwitz SR, Quinto RR: Diminished uptake of ^{67}Ga-citrate in a case of pseudarthrosis. J Nucl Med 16:167–170, 1975.

65. Jackson FI, Dierich HC, Lentle BC: Gallium-67 citrate scintiscanning in testicular neoplasia. J Canad Assoc Radiol 27:84–88, 1976.

66. Jackson FI, McPherson TA, Lentle BC: Gallium-67 scintigraphy in multisystem malignant melanoma. Radiology 122:163–167, 1977.

67. Javahari S, Levine BW, McKusick KA: Serial ^{67}Ga lung scanning in pulmonary eosinophilic granuloma. Thorax 34:822–823, 1979.

68. Jensen SR, Rao BR, Winebright JW, et al: Gallium-67 uptake in a benign thymic cyst. Clin Nucl Med 5:67, 1980.

69. Johnson PM, Berdon EW, Baker DH, et al: Thymic uptake of gallium-67 citrate in a healthy 4 year old boy. Pediatric Radiology 7:243–244, 1978.

70. Johnston GS, Go MF, Benua RS, et al: Gallium-67 citrate imaging in Hodgkin's disease: final report of Cooperative Group. J Nucl Med 18:692–698, 1977.

71. Johnston GS, Jones AE, Milder MS: The gallium-67 scan in clinical assessment of cancer. J Surg Oncol 5:529–538, 1973.

72. Johnston GS, Jones RE: Atlas of Gallium-67 Scintigraphy. New York: Plenum, 1973.

73. Jones AE, Kaslow M, Johnston GS, et al: ^{67}Ga-citrate scintigraphy of brain tumors. Radiology 105:693–697, 1972.

74. Joo KG, Landsberg R, Parthasarathy KL, et al: Abnormal gallium scan in regional enteritis. Clin Nucl Med 3:134–136, 1978.

75. Kan MK, Hopkins GB: Unilateral breast uptake of ^{67}Ga from breast feeding. Radiology 121:668, 1976.

76. Kaplan LR, Griep RJ, Schuffler MD, et al: Gallium-67 scanning at 6 hours in active inflammatory bowel disease. J Nucl Med 18:448–449, 1977.

77. Kaplan WB, Holman BL, Selenkow HA, et al: ^{67}Ga-citrate and the nonfunctioning thyroid nodule. J Nucl Med 15:424–427, 1974.

78. Karimeddini MK: Ga-67 scanning during peritoneal dialysis. J Nucl Med 22:479–480, 1981.

79. Kaufman JH, Cedermark BJ, Parthasarathy KL, et al: The value of ^{67}Ga scintigraphy in soft tissue sarcoma and chondrosarcoma. Radiology 123:131–134, 1977.

80. Kennedy TD, Martin NL, Robinson RG, et al: Identification of an infected pseudocyst of the pancreas with ^{67}Ga-citrate. J Nucl Med 16:1132–1134, 1975.

81. Kessler WD, Gittes RF, Hurwitz SR, et al: Gallium-67 scans in the diagnosis of pyelonephritis. West J Med 121:91–93, 1974.

82. Kim EE: Diffuse pulmonary gallium concentration. Sem Nucl Med 10:108–110, 1980.

83. Kim EE, DeLand FH: Uptake of ^{67}Ga citrate in pancreatic adenocarcinoma. Clin Nucl Med 3:302, 1978.

84. Kim EE, DeLand FH, Maruyama Y: Brain and lung involvement of mycosis fungoides demonstrated by radionuclide imaging. J Nucl Med 20:240–242, 1979.

84A. Kim EE, Gubuty A, Gutierrez C: Diffuse abdominal uptake of Ga-67 citrate in a patient with hypoproteinemia. J Nucl Med 24:508–510, 1983.

85. Kim YC, Brown ML, Thrall JH: Scintigraphic patterns of gallium-67 in the breast. Radiology 124:169–175, 1977.

86. Kinoshita F, Ushio T, Maekawa A, et al: Scintiscanning of pulmonary diseases with ^{67}Ga-citrate. J Nucl Med 15:227–233, 1974.

87. Kipper MS, Taylor A, Ashburn WL: Gallium-67-citrate uptake in a case of acne vul-

garis. Clin Nucl Med 6:409–410, 1981.

88. Kolyvas E, Rosenthall L, Ahronheim GA, et al: Serial ^{67}Ga-citrate imaging during treatment of acute osteomyelitis in childhood. Clin Nucl Med 3:461–466, 1978.

89. Kondo M, Hashimoto S, Kubo A, et al: [67]Ga scanning in the evaluation of esophageal carcinoma. Radiology 131:723–726, 1979.

90. Koutras DA, Pandos PG, Sfontouris J, et al: Thyroid scanning with gallium-67 and cesium-131. J Nucl Med 17:268–271, 1976.

91. Kramer RJ, Goldstein RE, Hirschfield JW, et al: Accumulation of gallium-67 in regions of acute myocardial infarction. Am J Cardiol 33:861–867, 1974.

92. Kumar B, Alderson PO, Geisse G: The role of Ga-67 citrate imaging and diagnostic ultrasound in patients with suspected abdominal abscesses. J Nucl Med 18:534–537, 1977.

93. Kumar B, Coleman RE: Significance of delayed ^{67}Ga localization in the kidneys. J Nucl Med 17:872–879, 1976.

93A. Lamki L, Holliday IR: Gallium uptake by a rare primary hepatic malignancy. Clin Nucl Med 8:129–130, 1983.

94. Langhammer H, Glaubitt D, Grebe SF, et al: [67]Ga for tumor scanning. J Nucl Med 13:25–30, 1972.

95. Larson SM, Graff KS, Tretner I-H, et al: Positive gallium-67 photoscan in myeloblastoma. JAMA 222:321–323, 1972.

96. Larson SM, Milder MS, Johnston GS: Interpretation of the ^{67}Ga photoscan. J Nucl Med 14:208–214, 1973.

97. Lavender JP, Lowe J, Barker JR, et al: Gallium-67 citrate scanning in neoplastic and inflammatory lesions. Br J Radiol 44:361–366, 1971.

98. Lentle BC, Castor WR, Khalig A, et al: The effect of contrast lymphangiography on localization of ^{67}Ga-citrate. J Nucl Med 16:374–376, 1975.

99. Lentle BC, Jackson FI, Dierich H: Gallium-67 citrate scintiscanning in the search for occult primary malignant tumors. Canad Med Assoc J 114:1113–1118, 1976.

100. Lentle BC, Jackson FI, McGowan DG: Localization of gallium-67 citrate in salivary glands following radiation therapy. J Canad Assoc Radiol 27:89–91, 1976.

101. Lentle BC, Ludwig R, Camuzzini G: Breast involvement in non-African Burkitt's lymphoma. J Canad Assoc Radiol 31:204–205, 1980.

102. Lentle BC, Scott JR, Noujaim AA, et al: Iatrogenic alterations in radionuclide biodistributions. Sem Nucl Med 9:131–143, 1979.

103. Leonard JC, Humphrey GB, Vanhoutte JJ: Positive ^{67}Ga-citrate scans in patients receiving *Corynebacterium parvum*. Clin Nucl Med 3:370–371, 1978.

104. Lepanto PB, Rosenstock J, Littman P, et al: Gallium-67 scans in children with solid tumors. Am J Roentgenol 126:179–186, 1976.

105. Line BR, Fulmer JD, Reynolds HY: Gallium-67 citrate scanning in the staging of idiopathic pulmonary fibrosis: correlation with physiologic and morphologic features and bronchoalveolar lavage. Am Rev Resp Dis 118:355–365, 1978.

106. Lisbona R, Rosenthall L: Observations on the sequential use of 99m-Tc-phosphate complex and ^{67}Ga imaging in osteomyelitis, cellulitis and septic arthritis. Radiology 123:123–129, 1977.

107. Littenberg RL, Alazraki NP, Taketa RM, et al: A clinical evaluation of gallium-67 citrate scanning. Surg Gyn Obstet 137:424–430, 1973.

108. Littenberg RL, Taketa RM, Alazraki NP, et al: Gallium-67 for localization of septic lesions. Ann Int Med 79:403–406, 1973.

109. Lomas F, Dibos PE, Wagner HN: Increased specificity of liver scanning with the use of [67]gallium citrate. New Eng J Med 286:1323–1329, 1972.

110. Lomas F, Wagner HN: Accumulation of ionic ^{67}Ga in empyema of the gallbladder. Radiology 105:689–692, 1972.

111. Lopez-Majano V, Schiff G: Cervico-facial actinomycosis. Eur J Nucl Med 7:143–144, 1982.

112. Lull RJ, Anderson JH, Telepak RH, et al: Radionuclide imaging in the assessment of lung injury. Sem Nucl Med 10:302–310, 1980.

113. Lunia S, Chodos RB, Goel V: Crohn's disease and ^{67}Ga-citrate scintigraphy. Clin Nucl Med 1:125–126, 1976.

114. Lunia S, Chodos RB, Sundaresh R: Actinomycosis of the liver and ^{67}Ga-citrate scintigraphy. Clin Nucl Med 1:263–264, 1976.

115. MacMahon H, Beckerman C: The diagnostic significance of gallium lung uptake in patients with normal chest radiographs. Radiology 127:189–193, 1978.

116. Madeddu G, Constanza C, Casu AR: Pulmonary hydatid cyst evidenced by Ga-67 citrate scan. J Nucl Med 21:599–600, 1980.

117. Manfredi OL, Quinones JD, Bartok SP, in Medical Radioisotope Scintigraphy, Vol. 2. Vienna: International Atomic Energy Agency, 1973, pp. 583–594.

118. Manning DM, Strimlan CV, Turbiner EH: Early detection of busulfan lung: report of a case. Clin Nucl Med 5:412–414, 1980.

119. Marta JB, Williams HJ, Smookler RA: Gallium-67 uptake in a stress fracture. J Nucl Med 23:271–272, 1982.

120. McCoombs RK, Singhi V, Olson WH: Positive Ga-67 citrate scan in retroperitoneal fibrosis. J Nucl Med 20:238–240, 1979.

121. Michal JA, Coleman RE: Localization of ^{67}Ga citrate in a mycotic aneurysm. Am J Roentgenol 129:1111–1113, 1977.

122. Milder MS, Frankel RS, Bulkey GB, et al: Gallium-67 scintigraphy in malignant melanoma. Cancer 32:1350–1356, 1973.

123. Milder MS, Glick JH, Henderson ES, et al: ^{67}Ga scintigraphy in acute leukemia. Cancer 32:803–808, 1973.

124. Miller JH: Accumulation of gallium-67 in costochondritis. Clin Nucl Med 8:362–363, 1980.

125. Mishkin FS, Maynard WP: Lacrimal gland accumulation of ^{67}Ga. J Nucl Med 15:630–631, 1974.

126. Miyamae T, Kan M, Fujioka M, et al: ^{67}Ga-citrate scanning in hypernephroma. Clin Nucl Med 3:225–228, 1978.

127. Miyamoto AT, Thadepalli H, Mishkin FS: ^{67}Gallium images of amebic liver abscesses. New Engl J Med 291:1363, 1974.

128. Moinuddin M, Rockett JF: Gallium imaging in inflammatory disease. Clin Nucl Med 1:271–278, 1976.

129. Myerson PJ, Berg GR, Spencer RP, et al: Gallium-67 spread to the anterior pararenal space in pancreatitis. J Nucl Med 18:893–895, 1977.

130. Myerson PJ, Myerson D, Spencer RP: Anatomic patterns of Ga-67 distribution in localized and diffuse peritoneal inflammation. J Nucl Med 18:977–980, 1977.

131. Myerson PJ, Myerson DA, Katz R, et al: Gallium imaging in pulmonary artery sarcoma mimicking pulmonary embolism. J Nucl Med 17:893–895, 1976.

132. Myerson PJ, Myerson DA, Spencer RP: Diffuse peritoneal uptake of Ga-67 in pancreatic disease: a possible prognostic indicator. J Nucl Med 19:1266–1267, 1978.

133. Myerson PJ, Myerson DA, Spencer RP, et al: ^{67}Ga-citrate identification of inflammation in the perirenal space. Clin Nucl Med 3:434–435, 1978.

134. Nash AG, Dance DR, McCready VR, et al: Uptake of gallium-67 in colonic and rectal tumours. Br Med J 3:508–510, 1972.

135. Newman RA, Gallagher JG, Clements CP, et al: Demonstration of Ga-67 localization in human placenta. J Nucl Med 19:504–506, 1978.

136. Niden AH, Mishkin FS, Khurana MML: [67]Gallium citrate lung scans in interstitial lung disease. Chest 69:266–268, 1976.

137. Niden AH, Mishkin FS, Khurana MML, et al: [67]Ga lung scan, an aid in the differential diagnosis of pulmonary embolism and pneumonitis. JAMA 237:1206–1211, 1977.

138. Norris S, Ehrlich MG, Keim DE, et al: Early diagnosis of disk-space infection using gallium-67. J Nucl Med 19:384–386, 1978.

139. O'Connell JB, Robinson JA, Henkin RE, et al: Gallium-67 citrate scanning for non-invasive detection of inflammation in pericardial diseases. Am J Cardiol 46:879–884, 1980.

140. O'Connell JB, Robinson JA, Henkin RE, Messmore HL: Muscles undergoing physiological adaption to stress take up gallium-67 citrate. Lancet 1:1083–1084, 1980.

141. Okuyama S, Ito Y, Awano T, et al: Prospects of ^{67}Ga scanning in bone neoplasms. Radiology 107:123–128, 1973.

142. Okuyama S, Ito Y, Awano T: Bone tumor imaging by scintigraphy of the skeleton, marrow reticuloendothelial system, and the proliferative tissue. Am J Roentgenol 125:965–971, 1975.

143. Olson WH, McCombs RK: Positive ^{99m}Tc-diphosphonate and ^{67}Ga-citrate scans in ameloblastoma: case report. J Nucl Med 18: 348–349, 1977.

144. Oren VO, Uszler JM, White J: Diagnosis of uveoparotid fever by ^{67}Ga-citrate imaging. Clin Nucl Med 3:127–129,1978.

145. Oster MW, Gelrud LG, Lotz M, et al: Psoas abscess localization by gallium scan in aplastic anemia. JAMA 232:377–379, 1975.

146. Page CP, Coltman CA, Robertson HD, et al: Candidal abscess of the spleen in patients with acute leukemia. Surg Gyn Obst 151:604–608, 1980.

147. Park CH, Miller PJ, Lipton A, et al: Incidentally detected thrombosed vein during ^{67}Ga citrate scanning. Am J Roentgenol 126:1249–1250, 1976.

148. Park H, Forry AE, Sagalowski RL: Localization of ^{67}Ga in renal abscesses. J Nucl Med 18:313–314, 1977.

149. Parthasarathy KL, Bakshi SP, Parikh S: Localization of metastatic adrenal carcinoma utilizing ^{67}Ga-citrate. Clin Nucl Med 3:24–26, 1978.

150. Patel D, Mitnick J, Braunstein P, et al: [67]Ga scan in thymoma. Clin Nucl Med 3:339, 1978.

151. Pechman R, Tetalman M, Antonmattei S: Diagnostic significance of persistent colonic gallium activity: scintigraphic patterns. Radiology 128:691–695, 1978.

152. Perez J, Rivera JV, Bermudez RH: Peritoneal localization of gallium-67. Radiology 123:695–697, 1977.

153. Pinsky SM, Bailey TB, Blom J, et al: ^{67}Ga-citrate in the staging of testicular malignancy (abstract). J Nucl Med 14:439, 1973.

154. Popa N, Lens E, Dubois JL, et al: Positive ^{67}Ga-citrate scintigraphy: vertebral, satellite lymph node and gallbladder foci in a case of gastroenteritis with *Salmonella*. Eur J Nucl Med 7:137–140, 1982.

155. Powers TA: Petit's hernia: an unusual cause of abnormality on Ga-67-citrate scintigraphy. Clin Nucl Med 5:61–62, 1980.

156. Que L, McCartney W, Hankins A, et al: Lymphomatous involvement of the stomach demonstrated by gallium-67 scanning. Am J Dig Dis 19:271–274, 1974.

157. RamSingh PS, Pujara S, Logic JR: ^{99m}Tc-pyrophosphate uptake in drug-induced gynecomastia. Clin Nucl Med 2:206, 1977.

158. Rao BR, Gerber FH, Greaney RB, et al: Gallium-67 citrate imaging of pyomyositis. J Nucl Med 22:836–837, 1981.

159. Rao GM, Garuprakash GH, Ghaskar G: Localization of gallium-67 in aspergilloma. J Nucl Med 20:900, 1979.

160. Rashad FA, Micaldi FD, Bellon EM: Gallium-67 uptake in tuberous sclerosis. Clin Nucl Med 4:242–243, 1979.

161. Reba RC, Poulose KP: Nonspecificity of gallium accumulation: gallium-67 concentration in cerebral infarction. Radiology 112:639–641, 1974.

162. Richman SD, Appelbaum F, Levenson SM, et al: [67]Ga radionuclide imaging in Burkitt's lymphoma. Radiology 117:639–645, 1975.

163. Richman SD, Ingle JN, Levenson SM, et al: Usefulness of gallium scintigraphy in primary and metastatic breast carcinoma. J Nucl Med 16:996–1001, 1975.

164. Richman SD, Levenson SM, Bunn PA, et al: [67]Ga accumulation in pulmonary lesions associated with bleomycin toxicity. Cancer 36:1966–1972, 1975.

165. Robinson JA, O'Connell J, Henkin RE, et al: Gallium-67 imaging in cardiomyopathy. Ann Int Med 90:198–200, 1979.

166. Rohatgi PK: Cutaneous localization of Ga-67 in systemic sarcoidosis. Clin Nucl Med 6:109–110, 1981.

167. Roos J, Shoot JB: The uptake of gallium-67 in euthyroid patients with multinodular goiter. Acta Med Scand 194:225–228, 1973.

168. Rose J: Increased salivary gland uptake of ^{67}Ga-citrate 36 months after radiation therapy. J Nucl Med 18:495–496, 1977.

169. Rosenthall L, Lisbona R: Role of radionuclide imaging in benign bone and joint diseases of orthopedic interest, in Freeman LM, Weissmann HS (eds): Nuclear Med Annual 1980 Ed. New York: Raven Press, 1980, pp. 267–301.

170. Russin LD, Staab EV: Radionuclide imaging of intestinal infarction. Radiology 122:171–172, 1977.

171. Sauerbrunn BJ, Andrews GA, Hubner KF: Ga-67 citrate imaging in tumors of the genito-urinary tract: report of the Cooperative Group. J Nucl Med 19:470–475, 1978.

172. Schor RA, Massie BM, Botvinick EH: Gallium-67 uptake in silent myocardial infarction. Radiology 129:117–118, 1978.

173. Scully RE: Editor Case Records of the Mass. Gen. Hosp. Case 40–1980, New Engl J Med 303:866–873, 1980.

174. Seder J, Hattner RS: Incidental localization of ^{67}Ga in an incarcerated inguinal hernia. Clin Nucl Med 3:411, 1978.

174AA. Shah PH, Shreeve WW: Uptake of ^{67}Ga in the cardiac region in hypersensitivity angiitis. Clin Nucl Med 6:547–549, 1981.

174A. Shigeno C, Morita R, Fukunaga M: Visualization of skeletal muscle involvement of mycosis fungoides on ^{67}Ga scintigraphy. Eur J Nucl Med 7:333–335, 1982.

175. Shimshak RR, Korobkin M, Hoffer PR, et al: The complementary role of gallium citrate imaging and computed tomography in the evaluation of suspected abdominal infection. J Nucl Med 19:262–269, 1978.

176. Siddiqui AR, Passu M: Accumulation of technetium-99m MDP and gallium citrate in soft tissues in a patient with polymyositis. Nucl Med Comm 2:165–169, 1981.

177. Siemsen JK, Grebe SF, Sargent EN, et al: Gallium-67 scintigraphy of pulmonary diseases as a complement to radiography. Radiology 118:371-375, 1976.

178. Silberstein EB: Cancer diagnosis: the role of tumor imaging radiopharmaceuticals. Am J Med 60:226–237, 1976.

179. Silberstein EB, Kornblut A, Shumrick DA, et al: [67]Ga as a diagnostic agent for the detection of head and neck tumors and lymphoma. Radiology 110:605–608, 1974.

180. Silva J, Harvey WC: Detection of infections with gallium-67 and scintigraphic imaging. J Infect Dis 130:125–131, 1974.
181. Sirotzky L, Memoli V, Roberts JL, et al: Recurrent *Pneumocystis* pneumonia with normal chest roentgenograms. JAMA 240:1513–1515, 1978.
182. Smith NJ, Teates CD, El-Mahdi AM, et al: The value of gallium-67 scanning in the evaluation of head and neck malignancy. Laryngoscopy 85:778–786, 1975.
183. Spies SM, Meyers SN, Barresi V, et al: A case of myocardial abscess evaluated by radionuclide techniques. J Nucl Med 18:1089–1090, 1977.
184. Stahly TL, Shoop JP: Plague and the gallium scan. J Nucl Med 16:1031-1032, 1975.
185. Steinbach JJ: Abnormal ^{67}Ga-citrate scan of the abdomen in tuberculous peritonitis. J Nucl Med 17:272–273, 1976.
186. Sty JR, Chusid MJ, Dorrington A: Ga-67 imaging: Kawasaki disease. Clin Nucl Med 6:112–113, 1981.
186A. Sty JR, Starshak RJ, Hubbard AM: Ga-67 scintigraphy: calcium gluconate extravasation. Clin Nucl Med 7:377, 1982.
187. Sty JR, Starshak RJ, Lauer SJ: Polymucositis, a cause of Ga-67 uptake. Clin Nucl Med 6:126, 1981.
188. Suzuki T, Honjo I, Hamamoto K, et al: Positive scintiphotography of cancer of the liver with Ga-67 citrate. Am J Roentgenol 113:92–103, 1971.
189. Swick HM, Preston DF, McQuillen MP: Gallium scans in myasthenia gravis. Ann NY Acad Sci 274:536–554, 1976.
190. Symmonds RE, Tauxe WN: Gallium-67 scintigraphy of gynecologic tumors. Am J Obstet Gyn 114:356–369, 1972.
190A. Taillefer R, Lemieux RJ, Picard D, et al: Gallium-67 imaging in pericarditis secondary to tuberculosis and histoplasmosis. Clin Nucl Med 6:413–415, 1981.
191. Tajima T, Naito T, Dohi Y, et al: Ga-67 and Tl-201 imaging in sarcoidosis involving the myocardium. Clin Nucl Med 6:120–121, 1981.
192. Tanaka T, Mishkin FS, Buozas J, et al: Pancreatic uptake of gallium-67 citrate in acute pancreatitis. Applied Radiol 7:163–164, 1978.
193. Teates CD, Bray ST, Williamson BRJ: Tumor detection with ^{67}Ga-citrate. Clin Nucl Med 3:456–459, 1978.
194. Teates CD, Preston DF, Boyd CM: Gallium-67 citrate imaging in head and neck tumors: report of Cooperative Group. J Nucl Med 21:622–627, 1980.
195. Teates CD, Hunter JG: Gallium scanning as a screening test for inflammatory lesions. Radiology 116:383–387, 1975.
196. Tedesco FJ, Coleman RE, Siegel BA: Gallium citrate Ga-67 accumulation in pseudomembranous colitis. JAMA 235:59–60, 1976.
197. Tenenzapf MJ, Thanawala S, Dunn EK, et al: Gallium scanning in rhabdomyolysis. Clin Nucl Med 6:425, 1981.
198. Tonami N, Seto H, Maeda T, et al: Increased concentration of ^{99m}Tc-methylene diphosphonate and ^{67}Ga-citrate in extracranial bone metastases from pinealoma. Clin Nucl Med 3:467–469, 1978.
199. Tonami N, Matsudo H, Oguchi M, et al: Ga-67 uptake in unilateral puberal gynecomastia. Clin Nucl Med 5:410–411, 1980.
200. Turbiner EH, Yeh SDJ, Rosen P, et al: Abnormal gallium scintigraphy in *Pneumocystis carinii* pneumonia with a normal chest radiograph. Radiology 127:437–438, 1978.
201. Vaidya SG, Chaudhri MA, Morrison R, et al: Localization of gallium-67 in malignant neoplasms. Lancet 2:911–914, 1970.

202. Van der Schoot JB, Groen AS, DeJong J: Gallium-67 scintigraphy in lung diseases. Thorax 27:543–546, 1972.
203. Wahner H, Brown ML, Dickson ER: Gallium accumulation in the stomach: a false positive scan suggesting abscess. J Nucl Med 20: 577–578, 1979.
204. Wahner HW, Goellner JR, Hoagland HC: Giant lymph node hyperplasia resembling abdominal abscess on gallium scan. Clin Nucl Med 3:19–21, 1978.
205. Walk RB: Gallium-67 scanning in the evaluation of mesothelioma. J Nucl Med 19:808–809, 1978.
206. Wallner RJ, Croll MN, Brady LW: [67]Ga localization in acute cerebral infarction. J Nucl Med 15:308–309, 1974.
207. Waxman AD, Lee G, Wolfstein R: Differential diagnosis of brain lesions by gallium scanning. J Nucl Med 14:903–906, 1973.
208. Waxman AD, Lee G, Wolfstein RS, et al: Further observations of gallium-67 evaluation of cerebral lesions. J Nucl Med 15:542–543, 1974.
209. Waxman AD, Siemsen JK: Gallium gallbladder scanning in cholecystitis. J Nucl Med 16:148–150, 1975.
210. Waxman AD, Siemsen JK: Gallium scanning in cerebral and cranial infections. Am J Roentgenol 127:309–314, 1976.
211. Weiner SN, Patel BP: ^{67}Ga-citrate uptake by the parotid glands in sarcoidosis. Radiology 130:753–755, 1979.
212. Winchell HS, Sanchez PD, Watanabe CK: Visualization of tumors in humans using ^{67}Ga-citrate and the Anger whole-body scanner, scintillation camera and tomographic scanner. J Nucl Med 11:459–466, 1970.
213. Winston MA, Retzky M: [67]Ga concentration in mesenteric adenitis. Clin Nucl Med 2:427–428, 1977.
214. Winzelberg G, Rabinowitz J: Scintigraphic evaluation of Legionnaire's disease. Clin Nucl Med 6:544–546, 1981.
215. Wiseman J, Rouleau J, Rigo P, et al: Gallium-67 myocardial imaging for the detection of bacterial endocarditis. Radiology 120:135–138, 1976.
216. Wolfe JA, Jr., Tuomaner EL, Greenberg ID: Radionuclide joint imaging: acute rheumatic fever simulating septic arthritis. Pediatrics 65:339–341, 1980.
217. Wood BC, Sharma JN, Germann DR, et al: Gallium citrate imaging in noninfectious interstitial nephritis. Arch Int Med 138:1665–1666, 1978.
218. Yang SL, Alderson PO, Kaizer HA, et al: Serial Ga-67 citrate imaging in children with neoplastic disease. J Nucl Med 20:210–214, 1974.
219. Yeh SDJ, Benua RS: Gallium-67-citrate accumulation in the heart with tumor involvement. Clin Nucl Med 3:103–105, 1978.

Part VI

Gastrointestinal System

Chapter 23

Salivary Glands

EDWARD B. SILBERSTEIN

I. Normal pattern with ^{99m}Tc-pertechnetate

    A. Parotid and submaxillary glands are visible at approximately 10 minutes (19)

    B. Oral cavity is seen 20 to 30 minutes (19)

    C. Sublingual and other minor salivary glands are not visualized (19)

II. Falsely normal salivary images

    A. Common

        1. Salivary tumors < 1–2 centimeters in diameter (14, 16)

        2. Certain mixed tumors (16)

        3. Sialoadenitis, convalescent phase (16)

    B. Uncommon

        1. Sjögren's syndrome—20%[1] (15)

        2. Sjögren's syndrome responding to cyclosphamide (16)

        3. Lipoid atrophy (8)

III. Focal increase in glandular uptake

    A. Common

        1. Warthin's tumor (papillary cystadenoma lymphomatosum)—67% (14, 16)

---

[1] Percentage refers to prevalence of scan finding

B. Uncommon
    1. Mixed tumor (only slight increase in concentration) (9, 16)
    2. Oncocytoma (oxyphilic granular cell adenoma) (2, 12)
    3. Carcinoma (9)
    4. Neurofibroma from facial nerve (20)

IV. Diffuse increase in glandular uptake

  A. Common
    1. Acute sialoadenitis (7, 16)
      a. bacterial, especially staphylococcal
      b. viral (mumps)
    2. Sialolithiasis with duct obstruction (unilateral and bilateral) (13)
    3. Sialosis
      a. endocrine, with malnutrition and cirrhosis (11)
      b. pharmacologic (11)
  B. Uncommon
    1. Mikulicz-Sjögren syndrome (17)
    2. After irradiation of 1000–2000 rads (11)
    3. Sarcoid (19)
    4. Chronic recurrent parotitis (5)
  C. Rare
    1. Masses compressing salivary ducts (14, 15)
    2. Congenital bilateral dilatation of parotid ducts with stasis of secretions (13)
    3. Hyperlipidemia (17)

V. Focal decrease in or unilateral absence of glandular uptake

  A. Common
    1. Tumors (8, 16)
      a. mixed salivary gland tumor
      b. squamous carcinoma
      c. cylindroma
      d. lipoma
      e. hemangioma
    2. Abscess (7, 16)
    3. Cysts, including bronchial cyst (8, 16)
    4. Post-surgical (16)
    5. Extrinsic masses, especially lymphadenopathy (14)
  B. Uncommon
    1. Warthin's tumor, especially cystic (8)
    2. Metastatic melanoma (8)
    3. Hyperplastic parotid lymph node (8)
    4. Carotid body tumor (8)

    5. Mycobacterial infection (4)

    6. Unilateral aplasia (9)

    7. Lymphoma (3)

    8. Other metastatic carcinoma (5)

    9. Invasion from facial osseous tumor and other adjacent tissues (5)

VI. Diffuse decrease in glandular uptake, unilateral or bilateral

  A. Common

    1. Physiological, with aging (15)

    2. Acute and chronic sialoadenitis, bacterial or viral (16)

    3. Recurrent sialoadenitis (7, 16)

    4. Sjögren's syndrome (16)

    5. Post radiotherapy over 4000 rads[2] (10, 15, 16)

    6. Surgical resection (5)

    7. Obstructive sialolithiasis (5)

  B. Uncommon

    1. Tumors, primary and secondary (15)

    2. Hypogammaglobulinemia (9)

    3. Neonatal hypothyroidism (18)

    4. Multicentric sialoangiectasis (15)

VII. Absent bilaterally glandular uptake

  A. Common

    1. Sjögren's syndrome, Schall class 4 (6)

    2. Chronic atrophic sialoadenitis (16)

    3. Salivary ductal obstruction (16)

    4. Surgical ablation (15)

  B. Rare

    1. Congenital aplasia (9)

VIII. Diminished oral activity (accompanying diminished glandular concentration)

  A. Common

    1. Sjögren's syndrome, Schall class 2 and 3 (15)

IX. Absent oral activity with absent glandular activity (a photopenic defect is usually seen)

  A. Common

    1. Sjögren's syndrome, Schall class 4 (15)

---

[2] but increased on Gallium-67 scan (3)

X. Absent oral activity with normal glandular activity

    A. Common

        1. Anticholinergic drugs

            a. atropine sulphate (1 mg intravenously) (6)

REFERENCES

1. Abramson AL, Levy LM, Goodman M, et al: Salivary gland scintiscanning with technetium 99m pertechnetate. Laryngoscope 79:1105–1117, 1969.
2. Ausband JR, Kittrell BJ, Cowan RJ: Radioisotope scanning for parotid oncocytoma. Arch Otolaryngol 93:628–630, 1971.
3. Bekerman C, Hoffer PB: Salivary gland uptake of ^{67}Ga citrate following radiation therapy. J Nucl Med 17:685–687, 1976.
4. Boedecker RA, Sty JR, Thompson N: Salivary gland scintigraphy in atypical mycobacterial infection. Clin Nucl Med 4:202, 1979.
5. Chaudhuri TK, Stadalnik RC: Salivary gland imaging. Sem Nucl Med 10:400–401, 1980.
6. Enfors B, Lind M, Soderburg B: Salivary gland scanning with 99m technetium. Acta Oto-laryngologia 67:650–654, 1969.
7. Fletcher MM, Workman JB: Salivary gland scintigram in inflammatory disease. Am Surg 35:765–772, 1969.
8. Gates GA: Current status of radiosialography in tumor diagnosis. Tr Am Acad Ophth and Otol 74:1183–1195, 1970.
9. Grove AS, DiChiro G: Salivary gland scanning with technetium-99m pertechnetate. Am J Roentgenol 102:109–116, 1968.
10. Higashi T, Fujimura T, Aoyama W, et al: Gamma camera images of the salivary gland using ^{99m}Tc. Oral Surg, Oral Med, Oral Path 40:804–810, 1975.
11. Housle RJ, Ritchard J, N'Goyen VT, et al: Differential diagnosis of xerostomia by quantitative salivary gland scintigraphy. Ann Otol 86:333–340, 1977.
12. Lunia S, Chodos RB, Lunia C, et al: Oxyphilic adenoma of the parotid gland. Radiology 128:690–693, 1978.
13. Parret J, Peyrin JO: Radioisotopic investigations in salivary pathology. Clin Nucl Med 4:250–261, 1979.
14. Schall GL: The role of radionuclide scanning in the evaluation of neoplasms of the salivary glands: a review. J Surg Oncol 3:699–714, 1971.
15. Schall GL, Anderson LG, Wolf RO, et al: Xerostomia in Sjögren's syndrome: evaluation by sequential salivary scintigraphy. JAMA 216:2109–2116, 1971.
16. Schall GL, DiChiro G: Clinical usefulness of salivary gland scanning. Sem Nucl Med 2:270–277, 1972.
17. Schall GL, Smith RR, Barsocchini LM: Radionuclide salivary imaging: usefulness in a private otolaryngology practice. Arch Otolaryngol 107:40–44, 1981.
18. Spencer RP, Karimeddini MK: Decreased salivary gland accumulation of pertechnetate in neonatal hypothyroidism. J Nucl Med 22:96, 1981.
19. Van Den Akker HP, Sokole EB, Van Der Schoot JB: Origin and location of the oral activity in sequential salivary gland scintigraphy with ^{99m}Tc-pertechnetate. Am J Roentgenol 102:109–116, 1968.
20. Wilkinson RH, Goodrich JK: A neurofibroma mimicking a parotid gland tumor both clinically and by scanning. J Nucl Med 12:646–648, 1971.

Chapter 24

Stomach

EDWARD B. SILBERSTEIN

I. Generalized increased Tc-99m-pertechnetate activity in the stomach

   A. Common

      1. Hypersecretion of gastric juice (40)

      2. Hyperchlorhydria (40, 82, 87)

      3. Duodenal ulcer (40, 81, 82)

   B. Uncommon

      1. Hypertrophic gastric mucosa (40)

      2. Pentagastrin and histamine injection (40, 81, 87)

II. Generalized decreased Tc-99m-pertechnetate activity in the stomach

   A. Common

      1. Achlorhydria (40)

      2. Hypochlorhydria (40)

      3. Pernicious anemia (3, 40, 81, 82)

      4. After vagotomy (81, 82)

      5. Gastric malignancy (81, 82)

      6. Gastric ulcer (81, 82)

      7. Chronic atrophic gastritis (3, 40)

   B. Uncommon

      1. Pre-treatment with perchlorate (33, 40)

      2. Gastric mucosal metaplasia (3)

III. Localized decreased radiopharmaceutical uptake in the stomach using Tc-99m-pertechnetate

   A. Common

      1. Gastric neoplasm (54, 82)

         a. carcinoma

         b. leiomyosarcoma

The use of an asterisk * in this chapter indicates that this entity has been observed by the author but the case report has not been published.

2. Large benign gastric ulcer with accompanying atrophy and edema of the gastric mucosa (55)
3. Food in the stomach (55)

B. Uncommon
1. Retained barium preventing emission of gamma photons from the stomach*
2. Previous gastrostomy (55)

References for this chapter may be found at the end of Chapter 26, page 153.

Chapter 25

Ectopic Gastric Mucosa

AMOLAK SINGH

EDWARD B. SILBERSTEIN

SUBHASH SAHA

I. Ectopic or malpositioned gastric tissue demonstrated by Tc-99m-pertechnetate scintigraphy

A. Common
1. Meckel's diverticulum (4, 29, 42, 56, 70)
2. Hiatal hernia with intrathoracic gastric activity (82)

B. Uncommon
1. Barrett's esophagus (5, 52, 82)
2. Retained gastric antrum following Billroth II gastrectomy (16)
3. Duplication (gastrogenic), communicating or noncommunicating (63)
   a. intrathoracic (53)
   b. intra-abdominal (77, 87, 88)
   c. associated with skeletal abnormalities of the pelvis and sacrum, often with meningomyelocele (23)
   d. intraluminal diverticula within ileal duplication (63)
4. Peptic ulceration of otherwise normal small bowel due to ectopic gastric mucosa (77)
5. Midgut malrotation (47)

The use of an asterisk * in this chapter indicates that this entity has been observed by one of the authors but the case report has not been published.

II. False positive scan for Meckel's diverticulum scintigraphic study using Tc-99m-pertechnetate (not due to ectopic gastric tissue)

   A. Common
   1. Activity secreted by the stomach filling loops of small bowel*
   2. Activity in the renal pelvis or proximal ureter due to obstructive uropathy (15)

   B. Uncommon
   1. Inflammatory lesions
      a. appendicitis (14, 19)
      b. intestinal obstruction (6, 23, 45)
         (1) intussusception (14, 23)
            (a) Peutz-Jeghers syndrome (24, 49)
         (2) volvulus (14, 46)
      c. abscess secondary to perforation of small bowel (24, 45)
      d. regional enteritis (29, 49)
         (1) Crohn's disease (39)
      e. ulcerative colitis (29)
   2. Activity in renal calyceal diverticulum (49)
   3. Vascular lesions
      a. A-V malformation of small bowel (75, 77)
      b. vascular tumor (hemangioma) (4, 15)
      c. aneurysm of intra-abdominal vessel (15)
      d. vascular ectasia (angiodysplasia) (15, 79)
   4. Accumulation of radioactivity around area of cecal fecal material (59)

   C. Rare
   1. Ulceration of small bowel, peptic and other (15, 77)
   2. Intestinal irritation secondary to repeated use of laxatives or Zarontin (ethosuximide) (24)
   3. Appendiceal stump (17)
   4. Parasitic infestation—ascariasis (89)
   5. Normal uterine blood pool (8)
      a. menstrual or secretory endometrium (27A)
   6. Tumors
      a. jejunal neurinoma (73)
      b. carcinoma of sigmoid colon (73)
      c. ileal lymphoma (78)
      d. leiomyosarcoma (36)
      e. carcinoid (66)

III. False negative scan for Meckel's diverticulum scintigraphic study using Tc-99m-pertechnetate

   A. Common
   1. No gastric mucosa in the diverticulum (70)
   2. Too little gastric mucosa exists to sequester a visible amount of Tc-99m-pertechnetate (29)

3. Scarring of the Meckel's diverticulum with minimal residual gastric mucosa (67)
4. Meckel's diverticulum obscured by the distended bladder (44, 76)

B. Uncommon
1. Stomach lies too close to the diverticulum to be visualized (67)
2. Residual barium in the bowel preventing emission of gamma photons to be detected by the scintillation camera (38, 60)
3. Pre-treatment with perchlorate (41)
4. Severe diverticulitis in the Meckel's diverticulum (61, 70)
5. Necrosis of Meckel's diverticulum (19)
6. Obstruction of sac outlet with back pressure preventing radiopharmaceutical uptake (70)

References for this chapter may be found at the end of Chapter 26, page 153.

Chapter 26

Gastric Emptying[†]

EDWARD B. SILBERSTEIN

I. Delayed emptying

  A. Common

    1. Gastric outlet obstruction (pyloric stenosis) (13)
    2. Vagotomy (13, 57)
    3. Gastric malignancy, especially linitis plastica (9, 13, 57)
    4. Gastric atony (25)
      a. diabetic autonomic neuropathy (10, 48)
    5. Post-operative period after vagotomy and/or pyloroplasty (13, 21, 50)
    6. Benign ulcers
      a. gastric (pyloric) ulcer (9, 13)
      b. duodenal ulcer (57)
    7. Celiac disease (30)

[†] ^{99m}Tc-sulfur colloid in solid food

    8. Gastric bypass surgery for obesity (64)
    9. Drug effects
        a. cholinergic blockage (1)
        b. opiates (57)
  10. Hypothyroidism (57)
  11. Gastroesophageal reflux (57)
  12. Other causes of ileus (57)
        a. post trauma
        b. from electrolyte imbalance
B. Uncommon
    1. Progressive systemic sclerosis (57)
    2. Bulbar poliomyelitis (57)
    3. Brain tumor (57)

II. Rapid gastric emptying

  A. Common
    1. Duodenal ulcer (13, 34, 40, 54)
    2. Vagotomy and pyloroplasty (34, 51)
    3. Post-gastrectomy syndrome (34, 35, 51)
    4. Metoclopramide (25, 31)
    5. Fatty meal (68)
    6. Fluid content of meal (1, 68)
    7. Erect posture (32)
    8. Small size of food particles (57, 68)
    9. Hyperthyroidism (57)
  10. Distension (57)
  B. Uncommon
    1. Gastrinoma (57)

REFERENCES[1]

1. Bandini P, Malmud L, Applegate G, et al: Dual radionuclide studies of gastric emptying using a physiological meal (abstract). J Nucl Med 21:66, 1980.
2. Basra GS, Teaford TL: Meckel's diverticulum. J Med Assoc Georgia 68:205–207, 1979.
3. Bartelink A, Woldring MG, Hoedemaeker J: Tc-99m in the scanning of the stomach. Lancet 2:420–421, 1967.
4. Berquist TH, Nolan NG, Adson MA, et al: Diagnosis of Meckel's diverticulum by radioisotope scanning. Mayo Clin Proc 48:98–102, 1973.
5. Berquist TH, Nolan NG, Carlson HC, et al: Diagnosis of Barrett's esophagus by pertechnetate scintigraphy. Mayo Clin Proc 48:276–279, 1973.
6. Berquist TH, Nolan NG, Stephens DH, et al: Specificity of Tc-99m-pertechnetate in scintigraphic diagnosis of Meckel's diverticulum: review of 100 cases. J Nucl Med 17:465–469, 1976.

[1] This list contains references for Chapters 24–26.

7. Bowden TA Jr., Hooks VH III, Teeslink CR, et al: Occult gastrointestinal bleeding: locating the cause. Am Surg 46:80–87, 1980.

8. Burt TB, Knochel JQ, Datz FL, et al: Uterine activity. A potential cause of false-positive Meckel's scan. J Nucl Med 22:886–887, 1981.

9. Calderson M, Sonnemaker RE, Hersh T, et al: Tc-99m-human albumin microspheres for measuring the rate of gastric emptying. Radiology 101:371–374, 1971.

10. Campbell IW, Heading RC, Tothill P, et al: Gastric emptying in diabetic autonomic neuropathy. Gut 18:462–467, 1977.

11. Chaudhuri TK: Can Tc-99m-pertechnetate be used to assess the secretion of gastric acid in pernicious anemia? J Nucl Med 18:121–122, 1977.

12. Chaudhuri TK, Polak JJ: Autoradiographic studies of distribution in the stomach of Tc-99m pertechnetate (abstract). J Nucl Med 17:559, 1976.

13. Chaudhuri TK: Use of Tc-99m DTPA for measuring gastric emptying time. J Nucl Med 15:391–395, 1974.

14. Chaudhuri TK: Detection of intestinal obstruction by radionuclide scan: case report. Military Med 141:793–794, 1976.

15. Chaudhuri TK, Chaudhuri TK, Christie J: False positive Meckel's diverticulum scan. Surgery 71:313, 1972.

16. Cobb JS, Bank S, Marks IN, et al: Gastric emptying after vagotomy and pyloroplasty. Am J Digest Dis 16:207–215, 1971.

17. Colbert PM: Problems with radioisotope scan for Meckel's diverticulum. Letter to the Editor, N Engl J Med 292:530, 1974.

18. Conte PJ: Demonstration of Meckel's diverticulum with and without perchlorate premedication. Clin Nucl Med 1:132, 1976.

19. Conway JJ, and the Pediatric Nuclear Club of the S.N.M.: The sensitivity, specificity and accuracy of radionuclide imaging of Meckel's diverticulum (abstract). J Nucl Med 17:553, 1976.

20. Cooper MM: Diagnosis of Meckel's diverticulum by sodium pertechnetate Tc-99m scan. JAMA 235:1471–1472, 1976.

21. Cowley DJ, Vernon P, Jones T, et al: Gastric emptying of solid meals after truncal vagotomy and pyloroplasty in human subjects. Gut 13:176–181, 1972.

22. Debois JM: Scintigraphic demonstration of a leiomyosarcoma of the stomach. Eur J Nucl Med 7:190–191, 1982.

23. Duszynski DO, Anthony R: Jejunal intussusception demonstrated by Tc-99m-pertechnetate and abdominal scanning. Am J Roentgenol 109:729–732, 1970.

24. Duszynski DO, Jewett TC, Allen JE: Tc-99m-Na-pertechnetate scanning of the abdomen with particular reference to the small bowel pathology. Am J Roentgenol 113:258–262, 1971.

25. Fajman WA, Perkel MS, Hersh T, et al: Assessment of gastric emptying of a solid meal utilizing a scintillation camera-computer system (abstract). J Nucl Med 19:734, 1978.

26. Feggi LM, Bighi SM: Technical note for scintigraphy of Meckel's diverticulum. J Nucl Med 20:888–889, 1979.

27. Ferguson A, Bemis J, Ross L, et al: Diagnostic possibilities for Tc-99m abdominal scanning. J Nucl Med Tech 4:146–147, 1977.

27A. Fink-Bennett D: The uterine blush. Clin Nucl Med 7:444–446, 1982.

28. Franken EA Jr.: Gastrointestinal bleeding in infants and children. Radiologic investigation. JAMA 229:10–11, 1974.

29. Gelfand MJ, Silberstein EB, Cox J: Radionuclide imaging of Meckel's diverticulum in children. Clin Nucl Med 3:4–8, 1978.

30. Hamlyn AN, McKenna K, Douglas AP: Gastric emptying in coeliac disease. Br Med J 1:1257–1258, 1977.
31. Hancock BD, Bowen-Jones E, Dixon R, et al: The effect of metoclopramide on gastric emptying of solid food. Gut 15:462–467, 1974.
32. Hancock BD, Bowen-Jones E, Dixon R, et al: The effect of posture on the gastric emptying of solid meals in normal subjects and patients after vagotomy. Br J Surg 61:945–949, 1974.
33. Harden RM, Alexander WD, Kennedy I: Isotope uptake and scanning of stomach in man with Tc-99m-pertechnetate. Lancet 1:1305–1306, 1967.
34. Harvey RF, Brown NJG, Mackie DB, et al: Measurement of gastric emptying time with a gamma camera. Lancet 1:16–18, 1970.
35. Heading RC, Tothill P, McLaughlin GF, et al: A double isotope scanning technique for simultaneous study of liquid and solid meal components of a meal. Gastroenterology 71:45–50, 1976.
36. Heyman S, Sacks B, Khettry J, et al: Localization of bleeding small intestinal lesions using scanning techniques. Surg 85:372–376, 1979.
37. Ho JE, Gleason WA, Thompson JS: The expanding spectrum of disease demonstrable by Tc-99m pertechnetate abdominal imaging (abstract). J Nucl Med 19:691, 1978.
38. Ho JE, Konieczny KM: The sodium pertechnetate Tc-99m scan: an aid in the evaluation of gastrointestinal bleeding. Pediatrics 56:34–40, 1975.
39. Holt S, Taylor TV, McLoughlin RC, et al: An evaluation of ^{99m}Tc pertechnetate scanning for the detection of coeliac disease and Crohn's disease. Eur J Nucl Med 6:361–364, 1981.
40. Irvine WJ, Stewart AG, McLoughlin GP, et al: Appraisal of the application of Tc-99m in the assessment of gastric function. Lancet 2:648–653, 1967.
41. Jaros R, Schussheim A, Levy LM: Preoperative diagnosis of bleeding Meckel's diverticulum utilizing Tc-99m pertechnetate scinti-imaging. J Pediatr 82:45–46, 1973.
42. Jewett TC Jr., Duszynski DO, Allen JE: The visualization of Meckel's diverticulum with Tc-99m-pertechnetate. Surg 68:567–570, 1970.
43. Kilburn E, Gilday DL, Ash J: Meckel's diverticula—serial multiple view imaging (abstract). J Nucl Med 17:553, 1976.
44. Kilpatrick AM: Scanning in diagnosis of Meckel's diverticulum. Hospital Practice 9:131–138, 1974.
45. Kilpatrick AM, Aseron CA Jr.: Radioisotope detection of Meckel's diverticulum causing acute rectal hemorrhage. N Engl J Med 287:653–654, 1972.
46. Lentle BC, Scott GW: A false-positive abdominal scan for Meckel's diverticulum. Br J Radiol 48:59–61, 1975.
47. Leonidas JC, Stuben JL, Ashcraft KW: Diagnosis of midgut malrotation with ^{99m}Tc-pertechnetate abdominal imaging. Radiology 115:143–144, 1975.
48. Lewis SE, Corbett DW, Richardson JS, et al: Gastric function in diabetic patients—gastric scanning and measurements of acid secretion (abstract). J Nucl Med 19:686, 1978.
49. Lunia S, Lunia C, Chandramouly B, et al: Radionuclide Meckelogram with particular reference to false-positive results. Clin Nucl Med 4:285–288, 1979.
50. MacGregor IL, Martin P, Meyer JH: Gastric emptying of solid food in normal man and after subtotal gastrectomy and truncal vagotomy with pyloroplasty. Gastroenterology 72:206–211, 1977.
51. MacGregor IL, Parent J, Meyer JH. Gastric emptying of liquid meals and pancreatic and biliary secretion after subtotal gastrectomy or truncal vagotomy in man. Gastroent 72:195–205, 1977.

52. Mangla JC, Brown M: Diagnosis of Barrett's esophagus by pertechnetate radionuclide. Am J Digest Dis 21:324–328, 1976.
53. Mark R, Young L, Ferguson C, et al: Diagnosis of intrathoracic gastrogenic cyst using pertechnetate-99m. Radiology 109:137–138, 1973.
54. Marsden DS, Alexander CH, Young PK, et al: The use of Tc-99m to detect gastric malignancy. Am J Gastroent 59:410–415, 1973.
55. Marsden DS, Alexander CH, Young P, et al: Autoradiographic explanation for use of Tc-99m in gastric scintiphotography (abstract). J Nucl Med 14:632, 1973.
56. Marsden DS, Priebe CJ: Preliminary appraisal of present Tc-99m-pertechnetate techniques for detecting ectopic gastric mucosa. Radiology 113:459–460, 1974.
57. Malmud LS, Fisher RS, Knight LC, et al: Scintigraphic evaluation of gastric emptying. Sem Nucl Med 12:116–125, 1982.
58. Martin GI, Kutner FR, Moser L: Diagnosis of Meckel's diverticulum by radioisotope scanning. Pediatrics 57:11–12, 1976.
59. Maxwell ME, Boggenstoss B: False-positive Meckel's diverticulum scan of non-pathologic origin. J Nucl Med Tech 1:16–17, 1973.
60. Meguid MM, Wilkinson RH, Canty T, et al: Futility of barium sulphate in diagnosis of bleeding Meckel diverticulum. Arch Surg 108:361–632, 1974.
61. Muroff LR, Casarella WJ, Johnson PM: Preoperative diagnosis of Meckel's diverticulum. JAMA 229:1900–1902, 1974.
62. Neale IA, Wright FW: Anemia caused by a giant Meckel's diverticulum and diagnosed by Tc-99m-pertechnetate. Br J Clin Pract 34:19–24, 1980.
63. Ohba S, Fukuda A, Kohno S, et al: Ileal duplication and multiple intraluminal diverticula: scintigraphy and barium meal. Am J Roentgenol 136:992–994, 1981.
64. Patton DD, Villar HV, Norton LW, et al: Measurement of gastric emptying rate (GER) after surgical treatment for obesity: use of Tc-99m tagged chopped chicken liver (abstract). J Nucl Med 21:P67, 1980.
65. Petrokubi RJ, Baum S, Rohrer V: Cimetidine administration resulting in improved pertechnetate imaging of Meckel's diverticulum. Clin Nucl Med 3:385, 1978.
66. Polga JP, Sargent J, Dickinson P: Positive intestinal scan caused by carcinoid tumor. J Nucl Med 15:365–366, 1974.
67. Rocha AFG, Harbert JC: Textbook of Nuclear Medicine: Clinical Application. Philadelphia: Lea and Febiger, 1979, p. 134.
68. Rock E, Malmud LS, Bandini P, et al: Combined gall bladder-gastric emptying in man: effects of varying meal composition (abstract). J Nucl Med 21:P66, 1980.
69. Rodgers BM, Youssef S: False positive scan for Meckel's diverticulum. J Pediatr 87:239–240, 1975.
70. Rosenthall L, Henry JN, Murphy DA, et al: Radiopertechnetate imaging of Meckel's diverticulum. Radiology 105:371–373, 1972.
71. Scarpello JHB, Barber DC, Hague RV, et al: Gastric emptying of solid meals in diabetics. Br Med J 2:671–673, 1976.
72. Sciarretta G, Malaguti P, Turba E, et al: Retained gastric antrum syndrome diagnosed by Tc-99m-pertechnetate scintigraphy in man: hormonal and radioisotopic study of two cases. J Nucl Med 19:377–380, 1978.
73. Seetz W, Keim HG, Hahn K: Abdominal scintigraphy for diagnosis of intestinal bleeding. World J Surg 2:613–619, 1978.
74. Shaw A: Guideline for diagnosing children who bleed through the rectum. Hospital Physician 8:36, 1974.
75. Siddiqui A, Ryo UY, Pinsky SM: Arteriovenous malformation simulating Meckel's diver-

ticulum on Tc-99m pertechnetate abdominal scintigraphy. Radiology 122:173–174, 1977.

76. Singh PR, Russell CD, Dubovsky EV, et al: Technique of scanning for Meckel's diverticulum. Clin Nucl Med 3:188–192, 1978.

77. Sfakianis GN, Conway JJ: Detection of ectopic gastric mucosa in Meckel's diverticulum and in other aberrations by scintigraphy. II. Indications and methods—a 10 year experience. J Nucl Med 22:732–738, 1981.

78. Tauscher JW, Bryant DT, Gruenther RC: False positive scan for Meckel's diverticulum. J Pediatr 92:1022–1023, 1978.

79. Tavormina A, Mousavi A, Gordon DH, et al: Extravasation of contrast material from vascular ectasia of cecum detected with Tc-99m-pertechnetate. Radiology 128:168–169, 1978.

80. Taylor AT, Alazraki N, Henry JE: Intestinal concentration of Tc-99m-pertechnetate into isolated loops of rat bowel. J Nucl Med 17:470–472, 1976.

81. Taylor TV, Bone D, Torrance B: A non-invasive test of gastric function. Br J Surg 64:702–708, 1977.

82. Taylor TV: Non-invasive investigation of the upper gastrointestinal tract using technetium-99m. Ann R Coll Surg 61:37–44, 1979.

83. Tothill P, McLoughlin GP, Heading RC: Techniques and errors in scintigraphic measurements of gastric emptying. J Nucl Med 19:256–261, 1978.

84. Treves S, Grand RJ, Eraklis AJ: Pentagastrin stimulation of technetium-99m uptake by ectopic gastric mucosa in a Meckel's diverticulum. Radiology 128:711–712, 1978.

85. Van Dam APM: The gamma camera in clinical evaluation of gastric emptying. Radiology 110:155–157, 1974.

86. Wilson JP, Wenzel WW, Campbell JB: Technetium scans in the detection of gastrointestinal hemorrhage. Preoperative diagnosis of enteric duplication in an infarct. JAMA 237:265–266, 1977.

87. Wine CR, Nahrwold DL, Rose RC, et al: Effect of histamine on technetium-99m excretion by gastric mucosa. Surgery 8:591–594, 1976.

88. Winter PF: Sodium pertechnetate Tc-99m scanning of the abdomen. Diagnosis of an ileal duplication cyst. JAMA 237:1352–1353, 1977.

89. Wynant GE: Pertechnetate abdomen scan in a patient with *Ascaris lumbricoides* infestation. J Nucl Med Tech 7:243–244, 1979.

Chapter 27

Liver Flow and Blood Pool[†]

EDWARD B. SILBERSTEIN

I. Abnormally early visualization of intrahepatic tissue

  A. Common
  1. Hepatoma (10, 11, 12, 21)
  2. Hepatic adenoma (6, 10, 13)
  3. Hemangioma (10, 12)
  4. Metastatic tumors (more often decreased flow) (2, 7, 11)
  5. Lymphoma (19)
  6. Cirrhosis (7, 19)

  B. Uncommon
  1. Hepatoblastoma (6, 10)
  2. Hepatitis with focal defect (18)
  3. Hamartoma (12)
  4. Focal nodular hyperplasia (13)
  5. Hepatic artery-portal vein fistula (17)
  6. Mycotic aneurysm of hepatic artery (16)

II. Decreased or absent flow with increased blood pool[1]

  A. Hemangioma (1, 6, 20)

III. Decreased to absent focal flow, blood pool not increased

  A. Common
  1. Hepatoblastoma (6, 10)
  2. Hepatoma (10, 12) especially with central necrosis (21)
  3. Cholangioma (3, 20)
  4. Metastatic tumors (10, 21)
  5. Pyogenic abscess (10, 11, 21)
  6. Amebic abscess (21)
  7. Hematoma (6, 10)
  8. Cirrhosis (5)

[†]^{99m} Tc-sulfur colloid
[1]^{199m}Tc-pertechnetate

B. Uncommon
  1. Tumor (primary or secondary) involuting on chemotherapy (10)
  2. Hepatic veno-occlusive disease (4)
  3. Hepatitis with focal defect (9)
  4. Hydatid cyst (8, 11)
  5. Congenital cyst (11, 21)
  6. Budd-Chiari syndrome (15)
  7. Cavernous hemangioma (1)
  8. Dilated, obstructed bile ducts (6)
  9. Hamartoma (6)

IV. Foci with increased blood pool peripherally, decreased centrally (flow not reported)

  A. Common
    1. Pyogenic abscess (19)
  B. Uncommon
    1. Amebic abscess (7)
    2. Cyst (2)

V. Extra-hepatic abnormalities seen on hepatic flow study (3, 14)

  A. Common
    1. Effusion
      a. pericardial
      b. pleural
    2. Cardiomegaly
    3. Decreased pulmonary perfusion
    4. Tortuous aorta or aneurysm
    5. Congestive heart failure
  B. Uncommon
    1. Non-perfused kidney
    2. Mediastinal shift
    3. Venous obstruction
      a. left subclavian vein
      b. superior vena cava
    4. Cholecystitis
    5. Abdominal mass lesions
  C. Rare
    1. Dextrocardia

REFERENCES

  1. Beal W, Soin JS, Burdine JA: Hepatic cavernous hemangioma presenting as an "avascular mass" in a newborn. J Nucl Med 15:902–903, 1974.

2. Coates G, Stadalnik RC, Palmer JM, et al: Hepatic scintiangiography in malignant parasitic tumors. J Nucl Med 15:137–139, 1974.

3. Echavarria RA, Bonanno C: Value of routine abdominal nuclide angiography as part of liver scan. Clin Nucl Med 4:66–78, 1974.

4. Fitzer PM: Technetium-99m-sulfur colloid and pertechnetate blood pool scan in hepatic veno-occlusive disease. J Nucl Med 16:1130–1131, 1975.

5. Freeman LM, Mandell CH: Dynamic vascular scintiphotography of the liver. Sem Nucl Med 2:133–138, 1972.

6. Gates GF: Scintiangiography of hepatic masses in childhood. JAMA 239:2667–2670, 1978.

7. Gordon F, Cuaron A, Muñoz JR, et al: Scanning of the hepatic blood pool in the differential diagnosis of space-occupying lesions of the liver. Ann Int Med 78:247–250, 1973.

8. Jain AN, Ramanathan P, Ganatra RD: Scan appearances in hydatid cysts of the liver: analysis of 55 cases. Clin Nucl Med 5:25–28, 1980.

9. Koenigsberg M, Freeman LM: Intrahepatic focal lesion in acute viral hepatitis. J Nucl Med 14:612–614, 1973.

10. Miller JH, Gates GF, Stanley P: The radiologic investigation of hepatic tumors in childhood. Radiology 124:451–458, 1977.

11. Muller-Brand J, Benz U, Kyg CA, et al: Triple radioisotope technique in etiologic evaluation of space-occupying lesions of the liver. Eur J Nucl Med 2:231–238, 1977.

12. Muroff LR, Johnson PM: The use of multiple radionuclide imaging to differentiate the focal intrahepatic lesion. Am J Roentgenol 121:728–734, 1974.

13. Myerson P, Prokop E, Sziklas JJ, et al: Scan findings in hepatic adenoma (focal nodular hyperplasia). Clin Nucl Med 1:108, 1976.

14. Siddiqui AR, Wellman HN: Diagnosis of extra-hepatic abnormalities on dynamic study over thoraco-abdominal region prior to hepatic imaging. Clin Nucl Med 3:214–216, 1978.

15. Singh A, Farrer PA, Grossman ZD, et al: Filling defects in Budd-Chiari syndrome. NY State J Med 80:801–802, 1980.

16. Sukerkar AN, Dulay CC, Anandappa E, et al: Mycotic aneurysm of the hepatic artery. Radiology 124:444, 1977.

17. Sziklas JJ, Spencer RP: Hepatic artery-portal vein fistula detected on hepatic flow study. J Nucl Med 16:910–911, 1975.

18. Valdez VA, Herrera NE: Granulomatous hepatitis: Spectrum of scintigraphic manifestations. Clin Nucl Med 3:393–396, 1978.

19. Waxman AD, Apau R, Siemsen JK: Rapid sequential liver imaging. J Nucl Med 13:522–524, 1972.

20. Wilcox NE, Joo KG: Sluggish perfusion in hepatic hemangioma. Clin Nucl Med 5:465–467, 1980.

21. Yeh S-H, Shih W-J, Liang J-C: Intravenous radionuclide hepatography in the differential diagnosis of intrahepatic mass lesion. J Nucl Med 14:565–567, 1973.

Chapter 28

Liver-Colloid Imaging

EDWARD B. SILBERSTEIN
RUPPERT DAVID

I. Hepatomegaly

  A. Common

    1. Metastatic tumors (95, 116, 120, 137, 163)

    2. Fatty infiltration (15, 60, 78, 116, 120, 163)

      a. diabetes mellitus

      b. obesity

      c. malnutrition

    3. Hepatitis (95, 116, 120, 195)

      a. granulomatous (101, 195, 200)

      b. viral (200)

      c. alcoholic (200)

    4. Cirrhosis (41, 68, 95, 116, 120)

    5. Congestive heart failure with chronic passive congestion (68, 95, 116, 120)

    6. Abscess (95, 116, 120, 140)

    7. Leukemia (78, 95, 120, 146)

    8. Lymphoma (78, 95, 116, 131, 146)

    9. Normal variants—Riedel's Lobe (116, 146)

  B. Uncommon

    1. Other infections (116, 120)

      a. tuberculosis

      b. infectious mononucleosis*

      c. hydatid cysts (120)

    2. Hemochromatosis (46, 116, 120 196)

    3. Trauma (58)

    4. Hemolysis

      a. erythroblastosis fetalis (209)

      b. chronic hemolytic anemia (116)

    5. Drugs (77, 93, 196)

      a. phenobarbital

The use of an asterisk * in this chapter indicates that this entity has been observed by one of the authors but the case report has not been published.

  b. phenytoin
  c. sulfonamides
  d. acetaminophen
  e. tetracycline
  f. corticosteroids
  g. methotrexate
  h. androgens
  6. Primary tumors
  a. hepatoma (120)
  b. hemangioendothelioma (186)
C. Rare
  1. Inherited metabolic disorders with hepatic involvement
  a. Wolman's disease (184)
  b. glycogen storage disease (78, 95, 146)
  c. Wilson's disease (95, 120)
  d. Gaucher's disease (95)
  e. mucopolysaccharidosis (78, 98)
  f. Niemann-Pick disease (120)
  g. gangliosidosis (120)
  h. alpha-1-antitrypsin deficiency (168)
  i. hepatic porphyrias*
  j. cystic fibrosis*
  k. histiocytosis X (19)
  l. galactosemia (120)
  m. acromegaly (149)
  n. hyperlipoproteinemia (160)
  2. Polycystic disease (116, 120, 163)
  3. Inflammatory non-infectious disorders
  a. sarcoidosis (116, 166)
  b. juvenile rheumatoid arthritis*
  4. Kwashiorkor (95); malnutrition (163)
  5. Biliary obstruction (116)
  6. Amyloidosis (95, 109, 116, 120, 188)
  7. Vascular disorders
  a. hereditary hemorrhagic telangiectasia*
  b. multinodular hemangiomatosis (51)
  c. cavernous hemangiomas (120)
  d. Budd-Chiari syndrome (86, 116)
  8. Acromegaly (149)
  9. Jamaican vomiting disease (199)
  10. Infection
  a. congenital or post-natal syphilis (52)
  b. schistosomiasis (120)
  c. amebiasis (116, 120)
  d. actinomycosis (120)

      e. hydatid cyst (116, 120)
      f. Weil's disease (120)
  11. Paroxysmal nocturnal hemoglobinuria (146)
  12. Post-jejunoileal bypass surgery with secondary fatty infiltration (12)

II. Small liver (116)

  A. Common
    1. Normal variation
    2. Cirrhosis
      a. Laennec's
      b. cardiac
      c. biliary
      d. hemochromatosis associated
    3. Artefact
    4. Metastatic disease
  B. Uncommon
    1. Collagen vascular disease
    2. Schistosomiasis
  C. Small or atrophic right lobe with/without left lobe hypertrophy (67, 208)
    1. Cirrhosis
    2. Congenital
    3. Post-surgical resection
    4. Post irradiation
    5. With tumor replacement
    6. Following right lobe trauma

III. Nonuniform and/or diffusely decreased uptake

  A. Common
    1. Metastasis (early) (78, 120)
    2. Hepatitis (9, 56, 104, 118)
      a. granulomatous hepatitis (195)
    3. Fatty infiltration (56)
    4. Cirrhosis (with or without esophageal varices) (41, 56, 89, 120, 155)
    5. Chronic passive congestion (120)
    6. Lymphoma (131, 200)
    7. Leukemia (120)
  B. Uncommon
    1. Fibrosis (56)
    2. Obstructive jaundice (120)
    3. Drugs (93)
      a. tetracycline
      b. phenobarbital
      c. phenytoin

       d. steroids

       e. acetaminophen

       f. chemotherapeutic agents

          (1) methotrexate

          (2) 6-mercaptopurine

    4. Statistical fluctuation at low counts (148)

C. Rare

    1. Primary tumors (69)

    2. Amyloidosis (4, 190, 201)

    3. Sarcoidosis (195)

    4. Focal nodular hyperplasia (150)

    5. Chemical hepatitis (95)

    6. Trauma (58)

    7. Congenital metabolic diseases

       a. cystic fibrosis*

       b. hemochromatosis*

       c. Wilson's disease (56)

       d. glycogen storage disease (78)

       e. Wolman's disease (184)

    8. Infection

       a. congenital syphilis (52)

       b. schistosomiasis (195)

       c. infectious mononucleosis*

       d. Coxsackie B included hepatic hemorrhagic necrosis (76A)

    9. Hyperlipoproteinemia (160)

   10. Vascular lesions

       a. periarteritis nodosa (111)

       b. Budd-Chiari syndrome (124, 191)

   11. Post-radiation therapy (26, 102)

   12. Post-jejunoileal bypass surgery with fatty infiltration (20)

   13. Pleural effusion (120)

IV. Single defect ("cold spot")

  A. Common

    1. Normal variants

       a. prominent porta hepatis (portal vein, hepatic artery, bile duct) (33, 118, 120, 173)

       b. prominent gallbladder fossa (32, 33, 45, 76)

          (1) after cholecystectomy (115)

       c. intra-hepatic gallbladder (167)

       d. prominent draining hepatic veins (33, 146)

          (1) in heart failure (115)

       e. costal margin imprint (33, 49, 121)

       f. localized thinning, especially left lobe (18, 33, 36, 115)

      (1) bipartite liver (109A)

  g. normal kidney, stomach, colon, adrenal, or pancreas imprint (33, 115, 129)

  h. anatomical variations in liver size, shape, and position (33, 116, 135, 187)

      (1) Riedel's lobe

      (2) atrophic left lobe

      (3) prominent quadrate lobe

      (4) ligamentum teres (32, 94, 124)

  i. inferior vena cava fossa (33)

  j. cardiac impression at the superior border of the left lobe (33, 209)

  k. hepatic flexure (of colon) imprint (115)

      (1) post-colectomy (115)

  l. flattened dome in upright view (128)

2. Artefact

  a. breast shadow (49, 143)

  b. barium in colon (120, 170)

  c. contrast medium in gallbladder (115)

  d. arm in field (198)

  e. ascites (204A)

3. Metastatic tumors (17, 33, 53, 78, 80, 120, 136)

4. Dilated bile ducts or gallbladder (50, 71, 115, 116, 118, 134)

5. Pyogenic abscess (14, 78, 140)

6. Post-radiation (75, 76, 88)

7. Hematoma (10, 86, 175)

8. Laceration (78, 116, 194)

9. Subphrenic abscess or hematoma (115, 116)

B. Uncommon

1. Idiopathic (38)

2. Anatomic variations of shape related to non-diseased surrounding structures

  a. diaphragmatic hernia, eventration, or elevation (78, 193)

  b. normal vertebral pressure on left lobe (32, 33)

  c. lordosis of spine (3, 174)

  d. kyphoscoliosis (79)

  e. pectus excavatum (84)

  f. falciform ligament (143)

  g. prominent portal vein or its bifurcation (152, 171)

  h. inferior vena cava (33)

  i. xiphoid process (115)

  j. pseudo-defect secondary to hepatodiaphragmatic interposition (143)

  k. changes in lateral liver view with patient position (207)

3. Neoplasia and hyperplasia

  a. focal nodular hyperplasia (85, 117, 122)

    b. adenoma (2, 7, 51, 83, 85, 123)

    c. hepatoma (3, 43, 47, 51, 66, 77, 78, 136, 159)

    d. regenerating nodules (78)

    e. benign cyst (123, 156)

4. Extra-hepatic compression from diseases (27, 44)

    a. renal tumors including Wilms' and hypernephroma (25, 49, 56, 113, 151, 176)

    b. supra or subdiaphragmatic fluid or abscess (33, 49, 107)

    c. emphysema with low diaphragm (33)

    d. splenomegaly (49)

5. Localized hepatitis (9, 12, 104, 146, 206)

6. Porta hepatis defects due to disease (118, 129)

    a. cirrhosis, fibrosis

    b. tumor

        (1) in lymph nodes

        (2) pancreatic tumor invasion

        (3) tumors of gallbladder, ampulla

        (4) hepatoma

        (5) hepatic artery, portal vein involvement

    c. hepatitis

    d. hepatic laceration

    e. bile duct dilatation

    f. cyst of falciform ligament

    g. ruptured gallbladder; empyema

    h. hepatoma (15)

    i. abscess

    j. infarction (23)

    k. choledochal cyst (142, 157, 205)

    l. dilated splenic vein (202)

    m. dilated portal vein (152)

    n. pancreatic pseudocyst (49)

7. Amebic abscess (141)

8. Artefacts

    a. post-surgical drains (115)

    b. foreign objects (metallic; breast prostheses) (115, 132, 198)

    c. devices to immobilize patient (115)

    d. brain scan the previous day with technetium in bowel (73)

C. Rare

    1. Metaplasia, hyperplasia and neoplasia

        a. hamartoma (51, 146, 171)

        b. drug-induced hepatoma

            (1) secondary to androgens (42, 66)

        c. angiosarcoma (13, 112, 114, 192, 203)

        d. cholangiosarcoma (87)

    2. Non-malignant infiltrative changes

      a. fibrosis (16, 118)
      b. amyloidosis (108, 188)
      c. cirrhosis (89, 103)
      d. hyperlipoproteinemia (160)
   3. Post-operative changes
      a. post-hepatojejunostomy (116)
      b. post-choledochojejunostomy (116)
      c. post-splenectomy (34)
      d. post-colectomy (24)
   4. Vascular
      a. dilated splenic vein (204)
      b. hemangioma (8, 48, 51, 116, 136, 144, 177, 189, 210)
      c. infarction (23, 201)
      d. aortic aneurysm (115)
      e. hemangioendothelioma (186)
   5. Congestive heart failure with cardiomegaly, pericardial effusion (6)
   6. Congenital alterations in shape
      a. situs inversus (120)
      b. malposition of liver with interposition of stomach (147)
      c. bipartite liver (109A)
   7. Phrenic nerve injury (143)
   8. Extra-hepatic compression
      a. pancreatic tumor (1, 49, 116, 154) and pseudocyst (49)
      b. common duct tumor (116)
      c. gallbladder tumor (116)
      d. adrenal tumor (49, 139)
      e. retroperitoneal tumor
         (1) liposarcoma (116)
         (2) lymphoma (116)
         (3) neuroblastoma (27)
      f. hypertrophy of psoas muscle (33)
      g. retroperitoneal lymph nodes (33)
      h. gastric duplication cyst (119)
      i. dextrogastria (26, 49, 115)
      j. leiomyosarcoma of ileum (91)
      k. lung abscess (54)
      l. perforated appendicitis with loculated extrahepatic abscess (183)
      m. splenic cyst (115)

V. Multiple defects

  A. Common
     1. Metastases (40, 78, 120, 136)
     2. Abscess (118)
       a. pyogenic

       b. amebic

       c. tuberculosis (213)

B. Uncommon

    1. Primary tumors (105, 116, 120, 123, 136)

       a. multiple adenomas

       b. hepatomas

       c. hemangiomas (177)

       d. focal nodular hyperplasia (85)

       e. multiloculated cystadenoma (125)

    2. Hepatitis (9, 104, 118, 120, 153, 206)

    3. Cirrhosis (89, 120)

    4. Fatty infiltration (116, 120)

C. Rare

    1. Post-radiation (88, 179)

    2. Cyst

       a. multiple simple cyst (116)

       b. multiple hydatid cysts (116)

       c. polycystic disease (116)

    3. Hematomas (116)

    4. Amyloidosis (116, 188)

    5. Extrinsic masses (59, 91)

       a. renal tumors

       b. renal cysts

       c. adrenal tumors

       d. aortic aneurysm (31)

       e. lymphoma

       f. peritoneal tumors (91)

    6. Periarteritis nodosa (111)

    7. Budd-Chiari syndrome (21, 81, 124, 191)

    8. Congestive heart failure (120)

    9. Caroli's disease (185)

    10. Glycogen storage disease, type I (65)

    11. Hypereosinophilic syndrome (204)

VI. Increased uptake ("hot spot") (70)

  A. Common

    1. Superior or inferior vena caval obstruction (30, 62, 74, 79, 92, 130, 197)

  B. Uncommon

    1. Budd-Chiari syndrome (81, 121, 146, 191)

    2. Innominate vein obstruction (126)

  C. Rare (14, 144)

    1. Liver abscess

    2. Hyperplasia, metaplasia and neoplasia

      a. primary or secondary hemangioma or hemangiosarcoma (14, 144, 197)

      b. hepatoma (62, 144, 172)

      c. hepatic hamartoma (28, 145, 169)

      d. focal nodular hyperplasia (162)

      e. hepatic adenoma (145, 161, 162)

   3. Vascular lesions

      a. caval-portal shunting (79, 133)

      b. arteriovenous malformation (144)

      c. hepatic veno-occlusive disease (68)

      d. tricuspid insufficiency (164)

      e. constrictive pericarditis (181)

   4. Hydatidiform mole (144)

   5. Artefact

      a. malposition of central venous catheter (72)

      b. free pertechnetate in stomach (120)

      c. ventral hernia (64)

   6. Pseudo Budd-Chiari syndrome (39)

   7. Cirrhosis (181)

   8. Idiopathic (3, 30, 72, 130)

VII. Diffuse lung uptake of colloid on liver scan

  A. Uncommon

    1. Liver disease often with poor prognosis (82, 96, 99)

      a. liver metastases (96)

      b. cirrhosis (96)

      c. lymphoma (96, 99)

      d. leukemia (96)

      e. hepatic abscess (96)

      f. subcapsular hepatic hematoma (96)

      g. myelofibrosis (96)

      h. amyloidosis (22)

      i. mucopolysaccharidosis type II (Hunter) (98)

      j. hepatoma (102)

      k. hepatic angiosarcoma (82)

      l. alcoholic hepatitis and gluteal abscess (82)

      m. histiocytosis X (19)

      n. malaria (212)

    2. Collagen-vascular disease (102)

    3. Endotoxin (animal model) (101)

    4. Disseminated intravascular coagulation (101, 178)

    5. Post trauma (22, 90)

    6. Androgen therapy for anemia due to marrow hypoplasia (164A)

  B. Rare

    1. Aluminum ion in plasma (5)
    2. With liver transplant (100)
    3. With spleen and marrow transplantation (same patient) (100)
    4. Sarcoid*
    5. Artefact from colloid aggregation*

VIII. Focal lung uptake of colloid on liver scan

    A. Rare
        1. Tuberculosis (82)
        2. Atelectasis (127)

IX. Renal uptake of sulfur colloid

    A. Uncommon
        1. Congestive heart failure (97)
        2. Disseminated intravascular coagulation (178)
        3. Rejection of renal transplant (55)
        4. Endotoxemia (in animal model) (101)
    B. Rare
        1. Liver transplant (106)

REFERENCES

1. Agnew JE, James O, Bouchier AD: Liver and pancreas scanning in extrahepatic obstructive jaundice (with special reference to tumors of the bile and hepatic ducts). Brit J Radiol 48:190–199, 1974.
2. Albritton DR, Tompkins RK, Longmire WP Jr.: Hepatic cell adenoma. Ann Surg 19:14–19, 1973.
3. Anderson JE, Perlmutter GS: Diagnosis of hepatoma using multiple radionuclide approach. Radiology 102:387–389, 1972.
4. Andujar MA, Valdez VA, Herrera NE: Abnormal distribution of Tc-99m-sulfur colloid in a patient with systemic amyloidosis. Clin Nucl Med 9:346–348, 1978.
5. Babinet DD, Sevrin R, Zurbriggen MT, et al: Lung uptake of ^{99m}Tc-sulfur colloid in patient exhibiting presence of Al^{3+} in plasma. J Nucl Med 15:1220–1222, 1974.
6. Barnett CA: Chronic passive congestion of the liver appearing as focal defect on liver image. Clin Nucl Med 2:52, 1977.
7. Baum JK, Holtz F, Bookstein JJ, et al: Possible association between benign hepatomas and oral contraceptives. Lancet 2:926–929, 1973.
8. Beal W, Soin J, Burdine JA: Hepatic cavernous hemangioma presenting as an "avascular mass" in a newborn. J Nucl Med 15:902–903, 1974.
9. Beauchamp JM, Belanger MA, Neitzchman HR: Intrahepatic focal lesion in acute viral hepatitis. J Nucl Med 15:356–357, 1974.
10. Beauchamp JM, Belanger MA, Neitzchman HR: The diagnosis of subcapsular hematoma of the liver by scintigraphy. South Med J 69:1579–1580, 1976.
11. Benedict IT Jr., Chen PS, Janower ML, et al: Contraceptive-associated hepatic tumor. Am J Roentgenol 132:452–454, 1979.

12. Bergmann P, Struyven J, Sommers G: Hepatic scintigraphic defect in viral hepatitis. J Nucl Biol and Med 19:162–163, 1975.

13. Berk PD: Vinyl chloride-associated liver disease. Ann Int Med 84:717–731, 1976.

14. Bess MA, Bartholomew LG, Wahner HW, et al: Radionuclide image patterns of hepatic metastasis and pyrogenic abscess: Difficulties in differential diagnosis. Clin Nucl Med 3:453–455, 1978.

15. Bieler EU, Meyer BJ, Jansen CR: Liver scanning as a method for detecting primary liver cancer. Am J Roentgenol 115:709–716, 1972.

16. Biersack JH, San Luis T Jr., Lange CE, et al: Scintigraphy of liver and spleen in vinyl chloride workers. Acta Hepato-Gastroenterol 24:357–361, 1977.

17. Blakeney CM, Cullum PA: A single hepatic metastasis from bronchial carcinoid treated by right hepatectomy. Brit J Surg 57:237–238, 1970.

18. Bolich PR, Tyson IB: False-positive liver image due to localized hepatic thinning. Radiology 109:139–140, 1973.

19. Bowen BM, Coates G, Garnett ES: Technetium-99m-sulfur colloid lung scan in patients with histiocytosis X. J Nucl Med 16:332, 1975.

20. Brown RG, O'Leary JP, Woodward ER: Hepatic effects of jejunoileal bypass for morbid obesity. Am J Surg 127:53–58, 1974.

21. Carulli N, Boraldi F, Roncal AR, et al: Liver scans in the Budd-Chiari syndrome. JAMA 223:1161, 1973.

22. Castleman B, Scully RE, McNeely BU: Case records of the Massachusetts General Hospital. N Eng J Med 290:1474–1481, 1974.

23. Chandra S, Laor YG: Liver scan in a case of hepatic infarct. J Nucl Med 14:858–860, 1973.

24. Chaudhuri TK: False-positive liver scan following colectomy. JAMA 234:705, 1975.

25. Chaudhuri TK: Caution in interpreting liver scan in presence of hypernephroma. J Urol 114:481–482, 1975.

26. Chaudhuri TK: False-positive liver scan caused by dextrogastria. J Nucl Med 17:1109, 1976.

27. Chaudhuri TK: Extra-hepatic lesions causing false-positive liver scans. VA Med Mon 103:129–165, 1976.

28. Chayes Z, Koenigsberg M, Freeman L: The hot hepatic abscess. J Nucl Med 15:305–307, 1974.

29. Clearfield HR: Anomalies of the liver, in Bockus HL (ed): Gastroenterology, Vol. III, Ed. 2. Philadelphia: W.B. Saunders, 1965, p. 124.

30. Coel M, Halpern S, Alazraki N, et al: Intrahepatic lesion presenting as an area of increased radiocolloid uptake on a liver scan. J Nucl Med 13:221–222, 1972.

31. Conte PJ: Aortic aneurysm causing multiple liver scan defects. Am J Roentgenol 128:516–517, 1977.

32. Covington EE: The gallbladder fossa in liver photoscans. Am J Gastroenterol 59:262–266, 1973.

33. Covington EE: Pitfalls in liver photoscans. Am J Roentgenol 109:745–758, 1970.

34. Custer JR, Shafer RB: Changes in liver scan following splenectomy. J Nucl Med 16:194–195, 1975.

35. DaCosta H, Gandhi R, Deshmukh S, et al: Hepatosplenic scintigraphy in children with obstructive jaundice. Clin Nucl Med 2:281–285, 1977.

36. DeLand PH, Wagner HN Jr. (eds): Atlas of Nuclear Medicine. Philadelphia: W.B. Saunders, 1972, pp. 68–86, 187–197.

37. DeNardo GL, Stadalnik RC, DeNardo SJ, et al: Hepatic scintiangiographic patterns.

Radiology 111:135–141, 1974.

38. DeRoo MJK: Scintigraphic appearance of necrotic liver metastasis identical with that of amebic abscesses. J Nucl Med 16:250–251, 1975.

39. Dhawan VM, Syiklas JS, Spencer RP: Pseudo-Budd-Chiari syndrome. Clin Nucl Med 3:30, 1978.

40. Drum DE, Beard J: Scintigraphic criteria for hepatic metastases from cancer of the colon and breast. J Nucl Med 17:677–680, 1976.

41. Drum DE, Beard JO: Liver scintigraphic features associated with alcoholism. J Nucl Med 19:154–160, 1978.

42. Farrell GC, Uren RF, Perkins KW, et al: Androgen-induced hepatoma. Lancet 1:430–432, 1975.

43. Farrell R, Steinman A, Green WH: Arteriovenous shunting in a regenerating liver simulating hepatoma. Radiology 102:279–280, 1972.

44. Fellow KE, Tefft M: Liver scans in children: Abnormal masses simulating metastatic disease. Am J Roentgenol 104:678–681, 1968.

45. Ferlin G: Focal and generalized hepatic lesions: a comparison of liver scans with anatomic and histologic findings. Int J Nucl Biol Med 19:135–144, 1975.

46. Finch SC, Finch CA: Idiopathic hemochromatosis, an iron storage disease. Medicine 34:381–430, 1955.

47. Franco J, Coppler M, Kovaleski R, et al: Diagnosis of hepatoma. J Nucl Med 13:644–645, 1972.

48. Freeman LM, Bernstein RG, Hayt DB: Diagnosis of hepatic hemangioma with combined scanning technique. Radiology 95:127–128, 1970.

49. Freeman LM, Meng CH, Johnson PM, et al: False-positive liver scans caused by disease processes in adjacent organs and structures. Br J Radiol 42:651–656, 1969.

50. Gammill SL, Maxfield WS, Font RG, et al: Filling defects on scintillation scans of the liver associated with dilation of the bile ducts. Am J Roentgenol 107:37–42, 1969.

51. Gates GF, Miller JH, Stanley P: Scintiangiography of hepatic masses in childhood. JAMA 239:2667–2670, 1978.

52. Gates GF, Stanley P, Gwinn JL, et al: Congenital syphilitic hepatitis. Radiology 128:163–164, 1978.

53. Geddes EW, Falskon G: Differential diagnosis of primary malignant hepatoma in 569 Bantu mineworkers. Cancer 31:1216–1221, 1973.

54. Genant HK, Hoffer PB: False-positive liver scan due to lung abscess. J Nucl Med 13:945–946, 1972.

55. George EA, Henry RE, Newton WT: Mechanisms of ^{99m}technetium sulfur colloid by the lung and kidney following disseminated intravascular coagulation. Clin Nucl Med 5:241–244, 1980.

56. Geslien GE, Pinsky SM, Poth RK, et al: The sensitivity and specificity of Tc-99m-sulfur colloid liver imaging in diffuse hepatocellular disease. Radiology 118:115–119, 1976.

57. Ghadimi H, Sass-Kortsak A: Evaluation of the radioactive rose bengal test for the differential diagnosis of obstructive jaundice in infants. N Eng J Med 265:351–358, 1961.

58. Gilday DL, Alderson PO: Scintigraphic evaluation of liver and spleen injury. Sem Nucl Med 4:357–370, 1974.

59. Go RT, Tonami N, Schapiro RL, et al: The manifestations of diaphragmatic and juxtadiaphragmatic disease in the liver-spleen scintigraph. Radiology 115:119–127, 1975.

60. Goldberg M, Thompson CM: Acute fatty metamorphosis of the liver. Ann Int Med 55:416–432, 1961.

61. Good LI, Alavi A, Trotman BW, et al: Hemangiomas: Pitfalls in scintigraphic detection.

Gastroent 74:752–758, 1978.

62. Gooneratne NS, Buse MG, Quinn JL, et al: Hot spot on hepatic scintigraphy and radio-nuclide venacavography. Am J Roentgenol 129:447–459, 1977.

63. Gooneratne NS, Quinn JL: Hepatic left lobe lesions—clinical usefulness of multiple imaging techniques to increase lesion detectability. Clin Nucl Med 2:377–380, 1977.

64. Greditzer HG, Ho JE, Wolverson M, et al: A benign cause of increased radiocolloid accumulation on a liver scan. Am J Roentgenol 132:289–290, 1979.

65. Greenwald L, Fajman W, Massie JD: An unusual scintigraphic pattern in glycogen storage disease-type one. Clin Nucl Med 6:424, 1981.

66. Guy JT, Auslander MO: Androgenic steroids and hepatocellular carcinoma. Lancet 1:148, 1973.

67. Ham JM: Segmental and lobar atrophy of the liver. Surg Gyn Obst 139:840–844, 1974.

68. Hanelin LG, Uszler JM, Sommer DG: Liver scan "hot spot" in hepatic veno-occlusive disease. Radiology 117:637–638, 1975.

69. Hatfield PM: Scan appearance of the hilus of the liver. Lahey Clinic Foundation Bulletin 26:25–30, 1977.

70. Hattner RS, Shames DM: Non-specificity of the radiocolloid hepatic "hot spot" for superior vena caval obstruction. J Nucl Med 15:1041–1043, 1974.

71. Heck LL, Gottschalk A: The appearance of intrahepatic biliary duct dilation on the liver scan. Radiology 99:135–140, 1971.

72. Helbig HD: Focal iatrogenic increased radiocolloid uptake on liver scan. J Nucl Med 14:354–355, 1973.

73. Hernberg JG, Braunstein P, Chandra E, et al: Artifacts in ^{99m}Tc-sulfur colloid liver scan. J Nucl Med 12:697–698, 1971.

74. Henke CE, Wolff JM, Shafer RB: Vascular dynamics in liver scan "hot spot." Clin Nucl Med 3:267–270, 1978.

75. Herbst KD, Corder MP: Radiotherapy-induced liver scan defects. J Nucl Med 17:424–425, 1976.

76. Herbst KD, Corder MP, Morita ET: Hepatic scan defects following radiotherapy for lymphoma. Clin Nucl Med 3:331–333, 1978.

76A. Hinkle GH, Leonard JC, Krous HF: Absence of hepatic uptake of Tc-99m sulfur colloid in an infant with Coxsackie B_2 viral infection. Clin Nucl Med 8:246–248, 1983.

77. Holder LE, Nishiyama H: Hepatoma associated with anabolic steroid therapy. Am J Roentgenol 124:638–642, 1975.

78. Holder LE, Saenger EL: The use of nuclear medicine in evaluating liver disease. Sem Roentgenol 10:215–222, 1975.

79. Holmquist DL, Burdine JA: Caval-portal shunting as a cause of focal increase in radiocolloid uptake in normal livers. J Nucl Med 14:348–351, 1973.

80. Howell MG, Diddle AW, Jones FS: Hepatic metastases from genital cancer: Diagnosis by scanning with radioactive gold. Am J Obstet Gyn 100:1008–1011, 1968.

81. Hungerford GD, Hamlyn ADN, Lunzer MR, et al: Pseudo-metastases in the liver: A presentation of the Budd-Chiari syndrome. Radiology 120:627–628, 1976.

82. Imarisio JJ: Liver scan showing intense lung uptake in neoplasia and infection. J Nucl Med 16:188–190, 1975.

83. Ishak KG, Rabin L: Benign tumors of the liver. Med Clin North Am 59:995–1013, 1975.

84. Izahr M: Pectus excavatum causing a false-positive defect in the liver. Clin Nucl Med 2:392–394, 1977.

85. Jhingran SG, Mukhopadhyay AK, Ajamani SK, et al: Hepatic adenomas and focal nodu-

lar hyperplasia of the liver in young women on oral contraceptives: case report. J Nucl Med 18:263–266, 1977.

86. Jochimsen PR, Platz CE, Pearlman NW: Hematoma of liver: A lesion mimicking hepatic neoplasm. J Surg Oncol 9:579–586, 1977.

87. Johnson PK, Babb RR: Cholangiocarcinoma in a patient previously given Thorotrast. Am J Digest Dis 20:384–390, 1975.

88. Johnson PM, Grossman FM, Atkins HL: Radiation induced injury. Its detection by scintillation scanning. Am J Roentgenol 99:453–462, 1967.

89. Johnson PM, Sweeney WA: The false-positive hepatic scan. J Nucl Med 8:451–460, 1967.

90. Johnson RA, Hladik WB: Post-traumatic pulmonary accumulation of Tc-99m sulfur colloid. J Nucl Med 23:147–148, 1982.

91. Joo KG, Carter JE: Extrinsic lesions simulating hepatic metastases. Clin Nucl Med 3:108–129, 1978.

92. Joyner JT: Abnormal liver scan (radiocolloid "hot spot") associated with superior vena caval obstruction. J Nucl Med 13:849–851, 1972.

93. Kaplan WD, Drum DE, Lokich JJ: The effect of cancer chemotherapeutic agents on the liver-spleen scan. J Nucl Med 21:84–87, 1980.

94. Karohara SS, Swensson JL, Usselman JA, et al: Response and recovery of liver to radiation as demonstrated by photoscans. Radiology 89:229–235, 1967.

95. Kaude JV, DeLand F: Hepatomegaly. Med Clin North Am 59:145–167, 1975.

96. Keyes JW, Wilson GA, Quinones JD: An evaluation of lung uptake of colloid during liver imaging. J Nucl Med 14:687–691, 1973.

97. Klingensmith WC, Datu JA, Burdick DC: Renal uptake of ^{99m}Tc-sulfur colloid in congestive heart failure. Radiology 127:185–187, 1978.

98. Klingensmith WC, Eikman EA, Maumenee I, et al: Widespread abnormalities of radiocolloid distribution in patients with mucopolysaccharidosis. J Nucl Med 16:1002–1004, 1975.

99. Klingensmith WC, Ryerson TW: Lung uptake of ^{99m}Tc-sulfur colloid. J Nucl Med 14:201–204, 1973.

100. Klingensmith WC, Ryerson TW, Corman JL: Lung uptake of ^{99m}Tc-sulfur colloid in organ transplantation. J Nucl Med 14:757–759, 1973.

101. Klingensmith WC, Tsan M-F, Wagner HN: Factors affecting the uptake of ^{99m}Tc-sulfur colloid by the lung and kidney. J Nucl Med 17:681–684, 1976.

102. Klingensmith WC, Yang SL, Wagner HN: Lung uptake of Tc-99m sulfur colloid in liver and spleen imaging. J Nucl Med 19:31–35, 1978.

103. Klion FM, Rudavsky AX: False-positive liver scans in patients with alcoholic liver disease. Ann Int Med 69:283–291, 1968.

104. Koenigsberg M, Freeman LM: Intrahepatic focal lesion in acute viral hepatitis. J Nucl Med 14:612–614, 1973.

105. Krell L, Jones EA, Tavill AS: Comparative study of arteriography and scintillation scanning in space-occupying lesions of liver. Br J Radiol 41:401–411, 1968.

106. Kuni CC, Klingensmith WC: Renal uptake of ^{99m}technetium sulfur colloid accumulation in canine renal allograft during hyperacute rejection. Int J Nucl Biol Med 19:213–220, 1975.

107. Lee HK, Jones L: Subphrenic abscess mimicking intrahepatic defect in a lung-liver scan. Clin Nucl Med 1:207, 1976.

108. Levine RA: Amyloid disease of the liver. Am J Med 33:349–357, 1962.

109. Levitt RG, Segal SS, Stanley RJ, et al: Accuracy of computed tomography of liver and

biliary tract. Radiology 124:123–128, 1977.

109A. Li YP, Morin ME, Tan A: Bipartite liver as a cause of ^{99m}Tc liver scan defect. Appl Radiol 11:97–98, 1982.

110. Lichtman SS, in: Disease of the Liver, Gallbladder and Bile Ducts. Philadelphia: Lea and Febiger, 1949, p. 169.

111. Lin CS, Lee HK: Abnormal liver scan in periarteritis nodosa. Mt Sinai J of Med 45:184–186, 1978.

112. Ludwig J, Hoffman HN: Hemangiosarcoma of the liver. Mayo Clin Proc 50:255–263, 1975.

113. Lunia S, Chodos RB, Chandrakanta L: Wilms' tumor simulating metastatic lesion in anterior hepatic scintigram. Clin Nucl Med 3:32, 1978.

114. Makk L, Creech JL, Whelan JG, et al: Liver damage and angiosarcoma in vinyl chloride workers. JAMA 230:64–68, 1974.

115. Mayle JE, Caldwell JH: False-positive liver scan due to a thin left hepatic lobe. J Clin Gastroent 2:165–167, 1980.

116. McAfee JG, Ause RG, Wagner HH: Diagnostic value of scintillation scanning of the liver. Follow-up of 1,000 studies. Arch Int Med 116:95–110, 1965.

117. McAvoy JM, Tompkins RK, Longmire WP Jr.: Benign hepatic tumors and their association with oral contraceptives. Arch Surg 111:761–767, 1976.

118. McClelland RR: Focal porta hepatis scintiscan defects: What is their significance? J Nucl Med 16:1007–1012, 1975.

119. McClelland RR, Kapsner AL, Uecker JH: Pulmonary sequestration associated with a gastric duplication cyst. Radiology 124:13–14, 1977.

120. McCready VR: Scintigraphic studies of space-occupying liver disease. Sem Nucl Med 2:108–127, 1972.

121. McDonald MW, Dubovsky EV, Luna RD, et al: Liver-kidney relationship in radioisotopic localization of retrohepatic and subhepatic masses. So Med J 71:389–391, 1978.

122. McLoughlin MJ, Colapinto RF, Gilday DL, et al: Focal nodular hyperplasia of the liver. Radiology 107:257–263, 1973.

123. McLoughlin MJ, Gilday DL: Angiography and colloid scanning of benign mass lesions of liver. Clin Radiol 23:377–391, 1972.

124. Meindok H, Langer B: Liver scan in Budd-Chiari syndrome. J Nucl Med 17:365–368, 1976.

125. Merchant FJ: Multiloculated cystadenoma of the liver. Illinois Med J 144:129–130, 1973.

126. Mettler FA, Christie JH: Another cause of the hepatic "hot spot": isolated innominate vein obstruction. Clin Nucl Med 5:514–515, 1980.

127. Mettler FA, Christie JH: Focal lung uptake of Tc-99m-sulfur colloid. Clin Nucl Med 6:332–333, 1981.

128. Mettler FA Jr., Shea WH Jr., Guiberteau MJ, et al: Improvement in visualization of hepatic lesions with upright views. J Nucl Med 18:1128–1130, 1977.

129. Myerson PJ: Focal porta hepatis defect on nuclide imaging. J Nucl Med 18:944–949, 1977.

130. Mikolajkow A, Jasinski WK: Increased focal uptake of radiocolloid by the liver. J Nucl Med 14:175, 1973.

131. Milder MS, Larson SM, Bagley CM, et al: Liver-spleen scan in Hodgkin's disease. Cancer 31:826–834, 1973.

132. Milder MS, Larson SM, Swann EJ, et al: False-positive liver scan due to breast prosthesis. J Nucl Med 14:189, 1973.

133. Morita ET, McCormack KR, Weisberg RL: Further information on a "hot spot" in the liver. J Nucl Med 14:606–608, 1973.

134. Morris JG, McRae J, Perkins KW, et al: Liver scanning in obstructive jaundice using a colloidal radiogold. J Coll Radiol Australasia 9:68–77, 1965.

135. Mouls RF: An investigation of the variations in normal liver shape. Br J Radiol 45:586–590, 1972.

136. Muroff LR, Johnson PM: The use of multiple radionuclide imaging to differentiate the focal intrahepatic lesion. Am J Roentgenol 121:728–734, 1974.

137. Murphy JF, Wade-Evans T: Drug resistant choriocarcinoma presenting with hepatomegaly. J Irish Med Assoc 66:350–353, 1973.

138. Nagler W, Bender MA, Blau M: Radioisotope photoscanning of liver. Gastroenterology 44:36–43, 1963.

139. O'Donnell TA: Liver scanning for extra-hepatic tumors. Am J Roentgenol 90:1063–1067, 1963.

140. O'Mara RE, McAfee JG: Scintillation scanning in the diagnosis of hepatic abscess in children. J Pediatr 77:211–215, 1970.

141. Otero E: ^{198}Au liver scanning in hepatic amebic disease. J Nucl Med 9:406, 1968.

142. Park CH, Garafola JH, O'Hara AE: Preoperative diagnosis of asymptomatic choledochal cyst by rose bengal liver scan. J Nucl Med 15:310–311, 1974.

143. Park CH, Mansfield CM: Pseudodefect in 99m-Tc-sulfur colloid liver scan caused by hepatodiaphragmatic interposition. J Natl Med Assoc 67:126–127, 1975.

144. Park FC, Bjelland JC, Patton DD, et al: Case of the Month #29. Arizona Med 35:185–186, 1978.

145. Pasquier J, Dorta T: Focal hyperfixation of radiocolloid by the liver. J Nucl Med 15:725, 1974.

146. Patton DD: Liver and spleen scanning in children. Recent advances in nuclear medicine: Technical and clinical aspects. Continuing Education Lectures, SE Chapter, Society of Nuclear Medicine, 1975, pp. 5–34.

147. Platthy A, Shah U: False-positive scintigrams due to malposition of the liver. J Nucl Med 15:717–719, 1974.

148. Popper H, Schaffner F, in: Liver: Structure and Function. New York: McGraw-Hill, 1957, p. 667.

149. Preisig R, Morris TO, Shaver JC: Volumetric, hemodynamic and excretory characteristics of liver in acromegaly. J Clin Invest 45:1379–1387, 1966.

150. Rabinowitz JG, Kinkabwala M, Ulreich S: Macro-regenerating nodule in the cirrhotic liver. Am J Roentgenol 121:401–411, 1974.

151. Raghavaiah NV: False positive findings on liver scans in carcinoma of kidney. Urology 12:733–734, 1978.

152. Ramsby GR, Henken EM, Spencer RP: Enlarged portal vein causing abnormality on hepatic dynamic and static images. Clin Nucl Med 3:301, 1978.

153. Raouf R, Stebner FC: Case report: Pseudo-tumor of the liver in hepatitis. JAMA 29:262–264, 1974.

154. Rockett JF, Miller KD: Multiple radionuclide demonstration of a pancreatic pseudocyst. So Med J 67:120–121, 1974.

155. Roger QI, Feiss JS: The application of liver scan to the diagnosis of esophageal varices. So Med J 63:950–953, 1970.

156. Rosch J, Mayer BS, Campbell JR, et al: "Vascular" benign liver cyst in children. Report of two cases. Radiology 126:747–750, 1978.

157. Rosenfield N, Griscom NT: Choledochal cysts: roentgenographic techniques. Radiology

114:113–119, 1975.

158. Rosenthal, SN: Are hepatic scans overused? Am J Digest Dis 21:659–663, 1976.

159. Ryo UY, Siddiqi A, Yu HA, et al: Focal defect due to renal impression in anterior liver imaging. Clin Nucl Med 1:64–69, 1976.

160. Sachs BA, Bardfeld PA, Bodian JE, et al: Liver scan in hyperlipoproteinemia. JAMA 227:907–910, 1974.

161. Sackett JF, Mosenthal WT, House RK, et al: Scintillation scanning of liver cell adenoma. Am J Roentgenol 113:56–60, 1971.

162. Salvo AP, Schiller A, Athanasoulis C, et al: Hepatoadenoma and focal nodular hyperplasia: Pitfalls in radiocolloid imaging. Radiology 125:451–455, 1977.

163. Salzman SH, Burke G: The differential diagnosis of giant liver. Am J Gastro 47:221–229, 1967.

164. Sandler MS, Park CH, Lin D: "Hot spot" on liver scan due to tricuspid insufficiency. Clin Nucl Med 5:494–496, 1980.

164A. Sayle BA, Helmer RE, Balachandran S, et al: Lung uptake of ^{99m}Tc-sulfur colloid secondary to androgen therapy in patients with anemia. Nucl Med Communication 2:289–293, 1981.

165. Schiff L: Diseases of the Liver. Philadelphia: J.B. Lippincott, 1963, pp. 189–589, 618.

166. Schmitte E, Appleman H, Threatt B: Sarcoidosis in children. Radiology 106:621–625, 1973.

167. Schulz RC, Shields JB, Fletcher JW, et al: Liver scanning and the intrahepatic gallbladder. J Nucl Med 16:1029–1030, 1975.

168. Scott JH, Anderson CL, Shankar PS, et al: Alpha-antitrypsin deficiency with diffuse bronchiectasis and cirrhosis of the liver. Chest 71:535–538, 1977.

169. Seibert JJ, Soper RT: Preoperative diagnosis of benign hepatic hamartoma by correlation of radioisotope and angiographic studies. Ped Radiol 4:149–152, 1976.

170. Seymour QE, Puckett SE, Edwards J: Pseudo abnormal liver scan secondary to residual barium in the bowel. Am J Roentgenol 107:54–56, 1969.

171. Shanser JD, Korobkin M, Hattner RS, et al: Bifurcation of the portal vein appearing as a focal defect on the liver image. Radiology 114:399–401, 1975.

172. Sharp JD: Functional hepatoma demonstrated with rose bengal scanning. Am J Roentgenol 107:51–53, 1969.

173. Sherlock S, in: Disease of the Liver and Biliary System. Philadelphia: F.A. Davis Co., 1963, 3rd Ed., pp. 7, 436.

174. Shih W-J, Nolan NG: False-positive liver scan due to spine deformity. J Nucl Med 21:808–809, 1980.

175. Shirley H, Font RG, Bresler EH, et al: Perihepatic hematoma. Am J Gastroent 50:387–390, 1968.

176. Siegelman SS: Caution in interpreting liver scan in the presence of hypernephroma. J Urol 114:481–482, 1975.

177. Slivis TL, Berdon WE, Haller JO, et al: Hemangiomas of the liver in infants. Am J Roentgenol 123:791–801, 1975.

178. Smith FW, Brown RG, Ash JM, et al: Accumulation of Tc-99m-sulfur colloid by the lung and kidney following disseminated intravascular coagulation. Clin Nucl Med 5:241–244, 1980.

179. Spencer RP, Knowlton AH: Redistribution of radiocolloid uptake after focal hepatic radiation. Oncology 32:266–268, 1975.

180. Spencer RP, Turner JW, Sued IB: Residual splenic function in the presence of thorotrast-associated hepatic tumor. J Nucl Med 17:200–202, 1976.

181. Stadalnik RC: "Hot spots"—liver imaging. Sem Nucl Med 9:220–221, 1979.
182. Stanley P, Gates GP, Eto TR, et al: Hepatic cavernous hemangiomas in infancy. Am J Roentgenol 129:317–321, 1977.
183. Sty JR, Babbitt DP: Perforated appendicitis presenting as a focal hepatic defect. Clin Nucl Med 4:209–211, 1979.
184. Sty JR, Starshak RJ: Scintigraphy in Wolman's disease. Clin Nucl Med 3:395–396, 1978.
185. Sty JR, Sullivan P, Wagner R, et al: Hepatic scintigraphy in Caroli's disease. Radiology 127:732–746, 1978.
186. Sugahara K, Shirakura T, Kawano N, et al: Primary malignant hemangioendothelioma of the liver. Am J Gastroen 62:240–244, 1974.
187. Suzuki K, Okuda K, Mush H, et al: False-positive liver scan caused by anomalous quadrate lobe and right portal branch. Acta Hepato-Gastroenterol 24:27–29, 1977.
188. Suzuki K, Okuda K, Yoshida T, et al: False-positive liver scan in a patient with hepatic amyloidosis. J Nucl Med 17:31–32, 1976.
189. Taylor RD, Anderson PM, Winston MA, et al: Diagnosis of hepatic hemangioma using multiple radionuclide and ultrasound techniques. J Nucl Med 17:362–364, 1976.
190. Tefft M, Mitus A, Das L, et al: Irradiation of the liver in children: Review of experience in the acute and chronic phases, and in the intact normal and partially resected. Am J Roentgenol 108:365–385, 1970.
191. Thijs LG, Heidendal GAK, Huijgens PC, et al: The use of nuclear medicine procedures in the diagnosis of Budd-Chiari syndrome. Clin Nucl Med 3:389–392, 1978.
192. Thomas LB, Popper H, Berk PD, et al: Vinyl chloride-induced liver disease from idiopathic portal hypertension (Banti's syndrome) to angiosarcomas. N Eng J Med 292:17–24, 1975.
193. Tinglestad JB, Howell TR, Sharpe AR: Case report: Diagnosis of omphalocele and diaphragmatic hernia and hepatopericardium using 99m-Tc-sulfur colloid. J Nucl Med 15:42–44, 1974.
194. Vadas M, McLaughlan AF, Morris JG: Emergency evaluation of liver trauma using the gamma camera. M J Australia 1:56–58, 1973.
195. Valdez VA, Herrera NE: Granulomatous hepatitis: Spectrum of scintigraphic manifestations. Clin Nucl Med 3:393–395, 1978.
196. Vaugh WP, Wilcox PM, Alderson PD, et al: Hepatic toxicity of adjuvant chemotherapy for carcinoma of the heart. Med Pediatr Oncol 7:315–359, 1979.
197. Volpe JA, Johnston GS: "Hot" hepatic hemangioma. A unique radiocolloid-concentration liver scan lesion. J Surg Oncol 2:373–377, 1970.
198. Volpe JA, Morita ET, Johnston GS: The false-positive technetium-99m hepatic scintiscan. J Surg Oncol 1:345–350, 1969.
199. Walker WA, Mathis RK: Hepatomegaly: An approach to differential diagnosis. Ped Clin N Am 22:929–942, 1975.
200. Waxman AD: Scintigraphic manifestations of diffuse hepatic disease. Sem Nucl Med 12:75–85, 1982.
201. Weichert RP III, Cerise EJ, Travieso CR: Atrophy of the right lobe of the liver: Case report and review of the syndromes associated with atrophy or agenesis of the liver. Am Surg 36:667–673, 1970.
202. Weinraub JM: False-positive liver scan caused by dilated splenic vein. J Nucl Med 15:142–143, 1974.
203. Whelan JG, Creech JL, Tamburro CH: Angiographic and radionuclide characteristics of hepatic angiosarcoma found in vinyl chloride workers. Radiology 118:549–557, 1976.

204. White WL, Wahner HW, Brown ML, et al: Sequential liver imaging in the hypereosinophilic syndrome. Clin Nucl Med 6:75–77, 1981.

204A. Williams AG, Christie JH, Mettler FA: Ascites causing a false-positive radionuclide liver image. Clin Nucl Med 8:76–77, 1983.

205. Williams LE, Fisher JH, Courtney RA, et al: Preoperative diagnosis of choledochal cyst by hepatoscintography. N Eng J Med 283:85–86, 1970.

206. Winston MA: Pseudotumors in acute hepatitis. J Nucl Med 16:799–800, 1975.

207. Winston MA, Karelitz J, Weiss ER, et al: Variation in the appearance of the lateral liver scan with patient position. Radiology 102:665–666, 1972.

208. Yeh C, Strashun A, Goldsmith SJ: Severe atrophy of right hepatic lobe simulating right hepatic lobectomy. Clin Nucl Med 6:523–524, 1981.

209. Yeh EL, Pohlmann GP, Meade RC: Liver-heart imaging in evaluating hepatic focal defect. J Nucl Med 16:896–898, 1975.

210. Yeh SH, Shih WJ, Liang JC: Intravenous radionuclide hepatography in differential diagnosis of intrahepatic mass lesions. J Nucl Med 14:565–567, 1973.

211. Yeung WC, Haines JE, Larson SM: Diagnosis of posterolateral congenital diaphragmatic (Bochdalek) hernia by liver scintigram: case report. J Nucl Med 17:110–112, 1976.

212. Ziessman HA: Lung uptake of ^{99m}Tc-sulfur colloid in falciparum malaria. J Nucl Med 17:794–796, 1976.

213. Zipser RD, Rau JE, Ricketts RR, et al: Tuberculous pseudo-tumors of the liver. Am J Med 61:946–951, 1976.

Chapter 29

Hepatobiliary Imaging[†]

EDWARD B. SILBERSTEIN

RUPPERT DAVID

HIROSHI NISHIYAMA

I. Nonvisualized gall bladder (over 24 hours)

   A. Common

      1. Acute cholecystitis (13, 25, 47)

The use of an asterisk * in this chapter indicates that this entity has been observed by one of the authors but the case report has not been published.

[†]Hepatobiliary imaging with ^{99m}Tc-HIDA compounds or ^{131}I-rose bengal.

      2. Chronic cholecystitis (11, 13, 25)

B. Less common

      1. Other conditions related to cystic duct obstruction (25, 32, 37)

          a. sclerosing cholangitis with cystic duct obstruction

          b. biliary atresia

          c. pancreatic carcinoma (11, 13)

      2. Absent gall bladder (13, 41, 42)

          a. congenital

          b. post-surgical

      3. Acute pancreatitis (11, 12)

      4. Penetrating ulcer disease (11)

      5. Cancer of gall bladder*

      6. T-tube bypass of cystic duct*

      7. Alcoholism (35)

      8. With total parenteral nutrition (35)

C. Rare

      1. Rotor syndrome (1)

      2. Dubin-Johnson syndrome (1)

      3. Hydrops of gall bladder with Kawasaki disease (18)

      4. Nicotinic acid toxicity (50)

II. Delayed visualization of gall bladder (over 1 hour)

A. Common

      1. Cholecystitis

          a. chronic cholecystitis (12, 25, 26, 32, 47)

          b. acute cholecystitis (44)

      2. Hepatocellular disease (i.e., hepatitis, post necrotic cirrhosis) (13, 26)

      3. Partial biliary obstruction

          a. pancreatic carcinoma (11, 13)

          b. enlarged lymph nodes (lymphoma) (47)

          c. surgically altered biliary and gastrointestinal anatomy, (e.g., Billroth II) (31)

          d. alcoholic pancreatitis (26)

      4. After meals (within 1 hour) (25)

B. Uncommon

      1. Dubin-Johnson syndrome (1)

III. Delayed visualization of gastrointestinal tract (over 1 hour)

A. Common

      1. Partial obstruction

          a. pancreatic carcinoma (13)

          b. choledocholithiasis (13, 32)

          c. intrahepatic cholestasis (29)

    2. Hepatocellular disease (e.g., hepatitis) (13, 32)

    3. Preferential gall bladder filling (13, 14)

        a. post-vagotomy (13)

        b. prolonged fasting (13, 24)

        c. functional common duct obstruction

            (1) enhanced tone of sphincter of Oddi (14)

            (2) narcotics (codeine, meperidine, morphine) (2, 46)

        d. chronic cholecystitis (14)

        e. Gilbert's disease (13)

    4. Acute pancreatitis (12, 30)

    5. Ampullitis (14)

IV. Enlarged gall bladder

    A. Common

        1. Preferential gall bladder filling (see Section III,A,3 above)

        2. Partial common duct obstruction*

    B. Uncommon

        1. Acromegaly (8)

V. Nonvisualized gastrointestinal tract (over 24 hours)

    A. Common

        1. Common duct stone (48)

        2. Ascending cholangitis (48)

        3. Severe hepatitis (13, 32)

        4. Intrahepatic cholestasis (30, 43)

        5. Other severe hepatocellular disease (13, 26)

        6. Carcinoma of pancreas (48)

        7. Ligation of biliary duct during surgery (13, 30, 37)

        8. Common hepatic duct carcinoma (48)

        9. Common duct stricture (48)

    B. Uncommon

        1. Biliary atresia (37)

VI. Dilated common duct and normal visualization of gastrointestinal tract

    A. Common

        1. Partial obstruction (29)

        2. Post-cholecystectomy (48)

        3. Post-cholangiointestinal anastomosis (29)

    B. Uncommon

        1. Caroli's disease (32)

        2. Choledochal cyst (32)

    3. Oriental cholangiohepatitis with intrahepatic cholelithiasis (52)

    4. Congenital hepatic fibrosis (22)

    5. Falsely abnormal if concentration of ^{99m}Tc-IDA is unusually high (20)

VII. Focal defects in abnormal liver with ^{99m}Tc-IDA uptake in defect never seen

  A. Common
    1. Hepatoma (4, 49)
    2. Metastases (4, 49)
    3. Abscess (49)
    4. Cysts (4, 49)
    5. Hematoma (49)
  B. Uncommon
    1. Polycystic liver (4)
    2. Hemangioma (4)

VIII. Abnormal extrahepatic, non-intestinal foci of radioactivity

  A. Common
    1. Renal activity with failure of liver excretion (47)
      a. common duct obstruction
      b. severe hepatocellular disease
  B. Uncommon
    1. Choledochal cyst (53)
    2. Bile leakage (7, 30, 31, 45, 48)
      a. post-surgical (48)
      b. post-traumatic (45)
      c. bile leak secondary to malignant invasion (48)
      d. gall bladder perforation (5)
      e. into a hepatic abscess (16)
      f. bronchobiliary fistula (2A)
    3. Lung metastasis of hepatoma (6)
    4. Displaced common duct (e.g., secondary to uriniferous perirenal pseudocyst of kidney) (37)
    5. Pyeloureterectasis (17A)

IX. Abnormal intestinal location of radiopharmaceutical shortly before or after biliary excretion

  A. Uncommon
    1. Gastric reflux, especially post biliary-intestinal anastomosis (12)
    2. Cystic duct remnant (48)
    3. Ureter simulating common duct (36A)
  B. Rare
    1. Cholecysto-colic fistula (54)

   2. Duodenal diverticulum simulating gall bladder (3, 48)

X. Blood pool abnormalities on early imaging (49)

   A. Common
   1. Cardiomegaly
   2. Pericardial effusion
   B. Less common
   1. Aneurysm
   2. Splenomegaly
   3. Renal enlargement
      a. hydronephrosis
   4. Hydroureter

XI. Radiopharmaceutical uptake in areas of parenchymal liver tissue with little or no reticuloendothelial function

   A. Common
   1. Prominent or dilated hepatobiliary system (4, 17, 22)
      a. hepatic duct
      b. gall bladder
   2. Intra-hepatic gall bladder (34)
   3. Hepatic adenoma (2, 33)
   4. Hepatocellular carcinoma (39, 40)
   5. Cirrhosis with regenerative nodules (6)
   6. Focal nodular hyperplasia (33)
   7. Alcoholic liver disease (27)
   B. Uncommon
   1. Dilated hepatobiliary system (17)
      a. Caroli's disease
      b. choledochal cyst
      c. hepatic duct diverticulum
   2. Bile leak into liver laceration (17)
   3. Encapsulated extrahepatic bile (17)
   4. Hepatitis (17)
   5. Liver abscess communicating with biliary system (17)
   6. Hepatic cystadenoma (17)
   7. Following hepatic radiation (14A)
   8. Trisegmentectomy for removal of metastatic colon carcinoma (15B)
   9. *Schistosoma mansoni* infestation (37A)

XII. Adequate reticuloendothelial function with poor ^{99m}Tc-IDA uptake by parenchymal cells

   A. Uncommon

1. Obstructive jaundice
   a. metastatic cancer (15A)
   b. biliary atresia (15B)
      (1) with Kasai procedure (15B)
   c. biliary cirrhosis (15B)
2. Diffuse hepatocellular disorders
   a. right lobectomy following trauma (15B)
   b. liver transplant (15B)
   c. hepatitis (Type B; non-A, non-B) (7A)
   d. jaundice secondary to sepsis from a non-hepatic focus (7A)

REFERENCES

1. Bar-Mein S, Baron J, Seligson U, et al: ^{99m}Tc-HIDA cholescintigraphy in Dubin-Johnson and Rotor syndromes. Radiology 142:743–746, 1982.
2. Belter AJ, Grijm R, VanderSchout JB: Hepatic adenoma: imaging with different radionuclides. Clin Nucl Med 4:375–378, 1979.
2A. Blue PW, Versteeg HJ, Cole FN: Bronchobiliary fistula. Clin Nucl Med 8:272–273, 1983.
3. Brown JF, Buchanan JW, Wagner HN: Pitfalls in technetium-99m HIDA biliary imaging: duodenal diverticulum simulating the gall bladder. J Nucl Med 22:747–748, 1981.
4. Brown ML, Freitas JE, Wahner HW: Useful hepatic parenchymal imaging in hepatobiliary scintigraphy. Am J Roentgenol 136:893–895, 1981.
5. Brunnetti JC, Van Heentum RL: Preoperative detection of gall bladder perforation. Clin Nucl Med 5:348–349, 1980.
6. Cannon JR, Long RF, Berens SV, et al: Uptake of Tc-99m PIPIDA in pulmonary metastases from a hepatoma. Clin Nucl Med 5:22–24, 1980.
7. Cheng TH, Davis MA, Seltzer SE, et al: Evaluation of hepatobiliary imaging by radionuclide scintigraphy, ultrasonography, and contrast cholangiography. Radiology 133:761–767, 1979.
7A. Coel MN, Denzer S: Disparate images in acute hepatitis using E-HIDA and sulfur colloid. Clin Nucl Med 7:315–317, 1982.
8. Cohen GA, Smoak WM, Goldberg LD: Acromegalic cholecystomegaly. J Nucl Med 15:720–721, 1974.
9. Eaton SB, Ferrucci JT, Handmaker H, et al: Radiologic diagnosis of extrahepatic biliary obstruction in jaundiced patients. Am J Gastroenterology 58:477–490, 1972.
10. Eikman EA: Teaching Editorial: Radionuclide hepatobiliary procedures: when can HIDA help? J Nucl Med 4:358–361, 1979.
11. Fonseca C, Greenberg D, Rosenthall L, et al: Assessment of the utility of gall bladder imaging with ^{99m}Tc-IDA. Clin Nucl Med 3:437–441, 1978.
12. Fonseca C, Greenberg D, Rosenthall L, et al: ^{99m}Tc-IDA imaging in the differential diagnosis of acute cholecystitis and acute pancreatitis. Radiology 130:525–527, 1979.
13. Fonseca C, Rosenthall L, Greenberg D, et al: Differential diagnosis of jaundice by ^{99m}Tc-IDA hepatobiliary imaging. Clin Nucl Med 4:135–142, 1979.
14. Freitas JE: Cholescintigraphy in acute and chronic cholecystitis. Sem Nucl Med 12:18–26, 1982.
14A. Gelfand MJ, Saha S, Aron B: Imaging of irradiated liver with Tc-99m sulfur colloid and Tc-99m-IDA. Clin Nucl Med 6:399–402, 1982.

15. Jenner RE, Howard ER, Clarke MB, et al: Hepatobiliary imaging: the use of [99mTc]-pyridoxylidene glutamate scanning in jaundiced adults and infants. Br J Radiol 51:862–866, 1978.
15A. Kim EE, Domstad PA, Choy YC: Complementary role of reticuloendothelial and hepatobiliary imaging agents in the assessment of liver disease. Clin Nucl Med 7:64–66, 1982.
15B. Klingensmith WC, Fritzberg AR, Zerbe GO, et al: Relative role of Tc-99m-diethyl-IDA and Tc-99m-sulfur colloid in the evaluation of liver function. Clin Nucl Med 5:341–346, 1980.
16. Klingensmith WC, Koep LJ, Fritzberg AR: Bile leak into a hepatic abscess in a liver transplant: demonstration with [99mTc]-diethyl-iminodiacetic acid. Am J Roentgenol 131:889–891, 1978.
17. Lamki L: A dichotomy in hepatic uptake of [99mTc]-IDA and [99mTc]-colloid. Sem Nucl Med 12:92–94, 1982.
17A. Lecklither ML, Flournoy JG, Ware RW: Hepatobiliary imaging: Pyeloureterectasis. J Nucl Med 24:450–451, 1983.
18. Liebmann LI, Mikelic V, Joh MM, et al: Hydrops of the gall bladder in an adult with Kawasaki disease. JAMA 247:827–829, 1982.
19. Lim RE, Dubovsky EV, Tim LO, et al: Morphine-prostigmine test: effect on Tc-99m Disida cholescintigraphy. Clin Nucl Med 7:213–214, 1982.
20. Lisbona R, Wexler MJ, Novales-Diaz JA: Misleading appearance of biliary dilatation. J Can Assoc Radiol 31:67–68, 1980.
21. Mall JC, Ghahremani GG, Boyer JL: Caroli's disease associated with congenital hepatic fibrosis and renal tubular ectasia. Gastroenterology 66:1029–1035, 1974.
22. Masuda Y, Sawa H, Kim OH, et al: A case of congenital hepatic fibrosis. Clin Nucl Med 5:359–361, 1980.
23. Matolo NM, Stadalnik RC, Wolfman EF: Clinical evaluation of [99mTc]-pyridoxylidene-glutamate for hepatobiliary scanning. Am J Surg 132:716–719, 1976.
24. Nordyke RA: Metabolic and physiologic aspects of [131I] rose bengal in studying liver function. Sem Nucl Med 2:157–166, 1972.
25. Pare P, Shaffer EA, Rosenthall L: Nonvisualization of the gall bladder by [99mTc]-HIDA cholescintigraphy as evidence of cholecystitis. Canada Med Assoc J 118:384–386, 1978.
26. Pauwels S, Steels M, Piret L, et al: Clinical evaluation of Tc-99m-diethyl-IDA in hepatobiliary disorders. J Nucl Med 19:783–788, 1978.
27. Rao BK, Weir GJ, Lieberman LM: Dissociation of reticuloendothelial cell and hepatocyte functions in alcoholic liver disease. Clin Nucl Med 6:289–294, 1981.
28. Richards AG, Brighouse R: Nicotinic acid—a cause of failed HIDA scanning. J Nucl Med 22:746–747, 1981.
29. Rosenthall L: Cholescintigraphy in the presence of jaundice utilizing Tc-IDA. Sem Nucl Med 12:53–63, 1982.
30. Rosenthall LM: Clinical experience with the new hepatobiliary radiopharmaceuticals. Canadian J Surg 21:297–300, 1978.
31. Rosenthall L, Fonseca C, Arzoumanian A, et al: [99mTc]-IDA hepatobiliary imaging following upper abdominal surgery. Radiology 130:735–739, 1979.
32. Rosenthall LR, Shaffer EA, Lisbona R, et al: Diagnosis of hepatobiliary disease by [99mTc]-HIDA cholescintigraphy. Radiology 126:467–474, 1978.
33. Salvo AF, Schiller A, Athanasoulis C, et al: Hepatoadenoma and focal nodular hyperplasia: Pitfalls in radiocolloid imaging. Radiology 125:451–455, 1977.
34. Schulz RC, Shields JB, Fletcher JW, et al: Liver scanning and the intrahepatic gall bladder. J Nucl Med 16:1029–1030, 1975.

35. Shuman WP, Gibbs P, Rudd TG, et al: PIPIDA scintigraphy for cholecystitis: false positives in alcoholism and total parenteral nutrition. Am J Roentgenol 138:1–5, 1982.

36. Silberstein EB: Teaching Editorial: Still more applications of hepatobiliary scintigraphy. J Nucl Med 21:99–100, 1980.

36A. Strickler S, Park HM: Pitfalls of cholescintigraphy. Clin Nucl Med 7:558–559, 1982.

37. Sty JR, Babbitt DP, Boedecker RA, et al: ^{99m}Tc-PIPIDA biliary imaging in children. Clin Nucl Med 4:315–324, 1979.

37A. Suresh K, Turner JW, Spencer RP, et al: Hepatic reticuloendothelial ''failure'' in *Schistosoma mansoni* infestation. Clin Nucl Med 2:163–165, 1977.

38. Taavitsainen M, Jarvinen H, Tallroth K: Cholescintigraphy in the diagnosis of acute cholecystitis. Ann Clin Res 10:227–234, 1978.

39. Ueno K, Haseda Y: Concentration and clearance of Tc-99m pyridoxylidene isoleucine by a hepatoma. Clin Nucl Med 5:196–199, 1980.

40. Utz JA, Lull RJ, Anderson JH, et al: Hepatoma visualization with Tc-99m pyridoxylidene glutamate. J Nucl Med 21:747–749, 1980.

41. Vaalasti T, Tuohimaa E: Congenital absence of the gall bladder. Annales Chirurgiae et Gynaecologiae Fenniae 59:235–237, 1970.

42. Verow PW, Wisbey M: Sequential liver and biliary tract scanning with ^{131}I rose bengal. Clin Radiol 26:499–504, 1975.

43. Wang CS, Chen PH, Siauw CP: Diagnosis of intrahepatic stone by Tc-99m-pyridoxylidene glutamate cholescintigram. J Formosan Med Assoc 77:525–532, 1978.

44. Weissmann HS, Badia J, Sugarman LA, et al: Spectrum of ^{99m}Tc-IDA cholescintigraphic patterns in acute cholecystitis. Radiology 138:167–175, 1981.

45. Weissmann HS, Chun KJ, Frank M, et al: Demonstration of traumatic bile leakage with cholescintigraphy and ultrasonography. Am J Roentgenol 133: 843–847, 1979.

46. Weissmann HS, Frank MS, Bernstein LH, et al: Rapid and accurate diagnosis of acute cholecystitis with ^{99m}Tc-HIDA cholescintigraphy. Am J Roentgenol 132:523–528, 1979.

47. Weissmann HS, Frank M, Rosenblatt R, et al: Cholescintigraphy, ultrasonography and computerized tomography in the evaluation of biliary tract disorders. Sem Nucl Med 9:22–35, 1979.

48. Weissmann HS, Gliedman ML, Wilk PH, et al: Evaluation of the post-operative patient with ^{99m}Tc-IDA cholescintigraphy. Sem Nucl Med 12:27–52, 1982.

49. Weissmann HS, Sugarman LA, Frank MS, et al: Serendipity in technetium-99m dimethyl iminodiacetic acid cholescintigraphy. Radiology 135:449–454, 1980.

50. Whiting EG, Nusynowitz ML: Radioactive rose bengal testing in the differential diagnosis of jaundice. Surg Gyn & Obst 127:729–733, 1968.

51. Winston MA, Blahd WH: ^{131}I rose bengal imaging techniques in differential diagnosis of jaundiced patients. Sem Nucl Med 2:167–175, 1972.

52. Yeh SH, Liu OK, Huang MJ: Sequential scintiphotography with technetium-99m pyridoxylidene glutamate in the detection of intrahepatic lithiasis. J Nucl Med 21:17–21, 1980.

53. Yeh SH, Stadalnik RC, DeNardo GL, et al: Definitive diagnosis of choledochal cyst by ^{99m}Tc-pyridoxylidene glutamate sequential scintiphotography. Clin Nucl Med 3:49–52, 1978.

54. Zaw-Wing B, Darwish M, Dibos PE, et al : ^{131}I rose bengal scanning in the detection of cholecystocolic fistula. Am J Gastroenterology 68:396–398, 1977.

Chapter 30

Pancreas

AMOLAK SINGH

EDWARD B. SILBERSTEIN

I. Normal visualization of pancreas

  A. Common

    1. Normal pancreas (6, 9)

  B. Less common

    1. Acute pancreatitis (9)

    2. Chronic pancreatitis (4, 6, 9)

    3. Pancreatic adenocarcinoma (6)

    4. Bile duct carcinoma (8, 9)

    5. Metastatic carcinoma (8)

    6. Pancreatic adenoma (8)

    7. Ampullary carcinoma (9)

II. Filling defects in pancreas

  A. Common

    1. Anatomic (normal) thinning of midportion (5, 7)

    2. Adenocarcinoma of pancreas (4, 5, 9)

    3. Pancreatitis (5, 12)

    4. Previous barium administration (7)

  B. Uncommon

    1. Metastatic carcinoma (12)

    2. Pancreatic adenoma (12)

    3. Pancreatic pseudocyst (1, 12)

    4. Partial pancreatectomy (9)

    5. Islet cell tumor of pancreas (4, 5, 9)

    6. Periampullary duodenal tumor (8)

    7. Ampullary carcinoma (1)

    8. Common bile duct carcinoma (1, 8)

    9. Gall bladder carcinoma (8)

    10. Aortic aneurysm (9)

    11. Tortuous aorta (4)

    12. Histiocytic lymphoma (4)

    13. Retroperitoneal tumor (12)

C. Rare
1. Hemangiosarcoma (8)
2. Gardner's syndrome (9)

III. Faint or uneven uptake
   A. Common
1. Normal, especially from thinning where the pancreas passes over the spine (10)
2. Acute and chronic pancreatitis (1, 6, 7)
3. Pancreatic adenocarcinoma (6, 7, 10)
4. Diabetes mellitus (6, 9, 12)
   B. Uncommon or rare
1. Carcinoma of ampulla of Vater (9)
2. Periampullary duodenal tumor (8)
3. Pancreatic adenoma (8)
4. In granulation tissue after pancreatectomy (3)
5. Active peptic ulcer (7, 9)
6. Gastritis (7)
7. Nasogastric suction (7, 9)
8. Gastroenterostomy with vagotomy (7, 9)
9. Inanition (7)
10. Gastric carcinoma (7)
11. Cirrhosis (2)
12. Cholelithiasis (9)
13. Sarcoidosis (9)
14. Primary amyloidosis (9)
15. Hyperthyroidism (7)

IV. Nonvisualization of pancreas

   A. Common
1. Artefact from overlying liver, especially with hepatomegaly (6, 9)
2. Pancreatic adenocarcinoma (1, 7, 8)
3. Acute pancreatitis (1, 9)
4. Chronic pancreatitis (1, 2, 9)
   B. Uncommon
1. Normal pancreas (6)
2. Diabetes mellitus (12)
3. Fibrocystic disease of pancreas (9)
4. Pancreatic pseudocyst (1)
5. Periampullary duodenal tumors (8)
6. Ampullary carcinoma (1)
7. Metastatic tumor (12)
8. Retroperitoneal tumor (12)

    9. Chronic active hepatitis (9)
   10. Thyrotoxicosis (9)
   11. Atherosclerosis (9)
   12. Mucoviscidosis (cystic fibrosis) (9)
   13. Amyloidosis (9)
   14. Calcinosis (1)

V. Lesions showing increased uptake of ^{75}Se-selenomethionine

  A. Uncommon
     1. Functional islet cell tumor (11)
     2. Pancreatic pseudocyst (9)
     3. Extrapancreatic tumors in upper abdomen
       a. hepatoma (5, 8)
       b. lymphoma (5)
       c. melanoma (5)

REFERENCES

1. Bachrach WH, Birsner JW, Izenstark JL, et al: Pancreatic scanning: a review. Gastroenterology 63:890–908, 1972.
2. Fink S, Ben-Porath M, Jacobson B, et al: Current status of dual channel pancreas scanning. J Nucl Med 10:78–82, 1969.
3. Goel T, Dubovski E, McDonald M: Pancreatic visualization with ^{75}Se-selenomethionine after surgery. J Nucl Med 13:765–766, 1972.
4. Hatchette JB, Shuler SE, Murison PJ: Scintiphotos of the pancreas: analysis of 134 studies. J Nucl Med 13:51–57, 1972.
5. Haynie TP, Miale A: The pancreas, in Freeman LM, Johnson PM (eds): Clinical Scintillation Imaging, New York: Grune and Stratton, 1975, pp. 601–621.
6. Landman S, Polcyn RE, Gottschalk A: Pancreas imaging — is it worth it? Radiology 100:631–636, 1971.
7. Miale A, Rodriquez-Antuñez A, Gill WM: Pancreas scanning after ten years. Sem Nucl Med 2:201–219, 1972.
8. McCarthy DM, Brown P, Melmed RN, et al: ^{75}Se-selenomethionine scanning in the diagnosis of tumours of the pancreas and adjacent viscera: the use of the test and its impact on survival. Gut 13:75–87, 1972.
9. Melmed RN, Agnew JE, Bouchier IAD: The normal and abnormal pancreatic scan. Quart J Med 37:607–621, 1968.
10. Rodriquez-Antuñez A, Filson EJ, Sullivan BH, et al: Photoscanning in diagnosis of carcinoma of the pancreas. Ann Int Med 65:730–737, 1966.
11. Thomas RL, Robinson AE, Johnsrude IS, et al: The demonstration of an insulin and gastrin producing pancreatic tumor by angiography and pancreatic scanning. Am J Roentgenol 104:646–651, 1968.
12. Watanabe K, Kawahira K, Matsura K: Scintigraphy as a screening test for carcinoma of the pancreas. Acta Radiol Diagn 15:57–64, 1974.

Chapter 31

Bile Acid Breath Test

AMOLAK SINGH
EDWARD B. SILBERSTEIN

I. Causes of true positive test (increased $^{14}CO_2$ in breath from bacterial overgrowth in small intestine or malabsorption of bile salts) (6)

  A. Common
- **1.** Multiple jejunal or ileal diverticula with bacterial overgrowth (3, 5)
- **2.** Gastrectomy with bacterial overgrowth (Billroth II) (1)
- **3.** Post vagotomy or gastroenterostomy (5)
- **4.** Achlorhydria (1)
- **5.** Small bowel resection (3)
- **6.** Small bowel obstruction or pseudo-obstruction (5)
  - **a.** Crohn's disease with stricture (2)
- **7.** Diabetes (1, 5)

  B. Uncommon
- **1.** Biliary disease (5)
  - **a.** biliary cirrhosis
  - **b.** cholangitis
- **2.** Diarrhea with nodular lymphoid hyperplasia or hypogammaglobulinemia (5)
- **3.** Idiopathic chronic diarrhea (5)
- **4.** Staphylococcal enterocolitis (3)
- **5.** Abdominal irradiation with stricture (1)
- **6.** Jejuno-ileal bypass (3)
- **7.** Amyloidosis (1)
- **8.** Carcinoma of pancreas with steatorrhea (1)
- **9.** Cholestyramine therapy (1)
- **10.** Duodenal diverticulum (1)
- **11.** Tumors with partial obstruction (1)
- **12.** Scleroderma (1)

II. Causes of false negative test (4)

  A. Antibiotic therapy
- **1.** Metronidazole

B. Rapid colonic transit

C. Absence of deconjugating organisms in colon

REFERENCES

1. Coates G, Garnett ES, Webber CE: Detection of deconjugation of bile salts with a $^{14}CO_2$ breath test. Sem Nucl Med 12:99–100, 1982.
2. Glover SC, Mowat NAG: A comparison of the structure and function of the terminal ileum in Crohn's disease using radiology, the "Dicopac" Schilling test and [^{14}C] G.C.A. breath test. Eur J Nucl Med 3:121–124, 1978.
3. Hirschowitz BI, Beschi R, Bondi H, et al: Location of the site of bacterial bile-salt deconjugation by combining abdominal scintigraphy with expired C-14. J Nucl Med 18:542–547, 1977.
4. Hofmann AF, Thomas PJ: Bile acid breath test. Ann Int Med 79:743–744, 1973.
5. Lauterburg BH, Newcomer AD, Hofmann AF: Clinical value of breath test. Mayo Clin Proc 53:227–233, 1978.
6. Rabinowitz JL, Lopez-Majano V: $^{14}CO_2$ in breath. Eur J Nucl Med 6:213–219, 1981.

Chapter 32

Gastrointestinal Bleeding

EDWARD B. SILBERSTEIN

I. Esophagus

    A. Varices (10)

II. Stomach

    A. Gastric varices (10)

    B. Mallory-Weiss tear (13)

    C. Ulcer (13)

    D. Gastric stump after Billroth II (15)

    E. Gastritis (12)

    F. Hamartoma (17)

Detection with technetium-labeled sulfur colloid or erythrocytes.

III. Biliary system

    A. Hemobilia from false hepatic artery aneurysm (19)
    B. Varices of gallbladder (13)

IV. Duodenum

    A. Aortoduodenal fistula (20)
    B. Ulcer (11, 13)
    C. Duodenitis (4)
    D. Varices (14)
    E. Telangiectasia (17, 18)

V. Jejunum

    A. Leiomyoma (11)
    B. Angiodysplasia (16)
    C. Esophagojejunal anastomosis (13)
    D. Metastatic implants (18)
    E. Sarcoidosis (3)

VI. Ileum

    A. Regional enteritis (11)
    B. Intussusception (11)
    C. Leiomyosarcoma (7)
    D. Ulceration (ischemia) (9)
    E. Angiodysplasia (13)
    F. Iliac artery-ileal fistula (15)
    G. Tuberculous ileitis (3)
    H. Metastatic choriocarcinoma (3)

VII. Cecum

    A. Varices (1)
    B. Hamartoma (17)

VIII. Colon-rectum

    A. Diverticular bleeding (10, 13)
    B. Carcinoma (4, 10)
    C. Crohn's disease (4)
    D. Ischemic ulcer (13)
    E. Hemorrhagic proctitis (13)
    F. Adenoma (13)

G. Colonic interposition (5)
H. Angiodysplasia (17)
I. Hamartoma (17)
J. Pseudomembranous colitis (17)

IX. Artefact

    A. Accessory spleen (8)
    B. Penile activity (6)
    C. Asymmetric marrow uptake (2)
    D. Normal organs
        1. Colon (18)
        2. Kidney (18)
        3. Stomach (18)
        4. Bladder (18)

REFERENCES

1. Barry JW, Engle CV: Detection of hemorrhage in a patient with cecal varices using ^{99m}Tc-sulfur colloid. Radiology 129:489–490, 1978.
2. Baum S, Locko RC, Scheff AM: False-positive interpretation in technetium-99m sulfur colloid imaging for gastrointestinal bleeding. Nucl Med Comm 2:351–357, 1981.
3. Briley CA, Jackson DC, Johnsrude IS, et al: Acute gastrointestinal hemorrhage of small-bowel origin. Radiology 136:317–319, 1980.
4. Bunkeor SR, Brown JM, McAuley RJ, et al: Detection of gastrointestinal bleeding sites. JAMA 247:789–792, 1982.
5. Fisher M, Lipuma JP, Agnone J: Scintigraphic demonstration of acute gastrointestinal bleeding in a colonic interposition. Clin Nucl Med 7:225–226, 1982.
6. Haseman MK: Potential pitfalls in the interpretation of erythrocyte scintigraphy for gastro-intestinal hemorrhage. Clin Nucl Med 7:309–310, 1982.
7. Heyman S, Sacks B, Khettry J, et al: Localization of bleeding small intestinal lesions using scanning techniques. Surgery 85:372–376, 1979.
8. Heyman S, Sunaryo FP, Ziegler MM: Gastrointestinal bleeding: An accessory spleen causing a false-positive Tc-99m-sulfur colloid study. Clin Nucl Med 7:38–40, 1982.
9. Makhija MC, Rose WS, Schultz S: Detection of bleeding in the ileum by radionuclide imaging. Clin Nucl Med 6:584–585, 1981.
10. Markisz JA, Front D, Royal HD, et al: An evaluation of ^{99m}Tc-labeled red blood cell scintigraphy for the detection and localization of gastrointestinal bleeding site. Gastroen-terology 83:394–398, 1982.
11. McKusick KA, Froelich J, Callahan RJ, et al: ^{99m}Tc red blood cells for detection of gastrointestinal bleeding. Am J Roentgenol 137:1113–1118, 1981.
12. Miskowiak J, Nielsen SL, Munck O, et al: Acute gastrointestinal bleeding detected with abdominal scintigraphy using technetium-99m-labeled albumin. Scand J Gastroenterol 14:389–394, 1979.
13. Miskowiak J, Nielsen SL, Munck O: Scintigraphic diagnosis of gastrointestinal bleeding with ^{99m}Tc-labeled blood-pool agents. Radiology 141:499–504, 1981.
14. Royal HD, Papanicolaou N, Bettman M, et al: Scintigraphic identification of bleeding

duodenal varices. Am J Gastroenterol 74:173–175, 1980.

15. Smith RK, Arterburr G: Detection and localization of gastrointestinal bleeding using Tc-99m-pyrophosphate *in vivo* labeled red blood cells. Clin Nucl Med 7:225–226, 1982.

16. Tu'meh SS, Parker JA, Royal HD, et al: Detection of bleeding from angiodysplasia of the jejunum by blood pool scintigraphy. Clin Nucl Med 8:127–128, 1983.

17. Winzelberg GG, Froelich JW, McKusick KA, et al: Radionuclide localization of lower gastrointestinal hemorrhage. Radiology 139:465–469, 1981.

18. Winzelberg GG, McKusick KA, Strauss HW, et al: Evaluation of gastrointestinal bleeding by red blood cells labeled *in vivo* with technetium-99m. J Nucl Med 20:1080–1086, 1979.

19. Winzelberg GG, Wholey MH, Ismail-Beigi F: Hemobilia detected by Tc-99m labeled red blood cells. Clin Nucl Med 7:36–37, 1982.

20. Yen C-K, Pollycove M, Parker H, et al: Rupture of a spontaneous aortoduodenal fistula visualized with Tc-RBC scintigraphy. J Nucl Med 24:332–333, 1983.

Part VII

Genitourinary System

Chapter 33

The Kidney (Excluding Transplant)

JOHN G. McAFEE
EDWARD B. SILBERSTEIN

I. Unilateral decrease or absence of renal perfusion in first-pass dynamic studies

   A. Common

      1. Unilateral pyelonephritis (39)

      2. Renal artery stenosis (40)

      3. Obstructive uropathy (stone, tumor, fibrosis) (39, 40, 45)

      4. Contusion (4, 30)

      5. Tamponade from perinephric or subcapsular hematoma or abscess (4, 40)

      6. Artefactual decrease from ptosis (9, 54, 60)

      7. Artefactual from anterior renal displacement (40, 67)

   B. Less common

      1. Renal vein thrombosis (40, 43)

      2. Masses compressing renal hilar vessels (40)

      3. Hemorrhagic infarct (42)

      4. Post-nephrectomy (26)

      5. Transitional cell carcinoma of renal pelvis (47)

      6. Schistosomal uropathy (34)

II. Filling defects on renal perfusion study (70) (cf. Sections XV, XVI)

   A. Common

The use of an asterisk * in this chapter indicates that this entity has been observed by one of the authors but the case report has not been published.

       1. Cyst (70)

       2. Abscess (59, 70)

       3. Hematoma or fracture (30)

       4. Infarct (30)

       5. Pyelonephritis (38)

       6. Marked hydronephrosis (34, 39)

  B. Uncommon

       1. Hypernephroma, especially if necrotic or cystic (11, 45)

       2. Embryonal cell tumors (11)

       3. Wilms' tumor (11)

       4. Metastases (70)

       5. Xanthogranulomatous pyelonephritis (70)

III. Localized increase in renal perfusion: vascular areas on flow study with non-functioning renal parenchyma on static imaging

  A. Common

       1. Renal cell carcinoma (57, 70)

  B. Less common

       1. Recurrent renal cell carcinoma (62)

       2. Arteriovenous malformations and fistulas, congenital or acquired (11, 37, 58)

       3. Cysts with large cortical vessels (11)

       4. Angiolipomatosis (hamartoma) (5, 11)

       5. Renal artery aneurysm (70)

       6. Focal pyelonephritis (59)

       7. Abscess (59)

IV. Localized perirenal area of increased perfusion

  A. Common

       1. Simulation of kidney or vascular renal mass

          a. small bowel vascularity (23, 54)

          b. prominent mesenteric veins (23, 52, 62)

          c. "wandering" spleen (2, 72)

  B. Less common

       1. Metastatic or recurrent renal cell carcinoma (62)

  C. Rare

       1. Adrenal pheochromocytoma (48)

V. Displacement of kidneys (56)

  A. Common

       1. Ptosis (especially in upright and prone positions) (54, 58)

       2. Renal transplant (20)

       3. Splenomegaly (16)

       4. Hepatomegaly (16)

       5. Perirenal hematoma (51)

       6. Perirenal abscess (51)

       7. Cyst (16)

  B. Uncommon

       1. Tumors

           a. neuroblastoma (11)

           b. adrenal adenoma (16)

           c. adrenal carcinoma (16)

           d. Wilms' tumor (51)

           e. sarcoma (69)

       2. Adrenal hematoma (21, 51)

       3. Adrenal cyst (16)

  C. Rare

       1. Ectopic congenital pelvic kidney (58)

       2. Crossed fused kidney (58, 71)

       3. Horseshoe kidney (26, 58)

       4. Intrathoracic kidney (53)

VI. Abnormalities of renal contour or position (11, 49, 56)

  A. Common

       1. Fetal lobulation (49)

       2. Dromedary hump of lateral border of left kidney (49)

       3. Prominent columns of Bertin (lobar dysmorphism) (49)

       4. Cysts (49, 51)

       5. Tumors (49)

       6. Abscesses (70)

       7. Hematomas (30)

       8. Localized compensatory hypertrophy, as in pyelonephritis (3, 49)

       9. Hydronephrosis (51)

     10. Scarring, any etiology (3)

  B. Uncommon

       1. Post-nephrolithotomy deformity (45)

       2. Horseshoe kidney (51, 58)

       3. Ectopic kidney (51, 58)

       4. Polycystic kidneys (3, 18)

       5. Congenital dysplasia (1)

       6. Crossed fused kidney (58, 71)

VII. Bilateral renal enlargement without obvious focal abnormalities (56, 65)

  A. Common

       1. Bilateral duplication

      2. Hydronephrosis
      3. Polycystic disease
      4. Toxic nephrosis, especially from cancer chemotherapy drugs
      5. Acute pyelonephritis or glomerulonephritis

B. Less common
      1. Acute tubular necrosis
      2. Acute cortical necrosis
      3. Renal vein thrombosis
      4. Collagen-vascular disease
      5. Goodpasture's syndrome
      6. Lymphoma

C. Rare
      1. Acromegaly
      2. Amyloidosis (58)
      3. Glycogen storage disease
      4. Hyperuricemia associated with lymphoma or leukemia
      5. Medullary sponge kidney
      6. Sarcoidosis (58)

VIII. Unilateral large kidney without obvious focal abnormalities

A. Common
      1. Compensatory hypertrophy (3)
      2. Hydronephrosis, obstructive and non-obstructive (39)
      3. Renal vein thrombosis (43)

B. Uncommon
      1. Cross fused renal ectopia (71)
      2. Congenital mesoblastic nephroma (leiomyomatous hamartoma) (66)

IX. Unilateral small kidney (44)

A. Common
      1. Chronic pyelonephritis (38, 44)
      2. Obstructive nephropathy (post-obstructive atrophy) (39)
      3. Renal artery stenosis, unilateral (40)
      4. Partial nephrectomy*
      5. Tumor infiltration allowing visualization only of uninvolved remnant (58)

B. Uncommon
      1. Renal infarction (3)
      2. Radiation atrophy (61)
      3. Congenital hypoplastic kidney*
      4. Contusion (30)

C. Rare
      1. Hemangioendotheliomatosis (69)

X. Unilateral decreased uptake (cf. Section I)

   A. Common

      1. Unilateral chronic pyelonephritis (38)

      2. Renal artery stenosis, unilateral (40)

      3. Obstructive uropathy (39)

      4. Contusion (30)

   B. Uncommon

      1. Renal tumor especially near renal pedicle (11)

      2. Unilateral severe acute pyelonephritis, including emphysematous type (8)

      3. Radiation nephritis (61)

   C. Rare

      1. Hemangioendotheliomatosis (69)

XI. Bilaterally decreased uptake

   A. Common

      1. Chronic glomerulonephritis (58)

      2. Chronic end-stage pyelonephritis (58)

      3. Nephrosclerosis (58)

      4. Diabetic nephropathy (58)

      5. Acute tubular necrosis (58)

      6. Shock (58)

      7. Severe dehydration (58)

   B. Uncommon

      1. Acute bilateral obstructive uropathy (58) (see Section XIII,A,1)

        a. lymphadenopathy

        b. carcinoma (bladder, prostate, etc.)

        c. retroperitoneal fibrosis

        d. schistosomiasis (34)

      2. Bilateral renal artery stenosis (40)

      3. Acute glomerulonephritis*

      4. Acute tubular necrosis (58)

      5. Chronic interstitial nephritis

        a. phenacetin-induced (58)

      6. Nephrotic syndrome with end-stage renal failure (19)

      7. Hyperuricemic nephropathy (64)

      8. Amyloidosis (63)

      9. Sarcoidosis (58)

   C. Rare

      1. Congenital renal dysplasia, prune belly syndrome (1)

      2. Medullary sponge kidney, end-stage (58)

XII. Unilateral absence of renal function (non-visualization of one kidney)

A. Common
   1. Nephrectomy*
   2. False non-visualization due to anterior displacement, ptosis of kidney, ectopia (67)
   3. Obstructive uropathy (permanent or reversible non-visualization) (29)
   4. Avulsion or severe injury to pedicle with hematoma (4, 27)
   5. Congenital atresia (1)
B. Less common
   1. Massive infarction or renal artery embolus*
   2. Neoplasms compressing or invading renal vascular pedicle (11)
   3. Renal artery or vein thrombosis*
   4. Pyonephrosis, tuberculosis, and other severe infections*

XIII. Delayed parenchymal retention with impaired urinary excretion (best observed with I-131 hippuran, but also demonstrated with Tc-99m DTPA or Tc-99m glucoheptonate; not reliably demonstrated with Tc-99m dimercaptosuccinic acid)

A. Common
   1. Hydronephrosis, obstructive and non-obstructive (31, 39)
      a. ureteropelvic junction obstruction
      b. previous pyeloplasty
      c. urinary diversion
      d. posterior urethral valves
      e. calculus
      f. ureteral reimplantation
      g. tumor
      h. stricture
      i. ureterocele
      j. post-operative ureteral edema
      k. retrocaval ureter
      l. ligated ureter
      m. post-irradiation
      n. blood clots
      o. retroperitoneal fibrosis
      p. prune belly syndrome (1)
      q. schistosomiasis (34)
   2. Acute tubular necrosis, ischemic or toxic
   3. Secondary to dehydration in infants and young children (1)
   4. Renal artery stenosis (11)
   5. Chronic pyelonephritis (12, 38)
   6. Diffuse renal parenchymal disease (12)
B. Less common

      1. Hemorrhagic infarct (42)
      2. Myeloma (12)
      3. Normal renal columns of Bertin (6)
      4. Artefact due to free pertechnetate or radioiodide in stomach overlying left kidney (41, 60)
   C. Rare
      1. Parenchymal increased uptake in renal tubular adenoma (11)

XIV. Delayed pelvocalyceal retention without parenchymal retention (best observed with I-131 hippuran or Tc-99m DTPA)

   A. Common
      1. Physiological, especially in dehydrated state in supine position (28)
      2. Hydronephrosis, obstructive, post-infectious or neurogenic (28)
      3. Stasis in calyceal system from chronic pyelonephritis and/or pyonephrotic cavities (11, 38)
      4. Pseudo-obstruction (diagnosed by furosemide infusion) (31)
   B. Rare
      1. Congenital megacalices (1A)

XV. Multiple irregular parenchymal filling defects (cf. Sections II, XVI)

   A. Common
      1. Chronic pyelonephritis (18, 38)
      2. Multiple infarcts (38)
      3. Polycystic renal disease (3, 18)
      4. Multiple renal cysts (18)
      5. Contusion or hematomas (30)
      6. Nephrosclerosis (13)
   B. Less common
      1. Acute pyelonephritis (17)
      2. Metastatic tumors (26, 58)
      3. Lymphoma (64, 65)
   C. Rare
      1. Congenital dysplasia (1)
      2. Angiomyolipoma (5)

XVI. Solitary parenchymal filling defect (cf. Sections II, XV)

   A. Common
      1. Normal hilar defect from large intrarenal pelvis (11)
      2. Hilar defect from uretero-pelvic junction obstruction with hemihydronephrosis (1, 39)
      3. Hilar defect from pelvic ''renal sinus'' lipomatosis (11, 45)
      4. Cyst (16, 26)

     5. Malignant tumor, primary or secondary (including carcinoma, sarcoma, lymphoma, Wilms' tumor) (26, 45, 58, 64, 65)

     6. Abscess or "carbuncle" (16, 46)

     7. Post-surgical defects or scarring (32)

     8. Infarct (42, 58)

     9. Pyelonephritic scarring (18, 38)

   10. Hematoma, contusion and/or laceration (30, 58)

B. Less common

     1. Acute pyelonephritis (17, 59)

       a. emphysematous pyelonephritis (8)

     2. Radiation damage (61)

     3. Segmental renal artery stenosis (40)

     4. Xanthogranulomatous pyelonephritis (25)

     5. Benign tumor (65, 69A)

       a. adenoma

       b. hamartoma

       c. lipoma

       d. leiomyoma

     6. Adrenal tumors (48) including benign adrenal cell nest (58)

     7. Megalocytic interstitial nephritis (25)

     8. Large calculus*

     9. Falsely abnormal from anterior displacement of the upper pole in prone position (54, 58)

C. Rare

     1. Tuberculosis (58)

     2. Angiomyolipoma (hamartoma) with tuberous sclerosis (4, 7, 11, 58)

     3. A-V malformation (58)

     4. Artefact from distended gastric fundus overlying upper pole of left kidney (60)

     5. Oncocytoma (35)

     6. Mesoblastic nephroma (61A)

XVII. Parenchymal filling defects with minimal or absent contrast urographic changes

  A. Common

     1. Chronic pyelonephritis (18, 38)

     2. Acute pyelonephritis (17)

     3. Infarction (38)

     4. Septic emboli (38)

     5. Contusion (11)

  B. Less common

     1. Lymphoma (64)

XVIII. Perirenal extravasation and/or extrarenal distribution of renal agents

    A. Common

        1. Following trauma (1, 4, 68)

        2. High grade obstructive uropathy (68, 73)

        3. Post-ureteral surgery (73)

        4. Normal (artefact) due to pertechnetate or free radioiodide in stomach or small bowel (41)

    B. Uncommon

        1. Ureteral duplication, blind ending (10)

        2. Gall bladder and bowel visualization, especially with renal insufficiency

            a. glucoheptonate (50)

            b. DMSA (22)

XIX. Renal parenchymal uptake of Tc-99m sulphur and other colloids

    A. Common

        1. Artefact due to impurities in Tc-99m generator eluate (24)

        2. Congestive heart failure (9)

    B. Uncommon

        1. Associated with liver transplant (33)

        2. Acute tubular necrosis (72)

        3. Sepsis (72)

REFERENCES

1. Alderson PO, Gilday DL, Wayne HN Jr.: Atlas of Pediatric Nuclear Medicine. St. Louis: C. V. Mosby, 1978.

1A. Atkins HL, Klopper JF, Ansari AN, et al: Lipid (cholesterol) granulomatosis (Chester-Erdheim disease) and congenital megacalices. Clin Nucl Med 3:324–327, 1978.

2. Ball JD, Cowan RJ, Maynard CD: Splenic simulation of a renal mass. J Nucl Med 17:1104–1105, 1976.

3. Ball JD, Maynard CD: Nuclear imaging in urology. Urol Clin North Am 6:321–342, 1979.

4. Berg BC Jr.: Radionuclide studies after urinary-tract injury. Sem Nucl Med 4:371–393, 1974.

5. Blatt CJ, Hayt DB, Freeman LM: Radionuclide imaging of the kidney in tuberous sclerosis. J Nucl Med 15:699–702, 1974.

6. Braunstein P, Hennberg JG: "Hot" renal pseudotumors (abstract). J Nucl Med 12:421, 1971.

7. Buse MG, Sibrens DF, Buse J: Scintillation scanning of kidneys in renal insufficiency. Ann Int Med 60:857–868, 1964.

8. Chaudhuri TK, Venkatesan R, Bobbitt JV: The monitoring of kidney dysfunction in renal emphysema by dual radiopharmaceutical scintiscanning. J Nucl Med 19:67–68, 1978.

9. Coleman RE: Renal colloid localization. J Nucl Med 15:367–368, 1974.

10. Dublin AB, Stadalnik RC, DeNardo GL, et al: Scintigraphic imaging of a blind-ending ureteral duplication. J Nucl Med 16:208–209, 1975.

11. Freeman LM: The kidney, in Freeman LM, Johnson PM (eds): Clinical Scintillation Imaging, Second ed. New York, Grune and Stratton, 1975, pp. 325–403.

12. Freeman LM, Goldman SM, Shaw RK, et al: Kidney visualization with ^{131}I-orthoiodohippurate in patients with renal insufficiency. J Nucl Med 10:545–549, 1969.

13. Friedman SA, Raizner AE, Rosen H, et al: Functional defects in the aging kidney. Ann Int Med 76:41–45, 1972.

14. George EA, Codd JE, Newton WT, et al: Further evaluation of ^{99m}Tc sulfur colloid accumulation in rejecting renal transplants in man and a canine model. Radiology 116:121–126, 1975.

15. Haden HT, Stacy WK, Wolf JS, et al: Scintiphotography in diagnosis of urinary fistula after renal transplantation. J Nucl Med 16:612–615, 1975.

16. Hamway SA, Schlegel JV: Radionuclides in the diagnosis of suprarenal masses. J Urol 114:797–801, 1975.

17. Handmaker H, Young B, Fay R: Nuclear renal imaging in acute pyelonephritis (abstract). J Nucl Med 20:623, 1979.

18. Handmaker H, Young BW, Lowenstein JM: Clinical experience with ^{99m}Tc-DMSA (dimercaptosuccinic acid), a new renal imaging agent. J Nucl Med 16:28–32, 1975.

19. Hatther RS, Maltz HE, Holliday MA: Differentiation of reversible ischemia from end-stage renal failure in nephrotic children with ^{131}I-hippuran dynamic scintigraphy. J Nucl Med 18:438–440, 1970.

20. Hayes M, Moore TC, Taplin GV: Radionuclide evaluation of renal transplant status, in Zumwinkel K, Blaufox MD, Funck-Brentano J-L (eds): Radionuclides in Nephrology. Littleton, Massachusetts: Thieme-Edition Publ. Sciences Group, Inc., 1974, pp. 207–240.

21. Heyman S, Treves S: Adrenal hemorrhage in the newborn: Scintigraphic diagnosis. J Nucl Med 20:521–523, 1979.

22. Hirsch JR, Fogel WM, Fratkin MJ: Localization of the renal cortical imaging agent ^{99m}Tc-DMSA in the bowel. Radiology 122:404, 1977.

23. Holmes ER III, Klingensmith WC, Kirchner PT, et al: Phantom kidney in technetium-99m DTPA studies of renal blood flow: case report. J Nucl Med 18:702–705, 1977.

24. Jackson GL: Renal accumulation of ^{99m}Tc-SC. Clin Nucl Med 2:176, 1977.

25. Jander HP, Pujara S, Murad TM: Tumefactive megalocytic interstitial nephritis. Radiology 129:635–636, 1978.

26. Kahn PC, Dewanjee MK, Brown SS: Routine renal imaging after ^{99m}Tc-glucoheptonate brain scans. J Nucl Med 17:786–787, 1976.

27. Kay CJ, Rosenfield AT, Armm M: Gray-scale ultrasonography in the evaluation of renal trauma. Radiology 134:461–466, 1980.

28. Kirchner PT, James AE Jr., Reba RC, et al: Patterns of excretion of radioactive chelates in obstructive uropathy. Radiology 114:655–661, 1975.

29. Kivet MD, Griep RJ: Pyonephrosis complicating ureteral obstruction, limitations of renal scintiscanning in predicting reversibility of renal damage. J Urol 109:393–395, 1975.

30. Koenigsberg M, Blaufox MD, Freeman LM: Traumatic injuries of the renal vasculature and parenchyma. Sem Nucl Med 4:117–132, 1974.

31. Koff SA, Thrall JH, Keyes JW: Assessment of hydroureteronephrosis in children using diuretic radionuclide urography. J Urol 123:531–534, 1979.

32. Kohn HD, Mostbeck A: Value of additional lateral scans in renal scintigraphy. Eur J Nucl Med 4:21–25, 1979.

33. Kuni CC, Klingensmith WC: Renal uptake of ^{99m}Tc sulfur colloid in liver transplant patients. Clin Nucl Med 4:335–337, 1979.

34. Lamki LM, Lamki N: Radionuclide studies of chronic schistosomal uropathy. Radiology 140:471–474, 1981.

35. Lautin EM, Gordon PM, Friedman AC, et al: Radionuclide imaging and computed tomography in renal oncocytoma. Radiology 138:185–190, 1981.

36. Levinson ED, Baldwin RD, Spencer RP: Renal sinus lipomatosis: a cause of medullary "nonfilling." J Nucl Med 20:1105–1106, 1979.

37. Maholi R, Soin JS: Congenital intrarenal arteriovenous fistula diagnosed by radionuclide study. J Nucl Med 19:440–441, 1978.

38. McAfee JG: Radionuclide imaging in the assessment of primary chronic pyelonephritis. J Nucl Med 18:669–675, 1977.

39. McAfee JG, Singh A, O'Callaghan JP: Nuclear imaging supplementary to urography in obstructive uropathy. Radiology 137:487–496, 1980.

40. McAfee JG, Thomas FD, Grossman Z, et al: Diagnosis of angiotensinogenic hypertension: the complementary roles of renal scintigraphy and the saralasin infusion test. J Nucl Med 18:669–675, 1977.

41. McKusick KA, Malmud LS, Kirchner PT, et al: An interesting artifact in radionuclide imaging of the kidneys. J Nucl Med 14:113–114, 1973.

42. Meringoff BN: Partial renal infarct simulating a collecting system tumor. J Nucl Med 13:125–126, 1972.

43. Mettler FA, Christie JH: The scintigraphic pattern of acute renal vein thrombosis. Clin Nucl Med 5:468–470, 1980.

44. Neiman HL, Korsower JM, Reeder MM: Unilateral small kidney. JAMA 224:585–590, 1973.

45. Norlander S, Asard P-E: Differential diagnosis of space-occupying lesions in the kidneys with the scintillation camera. Acta Radiol 15:630–638, 1974.

46. O'Reilly PH, Lupton EW, Testa HJ, et al: A case of renal carbuncle—the role of radionuclides. Br J Radiol 53:504–506, 1980.

47. O'Reilly PH, Osborn DE, Testa HJ, et al: Renal imaging: a comparison of radionuclide, ultrasound, and computed tomographic scanning in investigation of renal space-occupying lesions. Br Med J 202:943–945, 1981.

48. Petrocelli R, Wetzel RA: Radionuclide detection of pheochromocytoma. J Nucl Med 16:234–235, 1975.

49. Pollack HM, Edell S, Morales VO: Radionuclide imaging in renal pseudotumors. Radiology 111:639–644, 1974.

50. Prince JR, Dukstein WG, White WE: Gallbladder visualization with the renal imaging agent glucoheptonate. Clin Nucl Med 3:68, 1978.

51. Puyau FA, Meckstroth GR, Ho RD: Total body radionuclide localization in infants. Radiology 110:395–398, 1974.

52. Rambler LE, Winter PF, Johnson PM: Mesenteric vasculature masquerading as a kidney at renal imaging. Radiology 120:369–370, 1976.

53. Rao BR, Kirschenbaum AS, Winebright JW: Congenital intrathoracic kidney. Eur J Nucl Med 6:177–178, 1981.

54. Rao GM, Nagesh KG, Guruprakash GH: Position-related false-positive renal imaging. Clin Nucl Med 5:318–319, 1980.

55. Reba RC, Poulose KP, Kirchner PT: Radiolabeled chelates for visualization of kidney function and structure with emphasis in their use in renal insufficiency. Sem Nucl Med 4:151–168, 1974.

56. Reeder MM, Felson B: Gamuts in Radiology. Cincinnati, Ohio: Audiovisual Radiology of Cincinnati, Inc., 1975, pp. H-1–H-28.

57. Rosenthall L: Radionuclide diagnosis of malignant tumors of the kidney. Am J Roentgenol 101:662–668, 1967.

58. Rosenthall L: Nuclear medicine in renal imaging. Current Problems in Radiology 1:2–50, 1971.

59. Rosenthall L, Reid EC: Radionuclide distinction of vascular and non-vascular lesions of the kidney. Canad Med Assoc J 98:1165–1170, 1968.

60. Sarabella PA, Slovis TL, Fellows RA, et al: The distended gastric fundus: simulation of a left suprarenal mass. J Nucl Med 16:947–948, 1975.

61. Schulman N, Johnson PM: Scintillation imaging in generalized and localized reduction nephritis. Radiology 109:639–642, 1973.

61A. Siegel BA (ed): Nuclear Radiology (Second Series) Syllabus. Chicago: ACR 1978, pp. 182–183.

62. Simon H: Metastatic and recurrent hypernephroma demonstrated by isotope angiography. Clin Nucl Med 2:214–217, 1977.

63. Sostre S, Martin ND, Lucas RN, et al: Scintigraphic findings in primary amyloidosis. Radiology 115:675–677, 1975.

64. Sty JR, Babbit DP, Kumudchandra JS: Scintigraphy in pediatric urinary tract lymphoma. Clin Nucl Med 3:422–424, 1978.

65. Sty JR, Babbit DP, Kun L: Atlas of ^{99m}Tc-methylene diphosphonate renal images in pediatric oncology. Clin Nucl Med 4:122–127, 1979.

66. Sty JR, Oechler H: Tc-99m glucoheptonate renal imaging: congenital mesoblastic nephroma. J Nucl Med 21:809–810, 1980.

67. Suresh K, Puri S, Spencer RP: "Non-visualized" kidney during ^{99m}Tc-DTPA study due to anterior displacement by tumor. Clin Nucl Med 2:454, 1977.

68. Suzuki Y, Sugihara M, Kuribayashi S, et al: Uriniferous perirenal pseudocyst detected by ^{99m}Tc-dimerceptosuccinic acid renal scan. Am J Roentgenol 133:306–308, 1979.

69. Sy WM, Nissen AW: Radionuclide studies in hemangioendotheliomas: Case report. J Nucl Med 16:915–917, 1975.

69A. Tauxe WN, Dubovsky EV: The kidney, in Rocha AFG, Harbert JC (eds): Textbook of Nuclear Medicine: Clinical Applications. Philadelphia: Lea and Febiger, 1979, pp. 369–371.

70. Tori G, Marabini A, Frenchi R, et al: Angioscintiphotography with ^{99m}Tc in 310 cases of space-occupying kidney lesions. Nucl Med (Stuttg.) 14:133–143, 1975.

71. Trackler RT, Katzman DO, Coons HG: Diagnostic features of a unilateral fused kidney with a lower-pole inflamed, hemorrhagic cyst. Clin Nucl Med 4:289–290, 1979.

72. Webber MM, Pollak EW, Victery W, et al: Thrombosis detection by radionuclide particle (MAA) entrapment: correlation with fibrinogen uptake and venography. Radiology 111:645–650, 1974.

73. Yeh E-L, Chiang L-C, Meade RC: Radionuclide demonstration of urinary extravasation with ureteral obstruction. J Nucl Med 20:236–238, 1979.

74. Yeh E-L, Pohlmann G, Meade RC: Spleen simulating vascular renal mass in left renal agenesis. Clin Nucl Med:2:194–196, 1977.

75. Zum Winkel K, Harbst H, Das KB, et al: Application of radionuclides in renal transplantation. Sem Nucl Med 4:169–186, 1974.

Chapter 34

Renal Transplant

AMOLAK SINGH

EDWARD B. SILBERSTEIN

I. Decreased concentration in renal allograft
   A. 0–2 days
      1. Acute tubular necrosis (2, 7)
      2. Urinary extravasation (11)
      3. Hyperacute immune rejection (19)
      4. Renal artery occlusion (2, 6)
      5. Renal vein occlusion (19)
   B. 2–10 days
      1. Acute tubular necrosis (7)
      2. Acute rejection (22)
      3. Urinary extravasation (2, 11)
      4. Urinary obstruction (22)
      5. Accelerated rejection (21)
      6. Renal artery occlusion (7)
      7. Renal vein occlusion (16, 19)
   C. 10–40 days
      1. Acute rejection (12)
      2. Chronic rejection (6)
      3. Urinary extravasation (11)
         a. at uretero-vesical anastomosis (1)
         b. at cystotomy (1)
         c. mid-ureter (1)
         d. post-renal biopsy (1)
      5. Urinary obstruction (22)
      6. Renal vascular occlusion (21)
      7. Proliferative glomerulonephritis (12)
      8. Membranous glomerulonephritis (12)
   D. Beyond 40 days
      1. Chronic rejection (6, 12)
      2. Obstructive uropathy (23)
      3. Chronic pyelonephritis (12)

     4. Glomerulonephritis (12)
     5. Lipoid nephrosis (6)
     6. Papillary necrosis (14)
     7. Calculus formation (2)
     8. Vesicoureteral reflux (3)

II. Nonvisualization of renal allograft

  A. Common
     1. Hyperacute rejection (19)
     2. Accelerated rejection (21)
     3. Advanced rejection (22)
     4. Severe acute tubular necrosis (21)
     5. Renal artery thrombosis (1, 7)
     6. Renal vein thrombosis (1, 19)
     7. Complete obstructive uropathy (21)
  B. Uncommon
     1. Diffuse cortical necrosis (7, 22)
     2. Normal infant kidney (4)

III. Stasis and dilatation of calyces, pelvis or ureter

  A. Obstructive uropathy
     1. Postoperative edema (1)
     2. Lymphocele (1, 19)
     3. Urinary leak (urinoma) (11)
     4. Ureteric kinking (23)
     5. Ureteric stenosis (2)
     6. Ureteric rejection (2)
     7. Retroperitoneal fibrosis (2)
     8. Vascular insufficiency with intrinsic ureteric fibrosis (2)
     9. Clot in the ureter (17, 19)
    10. Pregnancy (2)
  B. Artefactual appearance of obstruction
     1. Pseudo-obstruction with dilated ureter and pelvis (1)
     2. Dehydration (1)

IV. Focal inhomogeneous activity in or around the transplant

  A. Common
     1. Advanced rejection (24)
     2. Acute tubular necrosis in cadaver donor transplant (24)
     3. Segmental ischemia or infarction (7, 19, 22)
  B. Uncommon

    1. Segmental tubular necrosis in live donor transplant (20)
    2. Arterial spasm (1)
    3. Abscesses (1)

V. Autologous kidney or transplant with photopenic areas in or around organ

  A. Common
    1. Hematoma (1, 4)
    2. Lymphocele (1, 4)
      a. lymphocutaneous fistula (13)
    3. Urinoma (4)
    4. Full bladder before injection (4)
    5. ''Mock'' lesions between kidney and large vessels or organs early in study (4)
    6. Infarct (1)
  B. Uncommon
    1. Abscess (3, 4)
    2. Bowel overlying kidney (4)
    3. Partial nonperfusion of kidney (4)
    4. Hydronephrosis, hydroureter before injection (4)
    5. Inflammatory edema (1)
    6. Ovarian cyst (3)

VI. Intrarenal accumulation of Tc-99m sulfur colloid

  A. Increased uptake
    1. Common
      a. acute rejection (8, 10, 15)
      b. chronic rejection (8, 15)
    2. Less common
      a. acute tubular necrosis (8)
      b. sepsis (8)
      c. impending rejection (15)
    3. Rare
      a. nephrotic syndrome (8)
  B. Accumulation of Tc-99m sulfur colloid not noted
    1. Common
      a. normal function (8, 10, 15)
      b. acute tubular necrosis (10, 15)
      c. sepsis (8)
    2. Less common
      a. acute rejection with necrosis (10, 15)
      b. acute rejection with heparin therapy (10)
      c. end stage chronic rejection (10)

    3. Rare

        a. renal artery thrombosis (15)

        b. renal vein thrombosis (15)

VII. Gallium-67 accumulation in allograft

    A. Increased uptake

        1. Common

            a. normal function, 0–30 days (5)

            b. acute rejection (10)

        2. Less common

            a. chronic rejection (10)

            b. acute tubular necrosis with anuria (10)

    B. No significant accumulation of gallium-67 in allograft

        1. Common

            a. normal function, beyond 60 days (5, 10)

            b. acute rejection with heparin therapy (10)

            c. acute rejection with necrosis (10)

            d. acute tubular necrosis (10)

VIII. Fibrinogen deposition in or around transplant

    A. Increased deposition

        1. Acute rejection (10, 25)

            a. acute rejection and infarction (18)

        2. Impending rejection (25)

        3. Hematoma (10, 18)

        4. Wound abscess (18)

        5. Urinary leaks (10)

        6. Subcutaneous ''seroma'' (18)

        7. Urinary tract infection (18)

        8. Artefact from retention of labeled fibrinogen split products in a hydronephrotic renal pelvis (9)

    B. No significant accumulation of labeled fibrinogen

        1. Normal function (25)

        2. Acute tubular necrosis (25)

        3. Stable or chronic rejection (10, 25)

        4. Recurring glomerulonephritis (25)

        5. Graft necrosis following rejection (10)

        6. Renal artery and vein thrombosis (10)

REFERENCES

    1. Ayres JG, Hilson AJW, Maisey MN: Complications of renal transplantation: appearance using Tc-99m-DTPA. Clin Nucl Med 5:473–480, 1980.

2. Becker J, Kutcher R: Urological complications of renal transplantation. Sem Roentgenology 13:341–351, 1978.

3. Burt RW, Reddy RF: Evaluation of nuclear imaging for detecting post-transplant fluid collection. Am J Roentgenol 133:91–95, 1979.

4. Corcoran RJ, Thrall JH, Kaminski RJ, et al: Body background defects with ^{99m}Tc-DTPA after renal transplantation: case reports. J Nucl Med 17:696–698, 1976.

5. Fawwaz RA, Johnson PM: Localization of gallium-67 in the normally functioning allograft kidney: concise communication. J Nucl Med 20:207–209, 1979.

6. Freedman GS, Schiff M, Zager P, et al: The temporal and pathological significance of perfusion failure following transplantation. Radiology 114:649–654, 1975.

7. Freeman LM: Clinical scintillation imaging, in Freeman LM, Johnson PM (eds): The Kidney. New York: Grune and Stratton, 1975, pp. 382–386.

8. Frick MP, Loken MK, Goldberg ME, et al: Use of ^{99m}Tc-sulphur colloid in evaluation of renal transplant complications. J Nucl Med 17:181–183, 1976.

9. George EA: Radionuclide diagnosis of allograft rejection. Sem Nucl Med 12:379–386, 1982.

10. George EA, Codd JE, Newton WT, et al: Comparative evaluation of renal transplant rejection with radio-iodinated fibrinogen, ^{99m}Tc-sulphur colloid and ^{67}Ga-citrate. J Nucl Med 17:175–180, 1976.

11. Haden HT, Stacy WK, Wolf JS, et al: Scintiphotography in diagnosis of urinary fistula after renal transplantation. J Nucl Med 16:612–615, 1975.

12. Hume DM: Kidney transplantation, in Rapaport F, Dausset J (eds): Human Transplantation. New York: Grune and Stratton, 1978, p. 127.

13. Jackson FI, Lentle BC, Higgins MR: Lymphocutaneous fistula following renal transplantation. Clin Nucl Med 5:19–21, 1980.

14. Kaude JV, Stone M, Fuller M, et al: Papillary necrosis in kidney transplant patients. Radiology 120:69–74, 1971.

15. Kim YC, Massari PU, Brown ML, et al: Clinical significance of ^{99m}Technetium sulphur colloid accumulation in renal transplant patients. Radiology 124:745–748, 1977.

16. Mandel SR, Mattern WD, Staab E: Venous embolus to a transplanted kidney. Arch Surg 3:1135–1148, 1976.

17. Pavel DG, Jonasson DM, Anderson O, et al: Improved diagnosis of post renal transplant collecting system abnormalities by radionuclide studies (abstract). J Nucl Med 16:557, 1975.

18. Quinlan JA, Dagher FJ, Loberg MD, et al: Early detection of acute rejection in renal allografts using radioiodinated autologous fibrinogen. Am J Surg 130:136–142, 1975.

19. Rosenthall L, Mangel R, Lisbona R, et al: Diagnostic applications of radiopertechnetate and radiohippurate imaging in post-renal transplant complications. Radiology 111:347–358, 1974.

20. Shimshak RR, Hattner RS, Tucker C, et al: Sequential acute tubular necrosis in kidneys with multiple renal arteries transplanted from living related donors. J Nucl Med 18:1074–1078, 1977.

21. Staab EV, Whittier F, Patton DD, et al: Early evaluation of cadaver renal allotransplant by means of radionuclide imaging. Radiology 106:147–151, 1973.

22. Weiss ER, Blahd WH, Winston MA, et al: Scintillation camera in the evaluation of renal transplants. J Nucl Med 11:69–77, 1970.

23. Weiss ER, Winston MA, Krishnamurthy GT, et al: Ureteral kinking and hydronephrosis in transplanted kidney mimicking the rejection phenomenon. J Nucl Med 12:43–46, 1971.

24. Winkel KZ, Harbst H, Das BD, et al: Application of radionuclides in renal transplantation. Sem Nucl Med 4:169–185, 1974.
25. Winston MA, Weiss ER, Blahd WH, et al: Use of ^{131}I-fibrinogen in detection of renal transplant rejection. Investigative Urology 9:119–123, 1971.

Chapter 35

Cystography

AMOLAK SINGH

I. Vesicoureteric reflux by direct radionuclide cystography (1–5)

   A. Common
- **1.** Recurrent urinary tract infections
- **2.** Neurogenic bladder with infection

   B. Uncommon
- **1.** Congenital anomalies of urinary tract
  - **a.** ureteric duplication
  - **b.** ureteric ectopia
  - **c.** congenital megaureter
  - **d.** extrophy of bladder
  - **e.** "prune belly" or Eagle-Barrett syndrome
  - **f.** "horse-shoe" kidney
- **2.** Bladder outlet obstruction
  - **a.** urethral valve
  - **b.** urethral stricture
  - **c.** bladder tumor
  - **d.** prostatic tumor
  - **e.** prostatic enlargement

   C. Rare
- **1.** Iatrogenic

      a. ureteric reimplantation
      b. ureteric meatotomy
      c. excision ureterocele
      d. traumatic manipulation of ureteric stone
      e. accidental surgical trauma to ureteric orifice
      f. radiation cystitis
  2. Infection
      a. tuberculosis
      b. bilharziasis
  3. Hirschsprung's disease

REFERENCES

1. Conway JJ, Kruglik GD: Effectiveness of direct and indirect radionuclide cystography in detecting vesicoureteral reflux. J Nucl Med 17:81–83, 1976.
2. Emmett JL, Witten DM: Clinical Urography. Philadelphia: W.B. Saunders, 1971, pp. 451, 839, 913, 1259, 1422.
3. Ransley PG: Vesicoureteric reflux: continuing surgical dilemma. Urology 12:246–255, 1978.
4. Rothwell DL, Constable AR, Albrecht M: Radionuclide cystography in the investigation of vesicoureteric reflux in children. Lancet 1:1072–1075, 1977.
5. Shopfner CE: Vesicoureteral reflux. Radiology 95:637–648, 1970.

Chapter 36

Testes

JOHN G. McAFEE
EDWARD B. SILBERSTEIN

I. Falsely normal scrotal perfusion and blood pool
  A. Common

1. Chronic, mild or resolving epididymitis (9, 18)
2. Torsion of appendix testis or appendix epididymis (12)
3. Undescended testis (9)
4. Minor but palpable enlargement of testis or cord (18)
5. Post-orchiopexy (1)

B. Less common

1. Testicular tumor (8, 13)
2. Incomplete testicular torsion (4, 7)
3. Testicular contusion (13)
4. Biliary orchiopexy with bilateral severance of the internal spermatic artery (18)

II. Increased perfusion (hyperemia) extending into scrotum without focal defects

A. Common

1. Acute epididymitis or epididymo-orchitis (10, 18)
2. Traumatic orchitis (4, 9, 10)
3. Torsion of appendix testis (7, 15)

B. Less common

1. Testicular tumor (9, 15)
2. Varicocele (6)
3. Reactive inflammation to missed torsion (12)

C. Rare

1. Reactive scrotal hyperemia secondary to torsion of redux testis (5)
2. Post-orchiopexy (1)

III. Focal area of decreased uptake in scrotum

A. Common

1. Testicular torsion (7, 8, 9, 14, 16)
2. Hydrocele (11, 17)
3. Abscess (17)

B. Less common

1. Testicular prosthesis (17)
2. Inguinal hernial sac (17)
3. Hematoma (17)
4. Spermatocele (9)
5. Hematocele (15)
6. Testicular tumor (with necrosis) (8)
7. Torsion of appendix testis (15, 17)
8. Chronic epididymitis (decreased but not absent uptake) (1, 9)
9. Acute epididymo-orchitis (decreased but not absent uptake) (13)
10. Post-varicocelectomy (1)

C. Rare
   1. Vasculitis (1)

IV. Increased scrotal activity surrounding focal defect
   A. Common
      1. Abscess (9)
      2. Missed torsion (>48 hours) (12, 17)
      3. Orchiectomy (12)
      4. Neoplasm (with necrosis) (9, 12)
         a. entodermal sinus tumor (3)
         b. seminoma (4)
      5. Hematoma (12, 17)
         a. infected hematoma (11)
   B. Less common
      1. Epididymo-orchitis (uptake decreased centrally but not absent) (10, 17)
      2. Hematocele (2, 12)
      3. Spermatocele (9)
   C. Rare
      1. Infarcted adrenal rest (12)
      2. Testicular infarction from infection (12)
      3. Vasculitis (1)

V. Decreased scrotal uptake with central nidus of activity
   A. Uncommon
      1. Hydrocele (8, 12)
      2. Scrotal hydrops (2)

REFERENCES

1. Abu-Sleiman R, Ho JE, Gregory JG: Scrotal scanning. Urology 13:326–330, 1979.
2. Barrett IR, Buozas DJ: The lady-bug sign of scrotal hydrops. Clin Nucl Med 1:35, 1976.
3. Boedicker RA, Glicklich M, Sty JR: Rim sign in entodermal sinus tumor. Clin Nucl Med 4:103–131, 1979.
4. Datta NS, Mishkin FS: Radionuclide imaging in intrascrotal lesions. JAMA 231:1060–1062, 1975.
5. Fink-Bennett D, Uppal TK, Conway GF: Redux testis: a potential pitfall in testicular imaging. J Urol 121:821–822, 1979.
6. Freund J, Handelsman DJ, Bautovich GJ, et al: Detection of varicocele by radionuclide blood-pool scanning. Radiology 137:227–230, 1980.
7. Gilday DC, Hitch D, Sherdling B, et al: Testicular imaging for testicular torsion in pediatric surgery. J Nucl Med 17:553–554, 1976.
8. Hahn LC, Nadel NS, Gitter MH, et al: Testicular scanning: a new modality for the preoperative diagnosis of testicular torsion. J Urol 113:60–72, 1975.

9. Holder LE, Martin JR, Holmes ER, et al: Testicular radionuclide angiography and static imaging: anatomy, scintigraphic interpretations and clinical indications. Radiology 125:739–752, 1977.

10. Lawrence D, Mishkin FS: Radionuclide imaging in epididymo-orchitis. J Urol 112:387–389, 1974.

11. Lutzker LG, Novich I, Perez LA, et al: Radionuclide scrotal imaging. Appl Radiol 6:187–194, 1977.

12. Mishkin FS: Differential diagnostic features of the radionuclide scrotal image. Am J Roentgenol 128:127–129, 1977.

13. Mukerjee MG, Vollero RA, Mittemeyer BT, et al: Diagnostic value of ^{99m}Tc in scrotal scan. Urology 6:453–455, 1975.

14. Nadel NS, Gitter MH, Hahn LC, et al: Preoperative diagnosis of testicular torsion. Urology 1:478–479, 1973.

15. Riley TW, Mosbaugh PG, Coles JL, et al: Use of radioisotope scan in evaluation of intrascrotal lesions. J Urol 116:472–475, 1976.

16. Skoglund RW, McRoberts JW, Magda H: Torsion of the spermatic cord: a review of the literature and analysis of 70 new cases. J Urol 104:604–607, 1970.

17. Stage KH, Schoenvogel R, Lewis S: Testicular scanning: clinical experience with 72 patients. J Urol 125:334–337, 1981.

18. Winston MA, Handler SJ, Pritchard JH: Ultrasonography of the testis—correlation with radiotracer perfusion. J Nucl Med 19:615–618, 1978.

Part VIII

Hematology

Chapter 37

Schilling Test

EDWARD B. SILBERSTEIN

AMOLAK SINGH

I. Causes of abnormal stage I Schilling Test (B-12 alone) (36)

    A. Intestinal malabsorption (31)

        1. Crohn's disease (30)

        2. Surgical resection or bypass of terminal ileum (30)

        3. Lymphoma of terminal ileum (30)

        4. Small bowel lesions with bacterial stagnation and B-12 utilization (6, 36)

            a. blind loop

            b. diverticula

            c. strictures

        5. Pancreatic insufficiency (30)

        6. *Diphyllobothrium latum* (23, 30)

        7. Drugs (23, 30)

            a. para-aminosalicylic acid

            b. colchicine

            c. calcium chelating agents

            d. neomycin

            e. bigaunides

            f. alcohol

        8. Zollinger-Ellison syndrome*

        9. Vitamin B-12 or folic acid deficiency induced malabsorption (9, 25, 44)

The use of an asterisk * in this chapter indicates that this entity has been observed by one of the authors but the case report has not been published.

       10. Tropical sprue (30)
       11. Celiac disease (30)
       12. Radiation ileitis (12)
       13. Fistula bypassing ileum (12)
  B. Absence of intrinsic factor (3)
       1. Total or partial gastrectomy (45)
       2. Addisonian pernicious anemia (38)
       3. Congenital absence of intrinsic factor secretion (37)
       4. Biologically inert intrinsic factor (27)
  C. Genetic abnormality of transport-protein (transcobalamin II) (21)
  D. Artefactual
       1. Incomplete urine collection or poor urinary output (45)
       2. Giving vitamin B-12 and intrinsic factor in separate capsules so that mixing is inadequate or intrinsic factor is antibody bound (33)
       3. Giving 3–21 mg. vitamin B-12 parenterally 3–5 days before the Schilling test (19)

II. Causes of abnormal stage II Schilling test (B-12 plus intrinsic factor) (36)

  A. Intestinal malabsorption as above (see Section I,A) (31)
       1. Vitamin B-12 deficiency induced B-12 malabsorption may not be corrected until several months after B-12 therapy has begun (9)
  B. Inactive intrinsic factor concentrate (25)
  C. Antibody to administered intrinsic factor (42)
  D. Genetic abnormality of transport protein (transcobalamin II) (21)
  E. Familial juvenile B-12 malabsorption with proteinuria and ileal receptor deficiency (18, 24)

III. Causes of normal stage III Schilling test (after antibiotics) with abnormal stage II

  A. Small bowel lesions with bacterial stagnation (6, 36)
       1. Jejunal diverticula
       2. Strictures
       3. Blind loops

IV. Causes of falsely normal Schilling test

  A. Recent radiopharmaceutical administration*
  B. Fecal contamination of collected urine*
  C. Contamination of contents or exterior of test tubes used for container*
  D. Administration of excessive radioactive B = 12 over $1\mu g$*

References for this chapter may be found at the end of Chapter 42, page 228.

Chapter 38

Shortened Chromium-51 Red Cell Survival (4, 13, 22, 29)

EDWARD B. SILBERSTEIN

AMOLAK SINGH

I. Intrinsic erythrocytic defects (4)

  A. Congenital

    1. Membrane disorders

      a. hereditary spherocytosis (32)

      b. hereditary elliptocytosis (39)

    2. Enzyme deficiencies (41)

      a. hereditary deficiency of enzymes of Embden-Meyerhof pathway (anerobic glycolysis)*

      b. abnormalities of the phosphogluconate oxidative pathway*

    3. Disorders of hemoglobin synthesis

      a. erythropoietic porphyria

      b. hemoglobinopathies S, C, etc.

      c. thalassemia syndromes (32)

  B. Acquired

    1. Folic acid deficiency (severe)

    2. Vitamin B-12 deficiency (severe)

    3. Iron deficiency (severe)

    4. Erythrocytes produced in response to hemorrhage (8)

    5. Paroxysmal nocturnal hemoglobinuria (32)

    6. Refractory hyperplastic anemia and other myeloproliferative disorders including leukemia (22)

II. Extra-erythrocytic factors (4)

  A. Antibodies

    1. Due to incompatible erythrocyte transfusions (22)

    2. Autoimmune hemolytic anemias (warm and cold antibodies) (2, 20)

  B. Chemical agents and drugs

    1. Related to the size of the dose of toxin, e.g. phenylhydrazine, toluene, benzene, acetanilid, aniline, lead, arsine, methyl chloride (41)

The use of an asterisk * in this chapter indicates that this entity has been observed by one of the authors but the case report has not been published.

  2. Secondary immunohemolytic anemia due to drugs, e.g. penicillin, quinidine, quinine, alpha-methyldopa, phenacetin (47)
C. Infectious agents*
  1. Malaria
  2. Septicemia
      a. *Clostridium welchii*
      b. *Bartonella*
      c. subacute bacterial endocarditis
D. Disseminated intravascular coagulation (41)
E. Vasculitis (41)
F. Anemia of chronic disease (15)
  1. Chronic inflammatory disease
      a. septic or aseptic
          (1) hepatitis and other liver disorders (14)
          (2) nephritis and other causes of uremia (15)
  2. Cancer, myeloproliferative and lymphoproliferative disorders
G. Mechanical causes
  1. Heart valve hemolysis (41)
H. Hypersplenism (17)

III. Artefactual

A. Blood loss or transfusion during the test*

References for this chapter may be found at the end of Chapter 42, page 228.

Chapter 39

Chromium-51 Red Cell Sequestration (26, 32, 43)

EDWARD B. SILBERSTEIN

AMOLAK SINGH

I. Rising spleen localization index, or spleen-to-liver or spleen-to-precordium ratio[1]

The use of an asterisk * in this chapter indicates that this entity has been observed by one of the authors but the case report has not been published.

[1] Splenomegaly alone may be associated with high initial spleen-to-liver ratio or spleen-to-precordium ratio, but no progressive rise is encountered unless increased splenic sequestration with cell destruction is present.

A. Common
    1. Acquired hemolytic anemia (2, 20, 32)
    2. Leukemia, chronic lymphocytic or monocytic (32)
B. Less common
    1. Hereditary spherocytosis (32)
    2. Anemia with ''spur cell'' membrane deformity (14)
    3. Myeloma (32)
    4. Myelosclerosis (17)
    5. Gaucher's disease (17)
    6. Felty's syndrome (17)
    7. Sickle thalassemia (32)
    8. Hodgkin's disease (32)
    9. Paroxysmal nocturnal hemoglobinuria (32)

II. Increased accumulation of labeled red cells in liver*

  A. Common
    1. Sickle cell disease
  B. Uncommon
    1. Alcoholic liver disease

References for this chapter may be found at the end of Chapter 42, page 228.

Chapter 40

Blood Volume

AMOLAK SINGH

EDWARD B. SILBERSTEIN

I. Elevated red cell volume with high, normal, or low plasma volume (7, 29)

  A. Polycythemia rubra vera
  B. Secondary polycythemia—causes:
    1. Hypoxia
      a. lung disease with chronic hypoxemia
        (1) chronic lung disease
          (a) obstructive
          (b) restrictive
        (2) pulmonary arteriovenous fistulae

   (3) cavernous hemangioma of lung
   (4) Pickwickian syndrome
   b. smokers' polycythemia from excess carbon monoxide
   c. congenital heart diseases with partial shunting of blood from pulmonary circulation
   (1) pulmonic stenosis with right-to-left shunt
   (2) transposition of great arteries
   (3) tricuspid atresia; Ebstein's anomaly
   (4) persistent truncus arteriosus
   (5) tetralogy of Fallot
   d. high altitude
   e. tissue hypoxia from cobalt toxicity
2. Cushing's syndrome
3. Hemoglobinopathies with increased oxygen affinity (over 20 described)
4. Lesions producing erythropoietin
   a. cerebellar hemangioblastoma
   b. renal
   (1) hypernephroma
   (2) adenoma
   (3) sarcoma
   (4) cysts
   (5) hydronephrosis
   c. hepatic carcinoma
   d. uterine leiomyoma
5. Familial erythrocytosis

II. Decreased plasma volume with normal red cell volume (relative polycythemia) (7)

   A. Common
   1. Fulminant diarrhea
   2. Protracted vomiting
   3. Extensive burns
   4. Dehydration
   B. Uncommon
   1. Idiopathic (''stress'' polycythemia; Gaisbock's syndrome)

III. Low whole body hematocrit: venous hematocrit ratio (1)

   A. Common
   1. Apprehension
   2. Vasopressors
   3. Hypertension
   4. Hypovolemia
   5. Shivering

      6. Chronic diseases
      7. Dehydration
      8. Intestinal obstruction
      9. Geriatric patients
     10. Hypothermia
  B. Uncommon
      1. Pheochromocytoma

IV. High whole body hematocrit: venous hematocrit ratio (1)

  A. Common
      1. Anesthesia
      2. Sedation
      3. Sympatholytic and ganglion blocking drugs
      4. Hypervolemia
      5. Cardiac decompensation
      6. Pediatric patients
      7. Late pregnancy
  B. Uncommon
      1. Neurogenic shock
      2. Marrow diseases
      3. Splenomegaly

References for this chapter may be found at the end of Chapter 42, page 228.

Chapter 41

Ferrokinetics

AMOLAK SINGH
EDWARD B. SILBERSTEIN

I. Transferrin-bound Fe-59 plasma disappearance curve (15, 34, 40, 48)

  A. Enhanced clearance and/or turnover

The use of an asterisk * in this chapter indicates that this entity has been observed by one of the authors but the case report has not been published.

   1. Iron deficiency anemia (15)
      a. recent blood loss
   2. Anemia of chronic diseases including infection and cancer (15)[1]
      a. myeloma (22)
   3. Some myeloproliferative disorders with or without extra-medullary hematopoiesis or ineffective erythropoiesis (15, 46)
      a. polycythemia vera (15)
   4. Hemolytic anemia (5, 13)
      a. hereditary spherocytosis (1, 38)
      b. autoimmune hemolysis (15)
      c. paroxysmal nocturnal hemoglobinuria (15)
   5. Pernicious anemia (5, 16)
   6. Hyperplastic refractory anemia (35)
   7. Hyperthyroidism (15)
   8. Folate deficiency (15)
   9. Hemoglobinopathy
      a. thalassemia (15, 46)
      b. sickle cell disease (5, 15)
B. Slow clearance
   1. Common
      a. renal failure (15)
      b. hypothyroidism (15, 28)
   2. Uncommon
      a. aplastic anemias (15, 46)
      b. hemochromatosis (5)
      c. some myeloproliferative disorders (11, 16)
         (1) leukemia
      d. marrow hypoplasia following chemotherapy or radiotherapy (10)

II. Daily external body organ counts (48)

   A. Persistently elevated marrow uptake (ineffective erythropoiesis) (15)
      1. Megaloblastic anemias (15)
         a. pernicious anemia
         b. folate deficiency anemia
      2. Hyperplastic (often sideroblastic) refractory anemias of unknown etiology*
      3. Many myeloproliferative syndromes*
      4. Thalassemia (22)
   B. Decreased marrow uptake with increased splenic and/or liver intake
      1. Myelofibrosis with splenic hematopoiesis (11, 15)
         a. myeloid metaplasia

---

[1] Iron turnover may be normal or slightly low with increased clearance since it is proportional to serum iron as well as being inversely proportional to the half time of serum iron clearance.

    b. chronic or acute leukemia (10)

    c. some solid tumors*

  2. Aplastic anemia (15)

  3. Hypoplasia secondary to chemotherapy, radiotherapy (45)

  4. Hemochromatosis (10)

III. Low Fe-59 utilization (15)

  A. Uncommon

    1. Aplastic anemia

    2. Any cause of erythroid hypoplasia

      a. chemotherapy

      b. radiotherapy

      c. idiopathic

    3. Hemochromatosis

    4. Myelofibrosis

    5. Pernicious anemia

    6. Leukemia

References for this chapter may be found at the end of Chapter 42, page 228.

Chapter 42

Shortened Chromium-51 Platelet Survival (3, 13, 29, 38)

AMOLAK SINGH

EDWARD B. SILBERSTEIN

I. Autoimmune disorders

  A. Autoimmune thrombocytopenic purpura

  B. Lupus erythematosus

  C. Lymphoproliferative disorders

II. Thrombotic thrombocytopenic purpura

III. Disseminated intravascular coagulation

    A. Cardiac prosthetic valves
    B. Extracorporeal circulatory devices
    C. Sepsis
    D. Neoplasia

IV. Drugs

    A. Acetazolamide
    B. Thiazides
    C. Sulfonylureas
    D. Phenytoin
    E. Gold salts
    F. Chloroquine
    G. Methyldopa
    H. Digitoxin, digoxin
    I. Sulfonamides

V. Artefactual

    A. Significant blood loss
    B. Transfusion of blood

REFERENCES[1]

1. Albert SN: Blood volume in clinical practice, in Rothfield B (ed): Nuclear Medicine In Vitro. Philadelphia: J.B. Lippincott Co., 1983, p. 360.
2. Allgood JW, Chaplin H: Idiopathic acquired autoimmune hemolytic anemia. Am J Med 43:254–273, 1967.
3. Aster RH: Clinical evaluation of thrombokinetics, in Williams WJ, Beutler E, Erslev AJ, et al (eds): Hematology. New York: McGraw-Hill, 1977, pp. 1221–1224.
4. Berlin N: Determination of red blood cell life span. JAMA 188:375–378, 1964.
5. Bothwell TH, Hurtado AV, Donahue DM, et al: Erythrokinetics IV. The plasma iron turnover as a measure of erythropoiesis. Blood 12:409–422, 1957.
6. Brandt LJ, Bernstein LH, Wagle A: Production of vitamin B-12 analogues in patients with small-bowel bacterial overgrowth. Ann Int Med 87:545–551, 1977.
7. Braunwald E: Cyanosis, hypoxia and polycythemia, in Isselbacher KJ, Adams RD, Braunwald E (eds): Harrison's Principles of Internal Medicine. New York: McGraw-Hill, 1980, pp. 166–171.
8. Card RT, McGrath MJ, Paulson EJ, et al: Life-span and autohemolysis of macrocytic erythrocytes produced in response to hemorrhage. Am J Physiol 216:974–978, 1969.
9. Carmel R, Herbert V: Correctable intestinal defect of vitamin B-12 absorption in pernicious anemia. Ann Int Med 67:1201–1207, 1967.
10. Chaudhuri TK: Marrow fibrosis studied by ferrokinetics. Sem Nucl Med 11:228–229, 1981.

[1] This list contains references for Chapters 37–42.

11. Chaudhuri TK, Chaudhuri TK: Marrow fibrosis studied by ferrokinetics. Sem Nucl Med 11:228–229, 1980.
12. Cohen MB: Vitamin B-12 deficiency. Sem Nucl Med 11:226–227, 1981.
13. Cooper RA, Buhn HF: Hemolytic anemias, in Isselbacher KJ, Adams RD, Braunwald E (eds): Harrison's Principles of Internal Medicine. New York: McGraw-Hill, 1980, pp. 1533–1546.
14. Cooper RA, Kimball DB, Durocher JR: Role of the spleen in membrane conditioning and hemolysis of spur cells in liver disease. N Engl J Med 290:1279–1284, 1974.
15. Finch CA, Deubelbeiss K, Cook DJ, et al: Ferrokinetics in man. Medicine 49:17–53, 1970.
16. Giblett ER, Coleman DH, Pirzio-Biroli G, et al: Erythrokinetics: Quantitative measurement of red cell production and destruction in normal subjects and patients with anemia. Blood 11:291–309, 1956.
17. Goldberg A, Hutchison HE, MacDonald E: Radiochromium in the selection of patients with haemolytic anemia for splenectomy. Lancet 1:109–114, 1966.
18. Goldberg LS, Fudenberg HH: Familial selective malabsorption of vitamin B-12. N Engl J Med 279:405–407, 1968.
19. Grames GM, Reiswig R, Jansen C, et al: Feasibility of consecutive day Schilling tests. J Nucl Med 15:949–952, 1974.
20. Habibi B, Homberg J-C, Schaison G, et al: Autoimmune hemolytic anemia in children. Am J Med 56:61–69, 1974.
21. Hakami N, Neiman PE, Canellos G, et al: Neonatal megoloblastic anemia due to inherited transcobalamin II deficiency in two siblings. N Engl J Med 285:1163–1170, 1971.
22. Haley TJ: Use of radioactive isotopes in hematology, in Szirmai E. (ed): Nuclear Hematology. New York: Academic Press, 1965, pp. 23–39.
23. Herbert V: Metformin and B-12 malabsorption. Ann Int Med 76:140–142, 1972.
24. Imerslung O: Idiopathic chronic megaloblastic anemia in children. Acta Pediatr (supp) 119:1–115, 1960.
25. Jacobson BE, Onstad GR: Misleading second stage Schilling test due to inactive intrinsic factor concentrate. Ann Int Med 91:570–580, 1979.
26. Jones NCH, Szur L: Determination of the sites of red-cell destruction using ^{51}Cr-labelled red cells. Br J Haemat 3:320–331, 1957.
27. Katz M, Lee SK, Cooper BA: Vitamin B-12 malabsorption due to a biologically inert intrinsic factor. New Engl J Med 287:425–429, 1972.
28. Kiely JM, Purnell DC, Owen CA: Erythrokinetics in myxedema. Ann Int Med 76:533–538, 1967.
29. Korst DR: Blood volume and red cell survival, in Wagner HN, Jr. (ed): Principles of Nuclear Medicine. Philadelphia: W.B. Saunders Co., 1968, pp. 429–443.
30. Lindenbaum J: Aspects of vitamin B-12 and folate metabolism in malabsorption syndromes. Am J Med 67:1037–1048, 1979.
31. Lindenbaum J, Pizzimenti JF, Shea N, et al: Small intestinal function in vitamin B-12 deficiency. Ann Int Med 80:320–331, 1974.
32. McCurdy PR, Rath CE: Splenectomy in hemolytic anemia. Results predicted by body scanning after injection of Cr-51 tagged red cells. N Engl J Med 259:459–463, 1958.
33. McDonald JWD, Barr RM, Barton WB: Spurious Schilling test results obtained with intrinsic factor enclosed in capsules. Ann Int Med 83:827–829, 1975.
34. McIntyre PA, Dibos PE: The blood, in Rocha AFG, Herbert JC (eds): Textbook of Nuclear Medicine: Clinical Applications. Philadelphia: Lea and Febiger, 1979, pp. 388–439.
35. McIntyre PA: Newer development in nuclear medicine applicable to hematology. Prog in

Hematol 10:361–409, 1977.

36. McIntyre PA: Use of radioisotope techniques in the clinical evaluation of patients with megaloblastic anemia. Sem Nucl Med 5:79–91, 1975.
37. Mollin DL, Baker SJ, Doniach I: Addisonian pernicious anemia without gastric atrophy in a young man. Br J Haematol 1:278–290, 1955.
38. Nossel HL: Platelet disorders, in Isselbacher KJ, Adams RD, Braunwald E (eds): Harrison's Principles of Internal Medicine. New York: McGraw-Hill, 1980, pp. 1555–1559.
39. Quaife MA, Gregorius C, Kelly R: Characteristics of red blood cell survival from subjects with hereditary elliptocytosis. Clin Nucl Med 3:398–400, 1978.
40. Ricketts C, Cavill I: Ferrokinetics: methods and interpretation. Clin Nucl Med 3:159–164, 1978.
41. Rogers J: Anemia thrombocytopenia, proteinuria and central nervous system dysfunction. Am J Med 63:789–798, 1977.
42. Schade S, Feick P, Muckerheide M, et al: Occurrence in gastric juice of antibody to complex of intrinsic factor and vitamin B-12. N Engl J Med 275:528–531, 1966.
43. Schloesser LL, Korst DR, Clatanoff DV, et al: Radioactivity over the spleen and liver following the transfusion of chromium-51 labeled erythrocytes in hemolytic anemia. J Clin Invest 36:1470–1485, 1957.
44. Scott RB, Kammer RB, Burger WF: Reduced absorption of vitamin B-12 in two patients with folic acid deficiency. Ann Int Med 69:111–114, 1968.
45. Silberstein EB: The Schilling test. JAMA 208:2325, 1969.
46. Sturgeon P, Finch C: Erythrokinetics in Cooley's anemia. Blood 12:64–73, 1957.
47. Swanson MA, Chanmougan D, Schwartz RS: Immunohemolytic anemia due to anti-penicillin antibodies. N Engl J Med 274:178–182, 1966.
48. Weinstein IM: Disorders of hematopoiesis, the reticuloendothelial system and the spleen, in Blahd WH (ed): Nuclear Medicine. New York: McGraw-Hill, 1971, pp. 416–452.

Chapter 43

Marrow

JOHN G. McAFEE
EDWARD B. SILBERSTEIN

I. Diffusely increased radiocolloid activity in central (axial) marrow

   A. Common

    1. Iron deficiency anemia (43)

      a. post-hemorrhage (43)

    2. Sickle cell anemia and other hemolytic anemias (43)

    3. Megaloblastic anemias (43, 49)

    4. Liver disease

      a. fatty metamorphosis; alcoholism (12)

      b. cirrhosis (20)

      c. chronic active hepatitis (3)

B. Uncommon

    1. Lymphoproliferative diseases (43)

      a. multiple myeloma (43)

      b. Hodgkin's disease, advanced (6)

    2. Myeloproliferative disorders (3)

      a. polycythemia vera (11, 43)

    3. Multiple hepatic abscesses (16)

    4. Hepatoma (22)

    5. Congestive heart failure (25)

C. Rare

    1. Following severe abdominal trauma (48)

II. Increase in colloid activity in extremities (distal to the proximal third of humeri and femora; decreased axial marrow may accompany this pattern, especially with myeloproliferative-myelofibrotic disease)

A. Common

    1. Normal in children under 10 years (47)

    2. Cirrhosis, alcoholic hepatitis (20)

    3. Marrow suppression following radiation or chemotherapy for malignancy (17, 19, 27, 32, 47)

    4. Stages III and IV lymphoma, Hodgkin's or non-Hodgkin's (27)

    5. Iron deficiency anemia (43)

    6. Folate deficiency anemia (43)

    7. Sickle cell disorders (1, 49)

      a. S-S disease

      b. sickle cell-thalassemia

      c. S-C disease

B. Less common

    1. Severe bacterial infection (17)

    2. Renal transplants with immunosuppressive therapy (17)

    3. Skeletal metastases, usually advanced and accompanied by anemia (5)

    4. Acute and chronic lymphocytic and nonlymphocytic leukemia (21, 28, 37, 41, 43)

    5. Myeloproliferative disorders

      a. refractory sideroblastic anemia (40)

      b. polycythemia vera (41)

      c. myeloid metaplasia with myelofibrosis (30)

      6. Chronic hemolytic anemias (other than sickle cell disorders)
        a. congenital spherocytosis (11, 41)
        b. autoimmune hemolytic anemia (11)
        c. Fanconi's anemia (9)
      7. Cystic fibrosis (40)
      8. Myeloma (27)
      9. Myelofibrosis associated with renal osteodystrophy (54)
      10. Aplastic anemia (31)
      11. Pernicious anemia (11, 26, 43)
   C. Rare
      1. Gaucher's disease (7)

III. Focal increase in radiocolloid uptake

   A. Juxta-articular, especially extremities
      1. Common
        a. normal in children (47)
      2. Uncommon
        a. synovitis (2)
   B. Localized vertebral increase in radiocolloid uptake
      1. Common
        a. recent compression fracture (46)
        b. degenerative joint disease (53)
   C. Extramedullary radiocolloid uptake in hematopoietic tissue
      1. Uncommon
        a. thalassemia (50)

IV. Generalized absence or decrease in marrow uptake

   A. Common
      1. Aplastic anemia (49)
   B. Uncommon
      1. Lymphoproliferative disease
        a. Hodgkin's disease, all stages (27, 43)
        b. lymphomas
          (1) after chemotherapy (20, 49)
        c. myeloma (37, 43)
      2. Acute and chronic leukemia (11, 34, 37, 43)
      3. Myeloproliferative disorders
        a. myeloid metaplasia with myelofibrosis (24, 43)
        b. polycythemia—late stage (27)
      4. Uremia (43)
      5. Marrow carcinomatosis (29, 44)
      6. Sickle cell disease-aplastic crisis (18)
   C. Rare

      1. Osteopetrosis (35)
      2. Mucopolysaccharidoses (26)
      3. Gaucher's disease (7)

V. Focal diminished or absent radiocolloid uptake in marrow

  A. Common
      1. Normal variant noted symmetrically in femoral heads (53)
      2. Avascular necrosis (33, 53)
         a. sickle cell disorders and arthropathy (usually juxta-articular in extremities) (1, 2)
         b. Legg-Perthes disease (10)
         c. hip dislocation (33, 41)
         d. femoral neck or head fracture (33)
         e. associated with alcoholism (33)
         f. associated with corticosteroids (33)
         g. idiopathic (33)
         h. lymphomatous (8)
      3. Tumor
         a. metastases (17, 29, 43)
         b. myeloma (11, 28, 43)
         c. lymphoma (27, 43)
         d. neuroblastoma (23, 47)
      4. Leukemia (28)
         a. acute
         b. chronic lymphocytic
      5. Paget's disease (15, 41)
      6. Radiation therapy portals after 2000–4000 rads (4, 41, 47)
      7. Osteomyelitis (14)
      8. Healed rib fractures (6)
  B. Uncommon
      1. Myeloid metaplasia with myelofibrosis (43)
         a. chronic renal failure with areas of myelofibrosis (39)
  C. Rare
      1. Gaucher's disease (7)

VI. Localized diminished radiocolloid marrow uptake with normal image by skeletal scanning agents

  A. Common
      1. Various malignancies (5%) (38, 41)
      2. Infarction in sickle cell disorders (1)
  B. Uncommon
      1. Acute osteomyelitis (14)

VII. Localized diminished radiocolloid marrow uptake with increased uptake by skeletal scanning agents

    A. Common
        1. Metastases (38, 41)
        2. Paget's disease (15)
        3. Healed or healing fractures (6)
        4. Sickle cell disease (1, 2)

VIII. Diffuse decrease in marrow uptake with diffuse increase in uptake with skeletal scanning agents

    A. Uncommon
        1. Myeloid metaplasia with myelofibrosis (24, 43)
    B. Rare
        1. Osteopetrosis (35)

IX. Normal marrow image associated with positive images with skeletal scanning agents

    A. Common
        1. Metastatic carcinoma (5)

X. Dissociation between marrow radiocolloid and radioiron activity (radioiron activity disproportionately decreased)

    A. Uncommon
        1. Aplastic or hypoplastic anemia, acquired or congenital (32, 36, 51)
        2. Hodgkin's disease treated with radiation or chemotherapy (36, 51)
        3. Radiation therapy or chemotherapy, especially early in the course of treatment (51)
        4. Polycythemia vera, usually after myelosuppression (36, 51)
        5. Myelofibrosis with myeloid metaplasia (51)

XI. Dissociation between marrow radiocolloid and ^{111}In-chloride activity (indium decreased). ^{111}In-transferrin distribution is usually similar to that of [59]Fe (30) but may also resemble that of colloids (32)

    A. Uncommon
        1. Leukemias with associated anemia (13)
        2. Radiation therapy (30)
        3. Preleukemia (36)
    B. Rare
        1. Chronic Thorotrast irradiation (36)

XII. Focal increase in marrow ^{111}In-chloride activity

    A. Uncommon

        1. Lymphomas (13)

XIII. Accelerated blood clearance of colloid

    A. Common

        1. Hemolytic anemias (17)

        2. Acute bacterial infections (52)

        3. Rheumatoid arthritis (42)

    B. Uncommon

        1. Lymphomas, especially advanced stages (17, 45)

        2. Acute rheumatic fever (42)

        3. Systemic lupus erythematosus (42)

XIV. Delayed blood clearance of colloid

    A. Common

        1. Viral infections (52)

        2. Cirrhosis and many other hepatocellular disorders (17)

    B. Uncommon

        1. Acute leukemia (17)

        2. Portal vein obstruction (17)

REFERENCES

1. Alavi A, Bond JP, Kuhl DE, et al: Scan detection of bone marrow infarcts in sickle cell disorders. J Nucl Med 15:1003–1007, 1974.

2. Alavi A, Schumacher HR, Dorwart B, et al: Bone marrow scan evaluation of arthropathy in sickle cell disorders. Arch Int Med 136:436–440, 1975.

3. Bekerman C, Gottschalk A: Diagnostic significance of the relative uptake of liver compared with spleen in ^{99m}Tc-sulphur colloid scintiphotography. J Nucl Med 12:237–240, 1971.

4. Bell EG, McAfee JG, Constable WC: Local radiation damage to bone and marrow demonstrated by radioisotopic imaging. Radiology 92:1083–1088, 1969.

5. Catane R, Kaufman JH, Bakshi S, et al: Indium chloride bone-marrow scanning in advanced prostatic carcinoma. NY State J Med 77:1413–1416, 1977.

6. Chafetz N, Slivka J, Taylor A, et al: Decreased ^{99m}Tc sulphur colloid activity in healed rib fractures. Radiology 126:735–736, 1978.

7. Cheng TH, Holman BL: Radionuclide assessment of Gaucher's disease. J Nucl Med 19:1333–1336, 1978.

8. Cowan JD, Rubin RN, Kies MS, et al: Bone marrow necrosis. Cancer 46:2168–2171, 1980.

9. Chu JH, Ho JE, Monteleone PL, et al: Technetium colloid bone marrow imaging in Fanconi's anemia. Pediatrics 64:635–639, 1979.

10. D'Angelis JA: Pinhole imaging in Legg-Perthes disease. Sem Nucl Med 6:69–82, 1976.

11. Dibos PE, Judisch JM, Spaulding MB, et al: Indium chloride bone marrow scanning in advanced prostatic carcinoma. NY State J Med 77:1413–1416, 1977.

12. Drum DE, Beard JO: Liver scintigraphic features associated with alcoholism. J Nucl Med 19:154–160, 1978.

13. Farrer PA, Saha GB, Katz M: Further observations on the use of ^{111}In-transferrin for the visualization of bone marrow in man. J Nucl Med 14:394–395, 1973.

14. Feigin DS, Strauss HW, James AE: Detection of osteomyelitis by bone scanning (abstract). J Nucl Med 15:490, 1974.

15. Fletcher JW, Butler RL, Henry RE, et al: Bone marrow scanning in Paget's disease. J Nucl Med 14:928–930, 1973.

16. Gates GF, Gwinn JL, Lee FA, et al: Excess extrahepatic uptake of radio-colloid associated with liver abscess. J Nucl Med 14:537–540, 1973.

17. Groch GS, Perillie PE, Finch SC: Reticuloendothelial phagocytic function in patients with leukemia, lymphoma and multiple myeloma. Blood 26:489–499, 1965.

18. Helmer RE, Sayle BA, Alperin JB, et al: [111]In chloride bone marrow scintigraphy and ferrokinetic studies in a case of sickle cell anemia with transient erythroid aplasia. Acta Haemat 61:330–333, 1979.

19. Henry RE, Fletcher JW, Solaric-George E, et al: Effect of granulocytopenia, marrow suppressive drugs and infection on marrow reticuloendothelial patterns. J Nucl Med 15:343–348, 1974.

20. Henry RE, George EA, Daly JL, et al: Marrow scanning with Tc-99m sulphur colloid in non-hematologic diseases (abstract). J Nucl Med 16:535, 1975.

21. Hoppin EC, Lewis JP, DeNardo SJ: Bone marrow scintigraphy in the evaluation of acute nonlymphocytic leukemia. Clin Nucl Med 4:296–301, 1979.

22. Johnson PM, Grossman FM: Radioisotope scanning in primary carcinoma of the liver. Radiology 84:868–872, 1965.

23. Judisch JM, McIntyre PA: Recognition of metastatic neuroblastoma by scanning the reticuloendothelial system (RES). Johns Hopkins Med J 130:83–86, 1972.

24. Kim EE, DeLand FH: Myelofibrosis presenting as hypermetabolic bone disease by radionuclide imaging in a patient with asplenia. Clin Nucl Med 3:406–408, 1978.

25. Klingensmith WC, Datu JA, Burdick DC: Renal uptake of ^{99m}Tc-sulfur colloid in congestive heart failure. Radiology 127:185–187, 1978.

26. Klingensmith WC, Eikman EA, Maumenee I, et al: Abnormalities of regional reticuloendothelial cell function in patients with mucopolysaccharidoses (abstract). J Nucl Med 16:542, 1975.

27. Kniseley RM, Andrews GA, Edwards CL, et al: Scanning of bone marrow in haematopoietic disorders, in Medical Radioisotope Scanning, Vol. II. Vienna: I.A.E.A., 1964, pp. 207–225.

28. Kniseley RM, Andrews GA, Tanido R, et al: Delineation of active marrow by whole-body scanning with radioactive colloids. J Nucl Med 7:575–582, 1966.

29. Larsson L-G, Jonsson L: Bone-marrow scanning after intravenous injection of colloidal [198]Au, in Medical Radioisotope Scanning, Vol. II. Vienna: I.A.E.A., 1964, pp. 193–206.

30. Lilien DL, Berger HG, Anderson DP, et al: ^{111}In-chloride: a new agent for bone marrow imaging. J Nucl Med 14:184–186, 1973.

31. McNeil BJ, Holman BL, Button LN, et al: Use of indium chloride scintigraphy in patients with myelofibrosis. J Nucl Med 15:647–651, 1974.

32. Merrick MJ, Gordon-Smith EC, Lavender JP, et al: A comparison of ^{111}In with [52]Fe and ^{99m}Tc-sulfur colloid for bone marrow scanning. J Nucl Med 16:66–68, 1975.

33. Meyers MH, Dowsey NT, Moore TM: Determination of the vascularity of the femoral head with technetium-99m sulfur colloid. J Bone Joint Surg 59A:658–664, 1977.
34. Nelp WB, Larson SM: Patterns in clinical bone marrow imaging. J Nucl Med 13:456–457, 1972.
35. Park HM, Lambertus J: Skeletal and reticuloendothelial imaging in osteopetrosis: a case report. J Nucl Med 18:1091–1095, 1977.
36. Parmentier C, Therain F, Charbord P, et al: Comparative study of ^{111}In and ^{59}Fe bone marrow scanning. Eur J Nucl Med 2:89–92, 1977.
37. Price DC: Bone marrow imaging in leukemia and multiple myeloma (abstract). J Nucl Med 12:387, 1971.
38. Price DC, Hattner RS: Comparison of bone and bone marrow scintigraphy in the evaluation of malignant disease (abstract). J Nucl Med 16:559, 1975.
39. Quint PA, Klingensmith WC, Datu JA: Multiple regions of absent bone mineral and marrow function in a patient with chronic renal failure. Radiology 130:751–752, 1979.
40. Ronai P, Winchell HS, Anger HO, et al: Whole body scanning of ^{59}Fe for evaluating body distribution of erythropoietic marrow, splenic sequestration of red cells and hepatic deposition of iron. J Nucl Med 10:469–474, 1969.
41. Rosenthall L, Chartrand R: Radionuclide imaging of the bone marrow. Canad Med Assoc J 100:54–61, 1969.
42. Salky NK, Mills D, DiLuzio NR: Activity of the reticuloendothelial system in diseases of altered immunity. J Lab Clin Med 66:952–960, 1965.
43. Schreiner DP: Reticuloendothelial scans in disorders involving the bone marrow. J Nucl Med 15:1158–1162, 1974.
44. Schreiner DP, Hsu Y: Comparison of reticuloendothelial scans with bone scans in malignant disease. Clin Nucl Med 6:101–104, 1981.
45. Sheagren JN, Block JB, Wolff SM: Reticuloendothelial system phagocytic function in patients with Hodgkin's disease. J Clin Invest 46:855–862, 1967.
46. Shook DR, Reinke DB: Increased uptake of ^{99m}Tc-sulfur colloid in vertebral compression fractures. J Nucl Med 16:92–94, 1975.
47. Siddiqui AR, Oseas RS, Wellman HN, et al: Evaluation of bone-marrow scanning with technetium-99m sulfur colloid in pediatric oncology. J Nucl Med 20:379–386, 1979.
48. Smith FW, Brown RG, Gilday DL, et al: Bone marrow uptake of [99m]technetium-sulfur colloid after severe abdominal trauma in children. Pediatr Radiol 10:169–171, 1981.
49. Staub RT, Gaston E: ^{111}In-chloride distribution and kinetics in hematological disease. J Nucl Med 14:456–457, 1973.
50. Stebner FC, Bishop CR: Bone marrow scan and radioiron uptake of an intrathoracic mass. Clin Nucl Med 7:86–87, 1982.
51. Van Dyke D, Shkurkin C, Price D, et al: Differences in distribution of erythropoietic and reticuloendothelial marrow in hematologic disease. Blood 30:364–374, 1967.
52. Wagner HN, Iio M, Hornick RB: Studies of the reticuloendothelial system (RES) I. Changes in the phagocytic capacity of the RES in patients with certain infections. J Clin Invest 42:427–434, 1963.
53. Webber MM, Wagner J, Cragin M, et al: Femoral blood supply demonstrated by radiotracers (abstract). J Nucl Med 15:543, 1974.
54. Weinberg SG, Lubin A, Weiner S, et al: Myelofibrosis and renal osteodystrophy. Am J Med 63:755–764, 1977.

Chapter 44

Fibrinogen Uptake†

JOHN G. McAFEE

I. No areas of increased uptake

   A. Common

     1. Normal

     2. Venous thrombosis false negatives [13% (1), 17% (2), 51% (3)]

       a. old inactive thrombi (2)

       b. small thrombi (3)

       c. femoral vein thrombi (5)

       d. anticoagulation more than 5 days (1)

II. Local or regional increased uptake

   A. Common

     1. Venous thrombosis (1–6)

     2. False positives (negative contrast venogram) [10% (1), 35% (5), 30% in total hip replacements (4)]

       a. early transient rise during first post-operative day (2)

       b. healing wounds less than 3 weeks old (6, 7)

       c. other inflammatory lesions (1)

       d. hematoma (1)

       e. varicosities (1)

       f. post-venogram, within 48 hours (7)

       g. post-arthrogram (7)

     3. True positive with negative venogram

       a. ? thrombi in soleus sinusoids (6)

REFERENCES

1. Browse NL, Clapham WF, Croft DN, et al: Diagnosis of established deep vein thrombosis with the ^{125}I fibrinogen uptake test. Brit Med J 4:325–328, 1971.

Difference in % uptake (normalized to heart counts) greater than 15–20% between adjacent points, or corresponding points on opposite limb.

2. Flanc C, Kakkar VV, Clarke MD: The detection of venous thrombosis of the legs using ^{125}I-labelled fibrinogen. Brit J Surg 55:742–747, 1968.
3. Harris WH, Salzman EW, Athanasoulis C, et al: Comparison of ^{125}I fibrinogen count scanning with phlebography for detection of venous thrombi after elective hip surgery. N Engl J Med 292:665–667, 1975.
4. Louden JR: ^{125}I-fibrinogen uptake test. Brit Med J 2:793–794, 1976.
5. McIvor J, Anderson DR, Britt RP, et al: Comparison of ^{125}I-labelled fibrinogen uptake and venography in the detection of recent deep-vein thrombosis in the legs. Brit J Radiol 48:1013–1018, 1975.
6. Negus D, Pinto DJ, LeQuesne LP, et al: ^{125}I-labelled fibrinogen in the diagnosis of deep-vein thrombosis and its correlation with phlebography. Brit J Surg 55:835–839, 1968.
7. Poulouse KP, Kapcar AJ, Reba RC: False positive I-125 fibrinogen test. Angiology 27:258–261, 1976.

Chapter 45

Platelet Imaging—Indium-111

EDWARD B. SILBERSTEIN

I. Cerebrovascular uptake

    A. Carotid arteriosclerosis (75%) (3, 11)
    B. Sagittal sinus thrombosis (13)
    C. Intracranial aneurysm (21)

II. Neck uptake

    A. Carotid artery atherosclerosis (3)

III. Cardiac uptake

    A. Left ventricular thrombi (8)
    B. Atrial thrombi (18)
    C. Bacterial endocarditis (23)

   D. Coronary bypass graft (6)
   E. Coronary thrombosis (1)
   F. Mitral valve prosthesis (7)
   G. Cardiac transplant (16)

IV. Pulmonary uptake

   A. Pulmonary embolism (10%) (4, 11)

V. Splenic uptake

   A. Increased
      1. Autoimmune thrombocytopenic purpura (19)

VI. Renal uptake

   A. Transplant
      1. Graft rejection (15)
      2. Peri-renal hematoma (9)
      3. Iliac vein thrombosis near transplant (9)
      4. Renal artery thrombosis (12)
   B. Renal vein thrombosis (2)

VII. Aortic uptake

   A. Abdominal aneurysm (20)
   B. Aortic graft (for up to 6 years) (20)
   C. Pseudoaneurysm at graft anastomotic site (20)

VIII. Peripheral vessels

   A. Trauma
      1. Femoral arterial puncture by platelets injected 24 hours previously (17)
      2. Platelets injected following femoral artery catheterization (22)
   B. Thrombosis
      1. Venous (85%) (2)
      2. Femoral artery (5)
   C. Femoropopliteal grafts (10)
   D. Vascular catheter (14)

REFERENCES

   1. Bergmann SR, Lerch RA, Mathias CJ, et al: Visualization of coronary thrombus in vivo with ^{111}In-platelets. Circulation 64(Suppl.IV):33, 1981.

2. Davis HH, Siegel BA, Joist JH, et al: Scintigraphic detection of atherosclerotic lesions and venous thrombi in man by indium-111-labelled autologous platelets. Lancet 1:1185–1187, 1978.
3. Davis HH, Siegel BA, Sherman LA, et al: Scintigraphic detection of carotid atherosclerosis with indium-111-labeled autologous platelets. Circulation 61:982–988, 1980.
4. Davis HH, Siegel BA, Sherman LA: Scintigraphy with ^{111}In-labeled autologous platelets in venous thromboembolism. Radiology 136:203–207, 1980.
5. Davis HH, Siegel BA, Welch MJ: Scintigraphic detection of an arterial thrombus with In-111-labelled autologous platelets. J Nucl Med 21:548–549, 1980.
6. Dewanjee MK, Fuster V, Kaye MP, et al: Imaging platelet deposition with ^{111}In-labeled platelets in coronary artery bypass grafts in dogs. Mayo Clin Proc 53:327–331, 1978.
7. Dewanjee MK, Kaye MP, Fuster V, et al: Noninvasive radioisotopic technique for detection of platelet deposition in mitral valve prosthesis and renal microembolism in dogs. Trans Am Soc Artif Internal Organs 26:475–479, 1980.
8. Ezekowitz MD, Leonard JC, Smith EO, et al: Identification of left ventricular thrombi in man using indium-111-labeled autologous platelets. Circulation 63:803–810, 1981.
9. Fenech A, Nicholls A, Smith FW: Indium (^{111}In)-labelled platelets in the diagnosis of renal transplant rejection. Br J Radiol 54:325–327, 1981.
10. Goldman M, Norcott HC, Hawker RJ: Femoropopliteal bypass grafts—an isotope technique allowing *in vivo* comparison of thrombogenicity. Br J Surg 69:380–382, 1982.
11. Goodwin DA, Bushberg JT, Doherty PW, et al: Indium-111-labeled autologous platelets for location of vascular thrombi in humans. J Nucl Med 19:626–634, 1978.
12. Grino JM, Alsina J, Martin J, et al: Indium-111 labeled autologous platelets as a diagnostic method in kidney allograft rejection. Transplant Proc 14:198–200, 1982.
13. Kessler C, Kniffert T, Botsch H: Der Nutzen der Plättchenszintigraphie zur Aufklärung intrakranieller vaskulärer. Prozesse Aktuel Neurol 7:27–29, 1980.
14. Lipton MJ, Doherty PW, Goodwin DA, et al: Evaluation of catheter thrombogenicity in vivo with indium-labeled platelets. Radiology 135:191–194, 1980.
15. Martin-Comin J, Roca M, Grino JM, et al: In-111 oxine autologous labeled platelets in the diagnosis of kidney graft rejection. Clin Nucl Med 8:7–10, 1983.
16. Oluwole S, Wang T, Rawwaz R, et al: Evaluation of cardiac allograft rejection with indium-111 labeled cells. Transplant Proc 13:1616–1619, 1981.
17. Peters AM, Lavender JP: Imaging vascular lesions with indium-111-labeled platelets. Circulation 64:1297–1298, 1981.
18. Piekarski A, Drouet L, Fauchet M, et al: Diagnosis of left atrial thrombi using non-invasive technics, in Raynaud C (ed): Proceedings of the Third World Congress of Nuclear Medicine and Biology. Paris: Pergamon Press, 1982, pp. 940–943.
19. Reiffers J, Vuillemin L, Broustet A, et al: Etude cinétique des plaquettes marquées à l'indium au cours des purpuras thrombopéniques idiopathiques. La Nouvelle Presse Med 11:2335–2338, 1982.
20. Ritchie JL, Stratton JR, Thiele B: Indium-111 platelet imaging for detection of platelet deposition in abdominal aneurysms and prosthetic arterial grafts. Am J Cardiol 47:882–889, 1981.
21. Sutherland GR, King ME, Peerless SJ, et al: Platelet interaction within giant intracranial aneurysm. J Neurosurg 56:53–61, 1982.
22. Terrier E, Forman J, Francois A, et al: Plaquettes marquées à l'indium-111. La Presse Medicale 4:239, 1983.
23. Thakur ML: New radionuclides in the diagnosis of obscure infections. Conn Med 45:302–304, 1981.

Chapter 46

Leukocyte Imaging—Indium-111[†] (Focal Accumulation at 4–24 Hours)

EDWARD B. SILBERSTEIN

I. Subdiaphragmatic disease

  A. Intra-abdominal infection

    1. Peritonitis (1)

    2. Diverticular abscess (14)

    3. Intestinal fistulas (1)

    4. Infected aortoiliac graft (22)

    5. Infected hematoma (10)

    6. Appendiceal abscess (5)

    7. Subphrenic abscess (13, 19)

    8. Subhepatic abscess (23)

    9. Suprarenal abscess (23)

    10. Right and left lower quadrant abscess (23)

    11. Gallbladder empyema (23)

  B. Liver infection

    1. Amebic liver abscess (15)

    2. Intrahepatic abscess (26)

  C. Pancreatic inflammation

    1. Pancreatitis (22)

    2. Pancreatic abscess (23)

  D. Intestinal inflammation

    1. Ulcerative colitis (12, 20)

    2. Crohn's disease (20, 24)

    3. "Diversion" colitis (28)

  E. Renal inflammation

    1. Renal cytomegalovirus infection (8)

    2. Pyelonephritis (6)

    3. Abscess (6)

    4. Rejection of transplanted kidney (acute or chronic) (3, 8, 16)

  F. Non-inflammatory intra-abdominal indium-WBC uptake

    1. Intestine

      a. swallowed granulocytes from lung, sinus, mouth disease (4, 15, 20)

[†]Indium-III oxine or tropolone-labeled leukocytes.

        b. gastrointestional bleeding (30)
        c. multiple enemas (3)
        d. intestinal infarction (9)
    2. Bile fistula (23)
    3. Retroperitoneal hematoma (23)
    4. Accessory spleen (3)

II. Intra-thoracic inflammation

  A. Pulmonary disease
    1. Adult respiratory disease syndrome (3)
    2. Bacterial pneumonia (3, 13)
    3. Viral pneumonia (8)
    4. Cystic fibrosis (4)
    5. Vasculitis (3)
    6. Infected cavitating bronchial carcinoma (20)
  B. Cardiac disease
    1. Pericardial-myocardial abscess (14)
    2. Myocarditis (16)
    3. Paracardiac abscess (26)
    4. Subacute bacterial endocarditis (16)
    5. Myocardial infarction, especially within 24 hours (31)

III. Disease of the skeletal system

  A. Septic
    1. Infected hip prosthesis (22)
    2. Septic arthritis (21)
    3. Osteomyelitis (21)
        a. acute (21)
        b. subacute (26)
  B. Aseptic skeletal disorders
    1. Fracture
        a. within 2 weeks (21)
    2. Post marrow aspirate (21)
    3. Bone graft donor site (21)
    4. Rheumatoid arthritis (29)

IV. Muscle, skin, subcutaneous disorders

  A. Septic
    1. Pyoderma gangrenosum (11)
    2. Subcutaneous abscess (1)
  B. Aseptic
    1. Arterial cannulation site (29)

   2. Intramuscular injection site (29)
   3. Surgical wounds (16)
   4. Jugular phlebitis (16)

V. Central nervous system
   A. Septic disease
      1. Brain abscess (19)
      2. Subdural empyema (17)
      3. Sinusitis (3)
   B. Aseptic disease
      1. Cerebral infarct (2)

VI. Neoplasia
   A. Intrahepatic or perihepatic metastases (23)
   B. Gallbladder carcinoma (23)
   C. Skeletal metastasis from lung carcinoma (27)
   D. Histiocytic lymphoma (16)
   E. Renal transitional cell carcinoma (6)

VII. Technical artefacts
   A. Spectral overlap from a recent Tc-99m study (7)

REFERENCES

1. Ascher NL, Ahrenholz DH, Simmons RL, et al: Indium-111 autologous tagged leukocytes in the diagnosis of intraperitoneal sepsis. Arch Surg 114:386–392, 1979.
2. Coleman RE, Black RE, Welch DM, et al: Indium-111 labeled leukocytes in the evaluation of suspected abdominal abscesses. Am J Surg 139:99–104, 1980.
3. Coleman RE, Welch D: Possible pitfalls with clinical imaging of indium-111 leukocytes. J Nucl Med 21:122–125, 1980.
4. Crass JR, L'Heureux P, Loken M: False-positive ^{111}In-labeled leukocyte scan in cystic fibrosis. Clin Nucl Med 4:291–293, 1979.
5. Doherty PW, Bushberg JT, Lipton MJ, et al: The use of indium-111-labeled leukocytes for abscess detection. Clin Nucl Med 3:108–110, 1978.
6. Fawcett HD, Goodwin DA, Lantieri RL: In-111 leukocyte scanning in inflammatory renal disease. Clin Nucl Med 6:237–241, 1981.
7. Fernandez M, Hughes JA, Krugh KB, et al: Bone imaging in infections: artefacts from spectral overlap between a Tc-99m tracer and In-111 leukocytes. J Nucl Med 24:589–592, 1983.
8. Forstrom LA, Loken MK, Cook A, et al: In-111-labeled leukocytes in the diagnosis of rejection and cytomegalovirus infection in renal transplant patients. Clin Nucl Med 6:146–149, 1981.
9. Gray HW, Cuthbert I, Richards JR: Clinical imaging with indium-111 leukocytes: uptake in bowel infarction. J Nucl Med 22:701–702, 1981.

10. Hall FM, Griffiths NJ, Coakley AJ: Detection of an infected hematoma by an ^{111}In-labelled leukocyte scan. Nucl Med Comm 3:167–171, 1982.
11. Johnson MA, Wells J, Frankel A, et al: The role of In-111 leukocyte scanning in pyoderma gangrenosum. Clin Nucl Med 6:491, 1981.
12. Kipper MS, Williams RJ: The potential role of In-111 white blood cell scans in patients with inflammatory bowel disease. Clin Nucl Med 7:469–471, 1982.
13. Kriever DA, McDougall IR: Disparity between early and late In-111 white blood cell scans in a patient with proven abscess. Clin Nucl Med 8:243–245, 1983.
14. Martin WR, Gurevich N, Goris ML, et al: Detection of occult abscesses with ^{111}In-labelled leukocytes. Am J Roentgenol 133:123–125, 1979.
15. McDougall IR: The appearance of amebic abscess of liver on In-111-leukocyte scan. Clin Nucl Med 6:67–69, 1981.
16. McDougall IR, Baumert JE, Lantieri RL: Evaluation of ^{111}In leukocyte whole body scanning. Am J Roentgenol 133:849–854, 1979.
17. McKillop JH, Holtzman DS, McDougall IR: Detection of subdural empyema with radionuclides. Clin Nucl Med 5:263–267, 1980.
18. Mountford PJ, Hall FM, Coakley AJ, et al: Assessment of the painful hip prosthesis with ^{111}In-labelled leucocyte scans. Br J Radiol 55:378, 1982.
19. Peters AM, Lavender JP, MacDermot J: Diagnosing cerebral abscess with indium-111 labelled leucocytes. Lancet 2:309–310, 1980.
20. Peters AM, Saverymuttu SH, Reavy JH, et al: Imaging of inflammation with indium-111 tropolonate labeled leukocytes. J Nucl Med 24:39–44, 1983.
21. Propst-Proctor SL, Dillingham MF, McDougall IR, et al: The white blood cell scan in orthopedics. Clin Orthop 169:157–165, 1982.
22. Rövekamp MH, Hardeman MR, van der Schoot JB, et al: [111]Indium-labelled leucocyte scintigraphy in the diagnosis of inflammatory disease—first results. Br J Surg 68:150–153, 1981.
23. Rövekamp MH, van Royen EA, Reinders Folmer SCC, et al: Diagnosis of upper-abdominal infections by In-111 labeled leukocytes with Tc-99m colloid subtraction technique. J Nucl Med 24:212–216, 1983.
24. Saverymuttu SH, Peters AM, Hodgson HJ, et al: Indium-111 autologous leucocyte scanning: comparison with radiology for imaging the colon in inflammatory bowel disease. Br Med J 285:255–257, 1982.
25. Segal AW, Arnot RN, Thakur ML, et al: Indium-111-labelled leucocytes for localisation of abscesses. Lancet 2:1056–1058, 1976.
26. Sfakianakis GN, Al-Sheikh W, Heal A, et al: Comparison of scintigraphy with In-111 leukocytes and Ga-67 in the diagnosis of occult sepsis. J Nucl Med 23:618–626, 1982.
27. Sfakianakis GN, Mnaymneh W, Ghandur-Mnaymneh L, et al: Positive indium-111 leukocyte scintigraphy in a skeletal metastasis. Am J Roentgenol 139:601–603, 1982.
28. Stein DT, Paldi JH, Goodwin DA: In-111 leukocyte scan in "diversion" colitis. Clin Nucl Med 8:1–2, 1983.
29. Thakur ML: Indium-111: A new radioactive tracer for leucocytes. Exp Hematol 5 (Suppl): 145–150, 1977.
30. Wilson DG, Lieberman LM: Gastrointestinal bleeding in leukocyte scintigraphy. Clin Nucl Med 8:214–215, 1983.
31. Zaret BL, Davies RE, Thakur ML, et al: Imaging the inflammatory response to acute myocardial infarction, in Thakur ML, Gottschak A (eds): Indium-111 Labeled Neutrophils, Platelets and Lymphocytes. New York: Trivirum, 1981, pp. 151–157.

Chapter 47

Lymph Nodes[†]

EDWARD B. SILBERSTEIN

I. Failure to visualize lymphatic chain because of tumor involvement
   A. Common
      1. In ilioinguinal nodes (12)
      2. In para-sternal nodes (2)
      3. In axillary nodes following injection into the lateral areola (1)
      4. In axillary or inguinal nodes following injection around truncal mela-noma (6)
      5. In cervical nodes following retroauricular injection (13)

II. Non-neoplastic disorders causing failure of or decreased node visualization
   A. Common
      1. Physiologic variants showing apparent interruption of a chain of nodes
         a. most commonly in the iliac region (13)
         b. with xiphisternal or submanubrial cross drainage (3A)
      2. Extensive trauma or inflammation on the ipsilateral side (5)
      3. Post lymphadenectomy and surgical lymphatic interruption (7, 11)
      4. Lymphadenitis (13)
      5. Post-irradiation (13)
      6. Lymphedema, primary or secondary (12)
      7. Unsatisfactory injection (3A)
   B. Uncommon
      1. Particles in the peritoneal cavity blocking parasternal lymph flow (5)
      2. Retroperitoneal fibrosis involving inguinal nodes (13)
      3. After intensive chemotherapy (13)
      4. Unsuitable agent (3A)

III. Enhanced nodal colloid uptake and/or nodal enlargement
   A. Common
      1. Obstructed circulation (13)

[†]Regional visualization 3–24 hours after superficial interstitial injection of radiocolloid.

    a. lymphoma (4, 13)

  2. Minimal tumor invasion with lymphatic hyperplasia (3)

  3. Acute lymphadenitis (13)

IV. Nodal displacement

  A. Common

    1. Metastases (13)

    2. Collateral lymphatics (13)

  B. Uncommon

    1. Lymphadenitis (13)

V. Extra-nodal foci of colloid uptake

  A. Common

    1. Liver visualized normally if the lymphatic chain is patent (13)

    2. Retention in lymphatic vessels and/or injected extracellular space in primary and secondary lymphedema (12, 13)

  B. Uncommon

    1. Subcutaneous accumulation from "dermal backflow" (through dermal lymphatic collaterals with secondary lymphedema) (10, 12)

    2. Lymphaticocutaneous fistula (9)

  C. Rare

    1. From stasis, leakage secondary to lymphangiomyomatosis (8)

REFERENCES

1. Black RB, Taylor TV, Merrick MV, et al: Prediction of axillary metastases in breast cancer by lymphoscintigraphy. Lancet 2:15–17, 1980.

2. Ege GN: Internal mammary lymphoscintigraphy: the rational, technique, interpretation and clinical application: a review based on 848 cases. Radiology 118:101–107, 1976.

3. Ege GN: Internal mammary lymphoscintigraphy in breast carcinoma. Int J Rad Oncol Biol Phys 2:755–761, 1977.

3A. Ege GN: Lymphoscintigraphy—techniques and applications in the management of breast carcinoma. Sem Nucl Med 13:26–34, 1983.

4. Fairbanks VF, Tauxe WN, Kiely JM, et al: Scintigraphic visualization of abdominal lymph nodes with ^{99m}Tc-pertechnetate-labeled sulfur colloid. J Nucl Med 13:185–189, 1972.

5. Goranson LR, Jonsson K: External factors affecting parasternal scintigraphy with technetium-99m sulfide colloid. Acta Radiologica Diag 15:508–514, 1974.

6. Meyer CM, Lecklitner ML, Logic JR, et al: Technetium-99m sulfur colloid cutaneous lymphoscintigraphy in the management of truncal melanoma. Radiology 131:205–209, 1979.

7. Rees WV, Robinson DS, Holmes EC, et al: Altered lymphatic drainage following lymphadenectomy. Cancer 45:3045–3049, 1980.

8. Spies SM, Kruglik GD, Nieman HL, et al: ^{99m}Tc-sulfur colloid lymphangiography in lymphangiomyomatosis. Clin Nucl Med 2:189–191, 1977.

9. Stolzenberg J: Detection of lymphaticocutaneous fistula by radionuclide lymphangiography. Arch Surg 113:306–307, 1978.

10. Sty JR, Boedecker RA, Scanlon GT, et al: Radionuclide "dermal backflow" in lymphatic obstruction. J Nucl Med 20:905–906, 1979.

11. Sty JR, Thomas JP, Jr., Abrahams J: Radionuclide lymphography: a demonstration of surgical lymphatic interruption. Clin Nucl Med 3:412–413, 1978.

12. Vieras F, Boyd CM: Radionuclide lymphangiography in the evaluation of pediatric patients with lower-extremity edema. J Nucl Med 18:441–444, 1977.

13. Zum Winkel K, Hermann H-J: Scintigraphy of lymph nodes. Lymphology 10:107–114, 1977.

Chapter 48

Spleen†

JOHN G. McAFEE
EDWARD B. SILBERSTEIN

I. Diffuse splenomegaly (without filling defects) (length in posterior projection greater than 13.0 cm in adults) (26)

   A. Common

      1. Congestive

         a. portal hypertension from cirrhosis, usually alcoholic (4, 73)

            (1) from cystic fibrosis (53)

            (2) hemochromatosis*

         b. thrombosis of splenic or portal veins (2)

         c. infectious hepatitis (39)

      2. Systemic infections* (25)

         a. infectious mononucleosis

         b. bacterial endocarditis

         c. histoplasmosis

The use of an asterisk * in this chapter indicates that this entity has been observed by one of the authors but the case report has not been published.

†Visualized by radiocolloids or Tc-99m heat-denatured erythrocytes.

       d. malaria (81)
- **B.** Uncommon
    1. Polycythemia vera* (25)
    2. Leukemias (74)
    3. Lymphomas (18, 74), with or without lymphomatous splenic involvement
    4. Anemias (74)
        a. hemoglobinopathies (61)
    5. Extramedullary hematopoiesis and myelofibrosis (61)
    6. Collagen diseases (25)
        a. systemic lupus erythematosus*
        b. Felty's syndrome*
    7. Physiological: minimal enlargement within 30 minutes of fluid ingestion (46)
    8. Sarcoidosis (24, 61)
    9. Psoriasis (62)
- **C.** Rare
    1. Amyloidosis* (25)
    2. Gaucher's disease (74)
    3. Glycogen storage disease (41)
    4. Mucopolysaccharidoses (35)
    5. Wilson's disease (1)
    6. Kala-azar (42)
    7. Osteogenic sarcoma (64)

II. Small spleen (length in posterior view less than 7.0 cm in adults) (36, 60)

- **A.** Common
    1. Normal variation
    2. Accessory spleen or splenosis following splenectomy (38)
- **B.** Uncommon
    1. Hypoplasia (61)
        a. Fanconi's anemia
        b. immunological disorders
        c. malabsorption syndromes
    2. Replacement by hematoma or other masses (63)
    3. Slight contraction in response to epinephrine (69)
- **C.** Rare
    1. Previous administration of Thorotrast (72)

III. Changes in splenic size without focal abnormalities

- **A.** Decrease
    1. Splenic artery occlusion including ligation*
    2. Radiation response in leukemias or lymphomas (65)

    3. Pharmacologic (67)

      a. epinephrine

      b. corticosteroids in sarcoidosis

      c. malaria after therapy

    4. Hypertransfusion in thalassemia (67)

B. Increase (67)

    1. Sequestration crisis of sickle cell disease

    2. Obstruction of splenic venous outflow

    3. Hydration after dehydration (46)

IV. Increased uptake of radiocolloid in spleen, relative to hepatic uptake

A. Common

    1. Cirrhosis (4, 74)

    2. Cancer chemotherapeutic agents (reversible) (31)

    3. Soft tissue malignancies, particularly melanoma (20, 59, 61)

      a. remote from spleen (3A)

    4. Fatty metamorphosis (80)

      a. from alcoholism (78)

    5. Portal hypertension of any cause (73)

    6. Chronic passive congestion (21A)

    7. Felty's syndrome (13A)

    8. Budd-Chiari syndrome (3A)

B. Less common

    1. Acute (53) or chronic hepatitis (4, 80)

      a. granulomatous hepatitis (78)

    2. Diabetes mellitus (80)

    3. Iron deficiency anemia (4)

    4. Malaria (81)

    5. Pyelonephritis (54)

    6. Cholangitis with cholestasis (78)

C. Rare

    1. Osteogenic sarcoma, with or without splenic metastases (64)

    2. Hypolipidemic drugs (reversible) (13)

    3. Post hepatic lobectomy (80)

    4. Hepatic abscess or hematoma (80)

    5. Hepatic parasitic infestation (80)

    6. Hepato-renal multicystic disease (80)

    7. Myeloproliferative diseases*

      a. polycythemia vera (13A)

    8. Chronic granulomatous disease*

      a. sarcoid (13A)

      b. histoplasmosis (3A)

    9. Glycogen storage disease (41)

   10. Gaucher's disease (5)

   11. Mucopolysaccharidoses (35)

12. Wilson's disease (1)
13. Collagen-vascular disease (80)
14. Hemosiderosis (78)
15. Histiocytic lymphoma (38A)

V. Nonvisualization, hypofunction or atrophy of the spleen

A. Common

    1. Splenectomy (22)

    2. Functional asplenia, irreversible, or reversible by transfusion in sickle disease

        a. sickle cell anemia (homozygous SS) (47, 49)

        b. S-C disease (45)

        c. S-E disease (14)

        d. sickle-thalassemia (14)

    3. Lymphomas, extensive involvement (18)

        a. Sézary syndrome (3)

        b. post-radiation for Hodgkin's disease (6)

        c. histiocytic lymphoma (57A)

B. Less common

    1. Functional asplenia

        a. associated with cyanotic congenital heart disease (48)

        b. myelofibrosis (34)

        c. idiopathic thrombocytopenic purpura (9)

        d. malnutrition (68)

        e. adult celiac disease (15)

        f. ileitis (13)

        g. ulcerative colitis (76A)

        h. Thorotrast (52)

        i. chronic aggressive hepatitis (11)

        j. with fever of unknown origin (16)

        k. combined immuno-deficiency (71)

        l. amyloidosis (27)

        m. immunoblastic lymphoma (22A)

        n. mycosis fungoides (76A)

        o. discoid lupus (76A)

        p. lupus erythematosus (12)

        q. rheumatoid arthritis (30A)

        r. thyrotoxicosis (4A)

            (1) post-therapy (76A)

        s. metastases without complete replacement by tumor (7)

        t. β-thalassemia major (31A)

        u. dermatitis herpetiformis (49A)

        v. partial splenic infarction from *Pseudomonas* infection, splenic artery and vein intact (71A)

        w. during pneumococcal septicemia (4B)

C. Rare

    1. Congenital asplenia (57, 74)

        a. heterotaxy or Ivemark syndrome (cardiac anomalies, visceral heterotaxia, bronchopulmonary abnormalities, symmetrical liver) (29)

    2. Ectopic or "wandering" spleen with torsion (28)

    3. Vascular occlusion, partial or complete (65, 71A)

        a. arterial

        b. venous

    4. Supradiaphragmatic splenic transposition (68)

VI. Diffuse decrease in splenic uptake of radiocolloid (may be difficult to distinguish from normal)

  A. Common

    1. Lymphomas (Hodgkin's and non-Hodgkin's) and chronic leukemias (4)

        a. mycosis fungoides

    2. Sickle cell hemoglobinopathies (4)

    3. Functional hyposplenia (see Section V,B,1)

  B. Less common

    1. Subacute bacterial endocarditis (4)

    2. Transient, following splenic artery resection or ligation (8)

  C. Rare

    1. Sarcoidosis (24)

VII. Focal splenic defects, single or multiple (including peripheral defects)

  A. Common

    1. Laceration; hematoma (39)

    2. Infarct (32, 74, 75)

        a. post-pancreatitis

        b. subacute bacterial endocarditis

        c. sarcoidosis

        d. sickle cell anemia

        e. arteritis

        f. malaria

    3. Lymphoma: Hodgkin's and non-Hodgkin's (18)

    4. Leukemias (74)

    5. Normal variations

        a. congenital fissures, especially along superior and inferior borders (58)

        b. superior location of splenic hilus ("upside-down" or inverted spleen) (79)

    6. Artefacts

      a. superimposition of left lobe of liver (19)
      b. Miller-Abbott tube with mercury balloon overlying spleen (50)
      c. rib impression (19)
      d. Tc-99m pertechnetate in stomach or intestine (26)
      e. barium in colon (53, 82)
      f. overlying metallic objects (32)
B. Less common
    1. Abscess (38)
    2. Other tumors of spleen, primary or secondary (17, 32)
      a. metastatic bronchogenic carcinoma
      b. breast carcinoma
      c. malignant melanoma
      d. islet cell carcinoma
      e. hemangioma
      f. fibroma
      g. hamartoma
      h. hemangiosarcoma
      i. cystic lymphangiomatosis (51A)
    3. Congenital multilobulated spleen (74)
      a. focal decreased blood supply without infarction (54)
C. Rare
    1. Granuloma (43)
    2. Amyloidosis with infarct (33)
    3. Arteriovenous malformation (32)
    4. Intrasplenic pancreatic pseudocyst (51, 77)
    5. Splenic artery aneurysm (32)
    6. Splenic band (79A)

VIII. Misplaced or displaced spleen

  A. Common
    1. Ectopic or "wandering spleen" (anywhere in abdomen or pelvis, but often infero-medial to usual position in left upper quadrant) (28, 74)
    2. Displacement by extrinsic masses (74)
      a. gastric tumor
      b. pancreatic tumors or cysts
      c. mesenteric tumors or cysts
      d. aortic aneurysms
      e. retroperitoneal lymphadenopathy
      f. abscess
      g. tumors
    3. Eventration or herniation of left dome of diaphragm (74)
      a. "high riding" under a high diaphragm (70)
    4. Gastric dilatation
      a. due to gas (21, 35)

      b. water ingestion (46)
   5. Left subphrenic abscess (56)
   6. Large intracapsular splenic hematoma (60)
   7. Parasplenic hematoma (44)
 B. Rare
   1. Situs inversus abdominis (57, 76)
   2. Congenital splenogonadal fusion (23, 40)

IX. Multiple functioning splenic masses

 A. Common
   1. Fracture of spleen (61)
   2. Accessory spleen (61)
 B. Less common
   1. Post-operative splenic implants (splenosis) (30, 61)
 C. Rare
   1. Congenital polysplenia, often associated with congenital heart disease and situs inversus (74)

X. Splenic "hot spot"

 A. Redundant tissue (72A)

REFERENCES

1. Antar MA, Hsia YE, Spencer RP: Hepatic-splenic reticuloendothelial-function and blood flow in Wilson's disease (abstract). J Nucl Med 12:410, 1971.
2. Antar MA, Spencer RP, Freedman GS, et al: Portal vein obstruction: radionuclide studies of a cause of small liver and splenomegaly (abstract). J Nucl Med 12:411, 1971.
3. Balachandran S, Kumar R, Kup T: Functional asplenia in Sézary syndrome. J Nucl Med 5:149–151, 1980.
3A. Baum S, Vincent NR, Lyons KP, et al: Atlas of Nuclear Medicine. New York: Appleton-Century-Crofts, 1981, pp. 59–75.
4. Bekerman C, Gottschalk A: Diagnostic significance of the relative uptake of liver compared with spleen in ^{99m}Tc-sulphur colloid scintiphotography. J Nucl Med 12:237–240, 1971.
4A. Brownlie BEW, Hamer JW, Cook HB: Thyrotoxicosis associated with splenic atrophy. Lancet 2:1046–1047, 1975.
4B. Boughton BJ, Simpson A, Chandler S: Functional hyposplenism during pneumococcal septicemia. Lancet 1:121–122, 1983.
5. Cheng TH, Holman BL: Radionuclide assessment of Gaucher's disease. J Nucl Med 19:1333–1336, 1978.
6. Coleman CN, McDougall IR, Dailey MO, et al: Functional hyposplenia after splenic irradiation for Hodgkin's disease. Ann Int Med 96:44–47, 1982.
7. Costello P, Gramm HF, Steinberg D: Simultaneous occurrence of functional asplenia and

splenic accumulation of diphosphonate in metastatic breast carcinoma. J Nucl Med 18:1237–1238, 1977.

8. Crass JR, Frick MP, Loken MK: The scintigraphic appearance of the spleen following splenic artery resection. Radiology 136:737–739, 1980.

9. Dekker PT, Propp RP: Functional asplenia in idiopathic thrombocytopenic purpura. NY State J Med 77:2282–2285, 1977.

10. Dhawan VM, Antar MA, Spencer RP: Functional asplenia with few Howell-Jolly bodies. Clin Nucl Med 2:106–108, 1977.

11. Dhawan VM, Spencer RP, Sziklas JJ: Reversible functional asplenia in chronic aggressive hepatitis. J Nucl Med 20:34–36, 1979.

12. Dillon AM, Stein HB, English RA: Splenic atrophy in systemic lupus erythematosus. Ann Int Med 96:40–43, 1982.

13. Dujovhe CA, Strauss HW: Changes in liver and spleen scans of patients during treatment with two hypolipidemic drugs. Radiology 98:682–684, 1971.

13A. Eddleston AL, Blendis LM, Osborn SB, et al: Significance of increased ''splenic uptake'' on liver scintiscanning. Gut 10:711–714, 1969.

14. Engelstad BL: Functional asplenia in hemoglobin S-E disease. Clin Nucl Med 7:100–107, 1982.

15. Ferguson A, Hutton MM, Maxwell JD, et al: Adult coeliac disease in hyposplenic patients. Lancet 1:163–164, 1970.

16. Ferguson RP, Hoang GN: Transient functional hyposplenia and fever. J Nucl Med 22:748–749, 1981.

17. Freeman MC, Tonkin AK: Focal splenic defects. Radiology 121:689–692, 1976.

18. Fuzy M, Karika S, Tarjan G: The importance of spleen scintigraphy in malignant lymphomas. Neoplasma 16:447–450, 1969.

19. Gilday DL, Alderson PO: Scintigraphic evaluations of liver and spleen injury. Sem Nucl Med 4:357–370, 1974.

20. Goldman AB, Braunstein P, Song C: Augmented splenic uptake of Tc-99m sulphur colloid in patients with malignant melanoma. Radiology 112:631–634, 1974.

21. Gordon DH, Burrell MI, Levin DC, et al: Wandering spleen—the radiological and clinical spectrum. Radiology 125:39–46, 1977.

21A. Gould L, Collica C, Comprecht RF: Scintigraphy in congestive heart failure. JAMA 219:1734–1736, 1972.

22. Graves DS, Stadalnik RC: Anatomic and functional asplenia—absence of the splenic image during ^{99m}Tc-sulfur colloid scintigraphy. Sem Nucl Med 12:95–96, 1982.

22A. Gross DJ, Braverman AJ, Koran G, et al: Functional asplenia in immunoblastic lymphoma. Arch Int Med 142:2213–2215, 1982.

23. Guarin U, Dimitrieva Z, Ashley SJ: Splenogonadal fusion—a rare congenital anomaly demonstrated by ^{99m}Tc-sulphur colloid imaging: case report. J Nucl Med 16:922–924, 1975.

24. Habibian MR, Abernathy EM: Splenomegaly with uniformly decreased splenic uptake of ^{99m}Tc-sulfur colloid: a new observation in childhood sarcoidosis. J Nucl Med 15:45–46, 1974.

25. Harvey AM, Bordley J III: Causes of splenomegaly, in Differential Diagnosis, Second Ed. Philadelphia: W.B. Saunders, 1970, p. 502.

26. Hernberg JG, Braunstein P, Chandra R, et al: Artifacts in ^{99m}Tc-sulfur colloid liver scans. J Nucl Med 12:697–698, 1971.

27. Hurd WW, Katholi RE: Acquired functional asplenia. Arch Int Med 140:844–845, 1980.

28. Isikoff MB, White DW, Diaconis JN: Torsion of the wandering spleen, seen as a migratory abdominal mass. Radiology 123:36–38, 1977.
29. Ivemark BI: Implications of agenesis of spleen on pathogenesis of cono-truncus anomalies in children. Acta Paediat 44 (Supp):1–110, 1955.
30. Jacobson SJ, DeNardo GL: Splenosis demonstrated by splenic scan. J Nucl Med 12:570–572, 1971.
30A. Jardin DR: Asplenia and rheumatoid arthritis. Ann Int Med 97:616–617, 1982.
31. Kaplan WD, Drum DE, Lokich JJ: The effect of cancer chemotherapeutic agents on the liver-spleen scan. J Nucl Med 21:84–87, 1980.
31A. Karpathios TH, Dimitriou P, Giamouris J, et al: Effective RES blood flow changes in children with homozygous β-thalassemia in relation to blood transfusion. Eur J Nucl Med 8:15–18, 1983.
32. Kim EE: Focal splenic defect. Sem Nucl Med 9:320–321, 1979.
33. Kim EE, Mattar AG: Scan findings in a case of splenic infarction due to amyloidosis. J Nucl Med 17:902–903, 1976.
34. Kim EE, DeLand FH: Myelofibrosis presenting as hypermetabolic bone disease by radionuclide imaging in a patient with asplenia. Clin Nucl Med 3:406–408, 1978.
35. Klingensmith WC, Eikman EA, Maumenee I, et al: Widespread abnormalities of radiocolloid distribution in patients with mucopolysaccharidoses. J Nucl Med 16:1002–1006, 1975.
36. Landgarten S, Spencer RP: Splenic displacement due to gastric dilatation. J Nucl Med 13:223, 1972.
37. Larson SM, Tuell SH, Moores KD, et al: Dimensions of the normal adult spleen scan and prediction of spleen weight. J Nucl Med 12:123–126, 1971.
38. LePage JR, Pratt AD Jr, Miale A, et al: Diagnosis of splenic abscess by radionuclide scanning and selective arteriography. J Nucl Med 13:331–332, 1972.
38A. Lin DS: "Hot" spleen on Tc-99m sulfur colloid images. Clin Nucl Med 8:237–238, 1983.
39. McIntyre PA: Diagnostic significance of the spleen scan. Sem Nucl Med 2:278–287, 1972.
40. McLean GK, Alavi A, Zieglu MM, et al: Splenic-gonadal fusion. J Ped Surg 16:649–651, 1981.
41. Miller JH, Gates GF, Landing BH, et al: Scintigraphic abnormalities in glycogen storage disease. J Nucl Med 19:354–358, 1978.
42. Monio AL: Liver-spleen scintiscan in kala-azar: case report. J Nucl Med 16:1128–1129, 1975.
43. Morgan H, Johnson PM: Splenic masses detected by scintillation imaging and contrast tomography. Radiology 97:301–306, 1970.
44. Nebesar RA, Rabinov KR, Potsaid MS: Radionuclide imaging of the spleen in suspected splenic injury. Radiology 110:609–614, 1974.
45. Park CH, Wecsler PI, Lin D, et al: Splenic scan findings in sickle cell-hemoglobin C disease (abstract). J Nucl Med 21:P43, 1980.
46. Parker JD, Bennett LR: Effect of water ingestion on spleen size as determined by radioisotope scans. Acta Radiol (Diag) 11:385–392, 1971.
47. Pearson HA, Cornelius EA, Schwartz AD, et al: Transfusion reversible functional asplenia in young children. New Engl J Med 283:334–337, 1970.
48. Pearson HA, Schiebler GL, Spencer RP: Functional hyposplenia in cyanotic congenital heart disease. Pediat 48:277–280, 1971.

49. Pearson HA, Spencer RP, Cornelius EA: Functional asplenia in sickle-cell anemia. New Engl J Med 281:923–926, 1969.

49A. Pettit JE, Hoffbrand AV, Seah PP, et al: Splenic atrophy in dermatitis herpetiformis. Br Med J 2:438–440, 1972.

50. Preston D: Personal communication. 24 March 1976.

51. Ramer M, Diznoff SB, Heines AC: Intrasplenic pancreatic pseudocyst. Clin Radiol 25:525–529, 1974.

51A. Rao BR, Aubuchon J, Lieberman LM, et al: Cystic lymphangiomatosis of the spleen. Radiology 141:781–782, 1981.

52. Rao BR, Winebright JW, Dresser TP: Functional asplenia after Thorotrast administration. Clin Nucl Med 4:437, 1979.

53. Rao BR, Winebright JW, Dresser TP: Splenic artifact caused by barium in the colon. Clin Nucl Med 4:249, 1979.

54. Rosenfield N, Treves S: Liver-spleen scanning in pediatrics. Pediat 53:692–701, 1974.

55. Russell CD, Jones AE, Johnston GS, et al: Arteriographically confirmed focal defect in colloid spleen scan with no gross pathologic lesion. J Nucl Med 17:376–377, 1976.

56. Salamanca JE, Stadalnik RC, DeNardo GL: Clinical assessment of combined organ imaging in the diagnosis of subphrenic abscesses. Clin Nucl Med 3:113–115, 1978.

57. Shah KD, Neill CA, Wagner HN Jr., et al: Radioisotope scanning of the liver and spleen with dextrocardia and situs inversus with levocardia. Circulation 29:231–241, 1965.

57A. Shih W-J, Sauerbrunn BJL, Bates HR: Total non-visualization of the spleen on ^{99m}Tc-sulfur colloid and ^{113m}In-chloride blood pool images. Eur J Nucl Med 7:513–514, 1982.

58. Smidt KP: Splenic scintigraphy: a large congenital fissure mimicking splenic hematoma. Radiology 122:169, 1977.

59. Sober AJ, Mintzis MM, Lew RA, et al: The significance of augmented radiocolloid uptake by the spleen in patients with malignant melanoma. J Nucl Med 20:1232–1236, 1979.

60. Solheim K, Nerdrum HJ: Radionuclide imaging of splenic laceration and trauma. Clin Nucl Med 4:528–533, 1979.

61. Spencer RP: Spleen scanning as a diagnostic tool. JAMA 237:1473–1474, 1977.

62. Spencer RP: The spleen in psoriasis. Clin Nucl Med 2:119–120, 1977.

63. Spencer RP, Baskurt VM: "Small spleen" due to liquified hematoma. J Nucl Med 18:1146, 1977.

64. Spencer RP, Flannery JT: The spleen in osteogenic sarcoma: a scan and autopsy survey. Clin Nucl Med 2:315–317, 1977.

65. Spencer RP, Johnson PM, Sziklas JJ: Unusual scan presentation of splenic vasculature occlusion by tumor. Clin Nucl Med 2:197–199, 1977.

66. Spencer RP, Knowlton AH: Radiocolloid scans in evaluating splenic response to external radiation. J Nucl Med 16:123–126, 1975.

67. Spencer RP, Lange RC, Schwartz AD, et al: Radioisotopic studies of changes in splenic size in response to epinephrine and other stimuli. J Nucl Med 13:211–214, 1972.

68. Spencer RP, Pearson HA, Binder HJ: Identification of cases of "acquired" functional asplenia. J Nucl Med 11:763–766, 1970.

69. Spencer RP, Pearson HA, Lang RC: Human spleen: scan studies on growth and response to medications. J Nucl Med 12:466–467, 1971.

70. Spencer RP, Plante SM, Coombs HE: The "high riding" spleen. Int J Nucl Med Biol 7:61–62, 1980.

71. Spencer RP, Suresh K, Pearson HA: "Reversible" functional asplenia in combined im-

munodeficiency. Int J Nucl Med Biol 5:125–126, 1978.

71A. Spencer RP, Spiklas JJ, Turner JW: Functional obstruction of splenic blood vessels in adults: A radiocolloid study. Int J Nucl Med Biol 9:208–211, 1982.

72. Spencer RP, Turner JW, Syed IB: Residual splenic function in the presence of Thorotrast-associated hepatic tumor: case report. J Nucl Med 17:200–202, 1976.

72A. Spencer RP: Splenic "hot spot" due to redundant tissue. Clin Nucl Med 8:239–240, 1983.

73. Thivolle P, Bel A, Veillas G, et al: Valeur de l'index angioscintigraphique hepato-splenique dans l'hypertension portale. Lyon Medical 241:273–277, 1979.

74. Treves ST, Spencer RP: Liver and spleen scintigraphy in children. Sem Nucl Med 3:55–68, 1973.

75. Vagenakis AG, Abreau CM, Braverman LE: Splenic infarction diagnosed by photoscanning. J Nucl Med 13:563–564, 1972.

76. Vyas K, Haines JE, Holzgang C: Right-sided spleen with partial situs inversus of the abdominal viscera. Clin Nucl Med 4:425–426, 1979.

76A. Wardrop CAJ, Lee FD, Dyet JF, et al: Immunologic abnormalities in splenic atrophy. Lancet 2:4–7, 1975.

77. Warshaw AL, Chesney TM, Evans GW, et al: Intrasplenic dissection by pancreatic pseudocysts. New Engl J Med 287:72–75, 1972.

78. Wasnich R, Glober G, Hayashi T, et al: Simple computer quantitation of spleen-to-liver ratios in the diagnosis of hepatocellular disease. J Nucl Med 20:149–154, 1979.

79. Westcott JL, Krufky EL: The upside-down spleen. Radiology 105:517–521, 1972.

79A. Wilson DG, Lieberman LM: Unusual splenic band. Clin Nucl Med 8:270, 1983.

80. Wilson GA, Keyes JW Jr.: The significance of the liver-spleen uptake ratio in liver scanning. J Nucl Med 15:593–597, 1974.

81. Ziessman HA: Lung uptake of ^{99m}Tc-sulphur colloid in falciparum malaria: case report. J Nucl Med 17:794–796, 1976.

82. Zivas ST, Braunstein P: Splenic focal defect produced by barium in the colon. Clin Nucl Med 3:202–203, 1978.

Part IX

Peri-Diaphragmatic Disease

Chapter 49

Lung-Spleen Separation†

EDWARD B. SILBERSTEIN

I. Separation of spleen and lung
   A. Common
      1. Normal variant—15% (5).
      2. Ascites (5)
      3. Subphrenic abscess (8–33% of such abscesses are on the left) (1)
      4. Left pleural effusion (1)
      5. Cardiomegaly (1)
      6. Left lung atelectasis (1)
   B. Uncommon
      1. Gastric distension (4)
      2. Splenic infarction (2)
      3. Pancreatic pseudocyst (3)

REFERENCES

1. DeLuca SA, Kolodny GM: The spleen-lung interface as diagnostic information. J Nucl Med 16:822–824, 1975.
2. Go RT, Tonami N, Schapiro RL, et al: The manifestations of diaphragmatic and juxtadiaphragmatic diseases in the liver-spleen scintigraph. Radiology 115:119–127, 1975.
3. Grant RW, Ackery D: Displacement of the spleen in infected pancreatic pseudocyst. J Nucl Med 17:193–195, 1976.
4. Lo H-H, McKusick KA, Strauss HW: Gastric distension simulating a left subphrenic abscess. J Nucl Med 19:438–439, 1978.
5. Yeh E-L, Ruetz PP, Meade RC: Separation of lung-liver scintiphotos due to ascites—a false positive test for subdiaphragmatic abscess. J Nucl Med 13:249–251, 1972.

†Demonstrated with Tc-99m macroaggregated albumin or Tc-99m microspheres and radiocolloid.

Chapter 50

Lung-Liver Separation[†]

EDWARD B. SILBERSTEIN

I. Common causes of abnormal liver-lung separation

   A. Subphrenic abscess (2)
   B. Subphrenic hematoma (2)
   C. Bile leakage (2)
   D. Ascites; serous intra-abdominal effusion (2, 8)
   E. Infra-pulmonary effusion (1)
   F. Peridiaphragmatic tumor (8)
   G. Consolidation of the lower lobe of the right lung (pneumonia, infarction) (1)
   H. Atelectasis (4)
   I. Emphysematous bulla*

II. Uncommon causes

   A. High ectopic kidney (7)
   B. Polycystic liver with intrahepatic abscess (3)
   C. Liver metastases (3)
   D. Fibrous adhesions over the liver (3)
   E. Cirrhosis (6)
   F. Subdiaphragmatic adiposity (5)
   G. Subphrenic, suprahepatic tumor*

REFERENCES

1. Brown DW: Combined lung-liver radioisotope scan in the diagnosis of subdiaphragmatic abscess. Am J Surg 109:521–525, 1965.
2. Gold RP, Johnson PM: Efficacy of combined liver-lung scintillation imaging. Radiology 117:105–111, 1975.
3. Middleton HM, Patton DD, Hoyumpa AM, et al: Liver-lung scan in the diagnosis of right subphrenic abscess. Digest Dis 21:215–222, 1976.

The use of an asterisk * in this chapter indicates that this entity has been observed by the author but the case report has not been published.

†Demonstrated with Tc-99m macroaggregated albumin or Tc-99m microspheres and radiocolloid.

4. Passalaqua AM, Oster ZH, Chandra R, et al: Liver/pleural cavity scan for diagnosis of subphrenic abscess. Clin Nucl Med 3:209–211, 1978.
5. Pozderac R, Borlaza G, Green RA: Subdiaphragmatic adiposity mimicking ascites by liver-lung scintigraphy. Radiology 132:154, 1979.
6. Salamanco JE, Stadalnik RC, DeNardo GL: Clinical assessment of combined organ imaging in the diagnosis of subphrenic abscesses. Clin Nucl Med 3:113–115, 1978.
7. Strakosch CR, Cooper RA, Wiseman JC, et al: High ectopic kidney presenting as an abnormal liver-lung scan. J Nucl Med 18:274–275, 1977.
8. Yeh EL, Ruetz PP, Meade RC: Separation of lung-liver scintiphotos due to ascites—a false positive test for subdiaphragmatic abscess. J Nucl Med 13: 249–251, 1972.

Part X

Pulmonary System

Chapter 51

Lung Perfusion†

AMOLAK SINGH

EDWARD B. SILBERSTEIN

I. Segmental or lobar perfusion defects (vascular disorders are more likely to cause ventilation-perfusion mismatches than disorders of lung parenchyma)

  A. Common

    1. Pulmonary embolism (new or old) (1, 26, 52, 66, 92)

    2. Obstructive lung disease (1, 26, 27, 69)

      a. emphysema (73)

      b. mucus plugging (41)

      c. bronchitis (76)

    3. Bronchial asthma (20, 71, 86)

      a. mucus impaction (41)

    4. Pulmonary edema (66)

    5. Bronchogenic carcinoma (49, 71)

    6. Atelectasis (73)

    7. Pneumonia (52, 55)

      a. aspiration (39)

  B. Less common

    1. Lymphangitic carcinomatosis (29)

    2. Post inflammatory atrophy (5)

    3. Histoplasmosis (42)

The use of an asterisk * in this chapter indicates that this entity has been observed by one of the authors but the case report has not been published.

†Demonstrated with Tc-99m macroaggregated albumin or microspheres, commonly performed in combination with ventilation imaging (Chapters 52, 53).

    4. Sickle cell anemia (2)

    5. Empyema (15)

    6. Post radiation therapy (3, 49)

    7. Obliterative bronchiolitis (2)

    8. Sarcoidosis with pulmonary artery compression (33, 52, 74, 95)

    9. Cystic fibrosis (64)

    10. Fibrothorax (23)

    11. Alpha-one antitrypsin deficiency related emphysema (93)

    12. Pneumatocele after staphylococcal pneumonia (2)

    13. Lung displacement from hiatal hernia (44)

    14. Bronchiectasis (91)

    15. Tuberculosis (46)

C. Rare

    1. Primary or intrinsic vascular disease

        a. vascular tumors

            (1) pulmonary hemangioendotheliomatosis (87)

            (2) pulmonary artery sarcoma (59)

        b. arteritis

            (1) Takayasu arteritis (86)

            (2) lupus erythematosus (17)

            (3) polyarteritis (17)

        c. pulmonary artery anomaly

            (1) stenosis (82)

                (a) branch stenosis (70)

            (2) hypoplasia (15, 34)

            (3) agenesis (15, 34, 55, 90)

        d. systemic arterial blood supply (88)

            (1) with broncho-pulmonary sequestration (28, 40)

        e. tetralogy of Fallot repair with bronchial artery supply to a lobe (32)

        f. pulmonary veno-occlusive disease (8)

        g. dog heartworm (*Dirofilaria immitis*) infestation (52)

        h. arteriovenous malformation*

        i. dissecting aneurysm (95A)

    2. Vascular compression from parenchymal pulmonary disease

        a. fibrosing mediastinitis (63)

        b. broncholithiasis (45)

        c. pulmonary artery compression by hemorrhage from aorta (24)

        d. melanoma (metastatic) compressing pulmonary vein (53)

    3. Embolic disease

        a. air embolism (14)

        b. fat embolism (54)

        c. from right atrial myxoma (58)

        d. from intravenous drug abuse (80)

    4. Congenital lobar emphysema (2, 17)

    5. Influenza A (48)

    6. Inadvertent injection into pulmonary artery catheter (6)

    7. High diaphragm from supine position or from pathologic causes (75)

II. Non-segmental perfusion abnormalities

  A. Common

      1. Chronic obstructive lung disease (26, 69)

      2. Pulmonary edema (35)

      3. Congestive heart failure (37)

      4. Hypoventilation (17, 41)

      5. Mucus plugs (41)

      6. Asthmatic attack (17, 23, 82)

      7. Bronchogenic carcinoma (27, 48)

      8. Cystic fibrosis (64)

      9. Pleural fluid (38, 89)

      10. Azygos fissures (65)

      11. Sickle cell disease (2)

      12. Pneumonia (17, 23)

  B. Less common

      1. Fat embolism (54)

      2. Sarcoidosis (74)

      3. Intravenous drug abuse (80)

      4. Bronchiectasis (17, 91)

      5. Pneumoconiosis (17)

      6. Pulmonary hypertension (2, 79)

      7. Pulmonary fibrosis (23, 67)

      8. Pulmonary tuberculosis (46)

      9. Hyaline membrane disease (16, 17)

      10. Radiation pneumonitis and fibrosis (27, 50, 67)

      11. Alpha-one antitrypsin deficiency (22)

      12. Pneumothorax (18)

      13. Pulmonary veno-occlusive disease (8)

      14. Mitral stenosis (84)

      15. Cirrhosis (81)

  C. Rare

      1. Chemical tracheobronchitis (17)

        a. smoke inhalation (57, 68)

      2. Lymphangitic carcinomatosis (60)

      3. Alveolar proteinosis (17, 73)

      4. Hiatus hernia (25, 77)

      5. Kartagener syndrome (2)

      6. Obliterative bronchiolitis (2)

      7. Idiopathic pulmonary hemosiderosis (4)

      8. Pulmonary papillomatosis (21)

III. Total or near total lung perfusion defect

    A. Common
        1. Bronchogenic carcinoma (92, 94)
    B. Less common
        1. Pulmonary embolism (92, 94)
        2. Congenital heart diseases (2, 17, 31, 94) (See also Part I: Cardiovascular System)
            a. left-sided defect:
                (1) left pulmonary artery atresia
                (2) left pulmonary artery stenosis
                (3) superior vena cava–right pulmonary artery anastomosis (Glenn procedure)—upper extremity injection
                (4) tetralogy of Fallot with left pulmonic stenosis
                (5) ventricular septal defect with compression of left pulmonary artery due to enlarged left heart
                (6) stricture of left pulmonary artery after Pott's (descending aorta to left pulmonary artery) anastomosis
            b. right-sided defect:
                (1) right pulmonary artery atresia (34, 90)
                (2) right pulmonary artery stenosis (82)
                (3) patent right Blalock-Taussig shunt (right subclavian-pulmonary artery anastomosis)
                (4) nonfunctioning right Blalock-Taussig shunt with right to left shunt
                (5) tetralogy of Fallot with right pulmonic stenosis
                (6) patent Waterston (ascending aorta to right pulmonary artery) anastomosis
                (7) right Waterston shunt with post-operative pulmonary artery stenosis
                (8) transposition of great vessels, right to left shunt
                (9) superior vena cava (right pulmonary artery anastomosis–Glenn procedure)—lower extremity injection
        3. Pneumonectomy (94)
        4. Cystic bronchiectasis (94)
        5. Infection
            a. tuberculosis
                (1) bronchopleural fistula (94)
                (2) pleural effusion with atelectasis (73)
            b. empyema (1)
                (1) with pneumonia (94)
                (2) with subphrenic abscess (15)
            c. pneumonia (73)
        6. Bronchial obstruction
            a. foreign body in the bronchus (39, 43)

        b. mucus plugging (41)
   7. Lung displacement
        a. large pleural effusion (15)
        b. pneumothorax (15)
        c. emphysema (15)
        d. compressed lung (2)
        e. mesothelioma (2)
C. Rare
   1. Emboli from right atrial myxoma (58)
   2. Hypoplastic lobe plus lobectomy (15)
   3. Bronchial intubation (12)
   4. Swyer-James syndrome (hyperlucent lung) (61, 96)
   5. Bronchial adenoma (51)
   6. Pulmonary veno-occlusive disease (8)
   7. Pulmonary contusion (15)
   8. Takayasu's arteritis (80)
   9. Anomalous origin of left coronary artery (72)
  10. Histoplasmosis (42)
  11. Bronchogenic (mediastinal) cyst (2)
  12. Broncholithiasis (45)
  13. Inadvertent injection into pulmonary artery catheter (6)
  14. Pulmonary artery tumor—sarcoma; carcinosarcoma (62)

IV. Fissure sign (linear photopenic area between lobes)

  A. Common
     1. Pleural fluid (36)
     2. Pulmonary edema (10, 36)
     3. Pulmonary embolism (10, 36, 38)
  B. Less common
     1. Emphysema (10, 36)
     2. Bronchopneumonia (10)
     3. Carcinomatosis of the lung (10)
     4. Pleural thickening (36)
     5. Cystic fibrosis (36)
  C. Rare
     1. Sickle cell anemia (36)
     2. Collagen vascular disease (36)

V. Widened mediastinum

  A. Common
     1. Cardiomegaly (15)
     2. Congestive heart failure (26)
     3. Pulmonary edema (27)
     4. Hilar lymphadenopathy (15)

5. Scoliosis (15)
B. Less common
   1. Pectus excavatum (15)
   2. Enlargement of pulmonary arteries (15)
   3. Sarcoidosis (74)
   4. Aortic aneurysm (15)
   5. Hemopericardium (9)
   6. Congenital absence of left pericardium (13)

VI. Altered circulation pattern without perfusion defects

  A. Cephalocaudal reversal (17)
    1. Mitral stenosis with pulmonary hypertension
    2. Congestive heart failure
    3. Idiopathic pulmonary hypertension
  B. Relatively increased perfusion at bases (17)
    1. Injection while upright

VII. Visualization of other organs during perfusion lung study

  A. Common
    1. Physiologic shunt (normal 3%) with high intensity of CRT display*
    2. Poor radiopharmaceutical with free pertechnetate*
  B. Uncommon
    1. Right to left intracardiac shunt (30, 31)
      a. pulmonary arteriovenous fistulae (78)
      b. pulmonary hypertension with arteriovenous shunting (83)
    2. Anomalous origin of left coronary artery (72)
  C. Venous collaterals to portal vein (only seen following foot vein injection) (48A)

VIII. Increased focal uptake ("hot spots") inside the pulmonary parenchyma on a perfusion lung scan

  A. Common
    1. Faulty injection technique (19)
  B. Uncommon
    1. Radioactive embolization from upper extremity thrombophlebitis (47)
    2. Radioactive embolization following radioactive venography (11)
    3. Bad radiopharmaceutical preparation (7)
    4. Bronchiolo-alveolar cell carcinoma (70A)

IX. Increased focal uptake outside the pulmonary parenchyma

  A. Uncommon
    1. Site of endothelial injury on wall of injured vessel (92A)

  2. Compression of subclavian vein by tumor (34A)
  3. Concentration by clot in central venous catheter*

X. Artefacts causing areas of apparent defect*

   A. Common
   1. Elevated hemidiaphragm
   2. Diaphragm angulation in obesity
   3. Pacemaker
   4. Medallion or other jewelry
   5. Breast or breast prosthesis
   6. Shoulders on lateral view

REFERENCES

1. Alderson PO, Rujanavech N, Secker-Walker RH: The role of ^{133}Xe ventilation studies in the scintigraphic detection of pulmonary embolism. Radiology 120:633–640, 1976.
2. Alderson PO, Gilday DL, Wagner HN: Atlas of Pediatric Nuclear Medicine. St. Louis: C. V. Mosby, 1978.
3. Bateman NT, Coakley AJ, Croft DN, et al: Ventilation perfusion lung scans for pulmonary emboli. Eur J Nucl Med 2:201–202, 1973.
4. Bliek AJ, Bachynski JE: Two severe reactions following a pulmonary scan in a patient with idiopathic pulmonary haemosiderosis. J Nucl Med 12:90–92, 1971.
5. Bookstein JJ, Silver TM: The angiographic differential diagnosis of acute pulmonary embolism. Radiology 110:25–33, 1974.
6. Brachman M, Tanasescu D, Ramanna L, et al: False-positive lung imaging: Inadvertent injection into a pulmonary artery catheter. Clin Nucl Med 4:415–416, 1979.
7. Burdine JA, Ryder LA, Sonnemaker RE: ^{99m}Tc-human albumin microspheres (HAM) for lung imaging. J Nucl Med 12:127–130, 1971.
8. Calderon M, Burdine JA: Pulmonary veno-occlusive disease. J Nucl Med 15:455–457, 1974.
9. Chandra S, Laor YG: Lung scan and wide mediastinum. J Nucl Med 16:324–325, 1975.
10. Chandler HL: Fissure sign in lung perfusion scintigrams. J Nucl Med 12:326–327, 1971.
11. Conca DM, Brill DR, Schoop JD: Pulmonary radioactive microemboli following radionuclide venography. J Nucl Med 18:1140–1141, 1977.
12. Cowan RJ, Short DB, Maynard CD: Nonperfusion of one lung secondary to improperly positioned endotracheal tube. JAMA 227:1165–1166, 1974.
13. D'Altorio RA, Cano JY: Congenital absence of the left pericardium detected by imaging of the lung: case report. J Nucl Med 18:267–268, 1977.
14. Datz FL: Ventilation-perfusion mismatch: lung imaging. Sem Nucl Med 10:193–194, 1980.
15. DeLand FH, Wagner HN: Atlas of Nuclear Medicine, Vol. 1. Philadelphia: W.B. Saunders, 1969.
16. DeNardo GL, Blankenship WJ, Burdine JA, et al: Lung, in Nuclear Medicine in Clinical Practice. New York: Society of Nuclear Medicine Press, 1974.
17. DeNardo GL, DeNardo SL (eds): Clinical Scintillation Imaging. New York: Grune & Stratton, 1975, pp. 461–536.

18. Dhekne RD, Burdine JA: The diagnosis of pneumothorax by ventilation-perfusion imaging. Radiology 129:119–121, 1978.
19. Duffy GT, DeNardo GL, Abington RB: Origin and evolution of radioactive pulmonary emboli in man. Radiology 91:1175–1180, 1968.
20. Eaton SB, James AE, Potsaid MS, et al: Scintigraphic findings in pulmonary microembolism. Am J Roentgenol 106:778–786, 1969.
21. Espinolo D, Rupani H, Camargo EE: Ventilation-perfusion imaging in pulmonary papillomatosis. J Nucl Med 22:975–977, 1981.
22. Fallat RJ, Powell MR, Jueppers F, et al: ^{133}Xe ventilatory studies in alpha 1-antitrypsin deficiency. J Nucl Med 12:586–590, 1971.
23. Farmelant MH, Trainor JC: Evaluation of a ^{133}Xe ventilation technique for diagnosis of pulmonary disorders. J Nucl Med 12: 586–590, 1971.
24. Franklin DH, Jacques J: Pulmonary artery compression by hemorrhage from the aorta simulating pulmonary embolism. Thorax 29:142–144, 1974.
25. Friedman ML, Cantor RE, Sherman BP: Regional hypoperfusion secondary to a hiatal hernia. Clin Nucl Med 3:443–444, 1978.
26. Gilday DL, James AE: Lung scan patterns in pulmonary embolism versus those in congestive heart failure and emphysema. Am J Roetgenol 115:739–750, 1972.
27. Goldman SM, Freeman LM, Ghossein M, et al: Effect of thoracic irradiation on pulmonary arterial perfusion in man. Radiology 93:289–296, 1969.
28. Gooneratne H, Conway JJ: Radionuclide angiographic diagnosis of bronchopulmonary sequestration. J Nucl Med 17:1035–1037, 1976.
29. Green N, Swanson I, Kern W, et al: Lymphangitic carcinomatosis: Lung scan abnormalities. J Nucl Med 17:258–260, 1976.
30. Greenfield LD, Bennet LR: Detection of intracardiac shunt with radionuclide imaging. Semin Nucl Med 3:139–152, 1973.
31. Haroutuman LM, Neill CA, Wagner HN Jr: Radioisotope scanning of lung in cyanotic congenital heart disease. Am J Cardiol 23:387–395, 1969.
32. Heches WH, Wens FH, Park SC, et al: Pulmonary perfusion defects and bronchial artery collateral flow. JAMA 238:1842–1844, 1977.
33. Hietala SO, Stinnett RG, Faunce HF, et al: Pulmonary artery narrowing in sarcoidosis. JAMA 237:572–573, 1977.
34. Isawa T, Taplin GV: Unilateral pulmonary artery agenesis, stenosis, and hypoplasia. Radiology 99:605–612, 1971.
34A. Isawa T, Teshima T, Hirano T, et al: Increased focal activity on perfusion lung image. J Nucl Med 23:513–515, 1982.
35. James AE Jr: Perfusion lung scan changes associated with pulmonary edema, in Progress in Nuclear Medicine: Regional Pulmonary Function in Health and Disease, Vol. 3. Baltimore: University Park Press, 1973.
36. James AE, Conway JJ, Chang H, et al: The fissure sign: its multiple causes. Amer J Roentgenol 111:492–500, 1971.
37. James AE, Cooper M, White RI, et al: Perfusion changes in lung scan in patients with congestive heart failure. Radiology 100:99–106, 1971.
38. Johnson PM: Lung scanning in pulmonary embolism. Semin Nucl Med 1:161–184, 1971.
39. Kassner GE, Soloman NA, Steiner P, et al: Persisting perfusion defects after bronchoscopic removal or spontaneous expulsion of aspirated foreign objects. Radiology 121:139–142, 1976.
40. Kawakami K, Tada S, Katsuyama N, et al: Radionuclide study in pulmonary sequestration. J Nucl Med 19:287–289, 1978.

41. Kelly MJ, Elliott LP: The radiological evaluation of the patient with suspected pulmonary thrombo-embolic disease. Med Clin N Amer 59:3–36, 1975.

42. Kim EE, DeLand FH: V/Q mismatch without pulmonary emboli in children with histo-plasmosis. Clin Nucl Med 3:328–330, 1978.

43. Leonidas JC, Stuber JL, Radawaky AZ, et al: Radionuclide lung scanning in the diagnosis of endobronchial foreign bodies in children. J Pediatr 83:628–631, 1973.

44. Li DK, Seltzer SE, McNeil BJ: V/Q mismatches unassociated with pulmonary embolism: case report and review of the literature. J Nucl Med 19:1331–1333, 1978.

45. Lloyd TV: Decreased lung perfusion due to broncholithiasis. Clin Nucl Med 4:523–525, 1979.

46. Lopez-Majano V, Wagner HN Jr, Tow DE, et al: Radioisotope scanning of lung in pulmonary tuberculosis. JAMA 194:1053–1058, 1965.

47. Lutzker LG, Perez LA: Radioactive embolization from upper extremity thrombophlebitis. J Nucl Med 16:241–242, 1975.

48. Lynn DJ, Wyman AC, Varma VM: Influenza-A infection simulating pulmonary embolism. JAMA 238:1166–1168, 1977.

48A. Marcus CS, Parker LS, Rose JG, et al: Uptake of Tc-99m MAA by the liver during a thromboscintigram/lung scan. J Nucl Med 24:36–38, 1983.

49. Maynard CD, Cowan RJ: Role of the scan in bronchogenic carcinoma. Semin Nucl Med 1:195–205, 1971.

50. McCormack KR, Cantril ST, Kamenetsky S: Serial pulmonary perfusion scanning in radiation therapy for bronchogenic carcinoma. J Nucl Med 12:800–803, 1971.

51. McGuinnis EJ, Lull RJ: Bronchial adenoma causing unilateral absence of pulmonary perfusion. Radiology 120:367–368, 1976.

52. McNeil BJ: A diagnostic strategy using ventilation-perfusion studies in patients suspect for pulmonary embolism. J Nucl Med 17:613–616, 1976.

53. Mendelson DS, Train JS, Goldsmith SJ, et al: Ventilation-perfusion mismatch due to obstruction of pulmonary vein. J Nucl Med 22:1062–1063, 1981.

54. Milstein DM, Nusynowitz ML, Stein S, et al: Pulmonary scintigraphy in fat embolism syndrome (FES). J Nucl Med 15:517, 1974.

55. Moser KM, Guisan M, Cuomo A, et al: Differential diagnosis of pulmonary vascular from parenchymal disease by ventilation/perfusion scintiphotography. Ann Int Med 75:597–605, 1971.

56. Moses DC, Silver TM, Bookstein JJ: The complementary role of chest radiography, lung scanning and selective pulmonary angiography in the diagnosis of pulmonary embolism. Circulation 49:179–187, 1974.

57. Moylan JA Jr, Wilmore DW, Mouton DE, et al: Early diagnosis of inhalation injury using 133-xenon lung scan. Ann Surg 176:477–484, 1972.

58. Muroff LR, Johnson PM: Right atrial myxoma presenting as non-resolving pulmonary emboli: case report. J Nucl Med 17:890–892, 1976.

59. Myerson PJ, Myerson DA, Katz R, et al: Gallium imaging in pulmonary artery sarcoma mimicking pulmonary embolism: case report. J Nucl Med 17:893–895, 1976.

60. Nathan G, Swanson L, Kern W, et al: Lymphangitic carcinomatosis: lung scan abnormalities. J Nucl Med 17:258–260, 1976.

61. O'Dell CW, Taylor A, Higgins C, et al: Ventilation-perfusion lung images in the Swyer-James syndrome. Radiology 121:423–426, 1976.

62. Olsson HE, Spitzer RM, Erston WF: Primary and secondary pulmonary artery neoplasia mimicking acute pulmonary embolism. Radiology 118:49–53, 1976.

63. Park HM, Jay SJ, Brandt MV, et al: Pulmonary scintigraphy in fibrosing mediastinitis due

to histoplasmosis. J Nucl Med 22:349–351, 1981.

64. Piepsz A, Decostre P, Baran D: Scintigraphic study of pulmonary blood flow distribution in cystic fibrosis. J Nucl Med 14:326–330, 1973.

65. Polga JP, Drum DE: Abnormal perfusion and ventilation scan in azygos fissures. J Nucl Med 13:633–636, 1972.

66. Poulose KP, Reba RC, Gilday DL, et al: Diagnosis of pulmonary embolism. A correlative study of the clinical, scan and angiographic findings. Brit Med J 3:67–71, 1970.

67. Prato FS, Kurdyak R, Saibil EA, et al: Physiologic and radiographic assessment during the development of pulmonary radiation fibrosis. Radiology 122:389–397, 1977.

68. Putman CE: X-ray films often fail to show smoke damage to fire victim's lungs. JAMA 237:203, 1977.

69. Quinn JL III: Perfusion scanning in chronic obstructive lung disease. Semin Nucl Med 1:185–194, 1971.

70. Raju BL, Sakowitz M, Goldfarb R, et al: Lung-scan abnormality in pulmonary artery branch stenosis. J Nucl Med 21:495–496, 1980.

70A. Rao BR, Schillaci RF, Gerber FH, et al: "Hot spot" on perfusion lung scan produced by bronchiolo-alveolar cell carcinoma. Clin Nucl Med 7:282–283, 1982.

71. Secker-Walker RH, Alderson PO, Wilhelm BS, et al: Ventilation-perfusion scanning in carcinoma of the bronchus. Chest 65:660–663, 1974.

72. Sfakianakis GN, Damoulaki-Sfakianakis E, McClead RE, et al: Anomalous origin of left coronary artery diagnosed by a lung scan. New Eng J Med 296:675, 1977.

73. Shibel EM, Tisi GM, Moser KM: Pulmonary photoscan-roentgenographic comparison in sarcoidosis. Am J Roentgenol 106:770–777, 1969.

74. Sieniewicz DJ, Rosenthall L, Herba MJ, et al: Correlative assessment of the macroalbumin lung scan with the clinical and roentgenographic chest findings. Am J Roentgenol 100:822–834, 1967.

75. Silver FM, Moser DC, Bookstein JJ, et al: The effect of patient posture on the position of the diaphragm. Radiology 109:131–132, 1973.

76. Simon H: Ventilation perfusion mismatch lung scan without pulmonary emboli. Clin Nucl Med 2:124–127, 1977.

77. Slivka J, Taylor A, Nelson H: Abnormal perfusion scan due to an oesophageal hiatus hernia. Clin Nucl Med 2:389–391, 1977.

78. Snow RM, Wilson GA: Multiple pulmonary arteriovenous fistulae demonstrated by dynamic radionuclide pulmonary perfusion scanning. J Nucl Med 16:328–330, 1975.

79. Soin JS, James E Jr, Wagner HN: Detection of pulmonary hypertension by perfusion lung scan. Am J Roentgenol 118:792–800, 1973.

80. Soin JS, McKusick KA, Wagner HN Jr: Regional lung-function abnormalities in narcotic addicts. JAMA 224:1717–1720, 1973.

81. Stanley NN, Ackrill P, Wood J: Lung perfusion scanning in hepatic cirrhosis. Br Med J 4:639–643, 1972.

82. Stjernholm MR, Landis GA, Marcus FI, et al: Perfusion and ventilation radioisotope lung scans in stenosis of the pulmonary arteries and their branches. Am Heart J 78:37–42, 1969.

83. Suprenant EL, Wilson AF, Novey HS: Significance of regional ventilation and perfusion abnormalities in bronchial asthma. J Nucl Med 11:366–367, 1970.

84. Suprenant EL, Spellberg RD: Regional pulmonary function in supine patients with mitral valve disease. Radiology 17:99–104, 1975.

85. Sutherland JD, DeNardo GL, Brown D: Lung scan with ^{131}Ilabeled macroaggregated human serum albumin (MAA). Am J Roentgenol 98:416–426, 1966.

86. Suzuki Y, Konishi K, Hasada K: Radioisotope lung scanning in Takayasu's arteritis. Radiology 109:133–136, 1973.

87. Sy WM, Nissen AW: Radionuclide studies in hemangioendotheliomatosis: case report. J Nucl Med 16:915–917, 1975.

88. Sziklas JJ, Rosenberg R, Spencer RP: Ventilation-perfusion mismatch due to systemic arterial supply. Clin Nucl Med 4:231–232, 1979.

89. Tow DE, Wagner HN Jr: Effect of pleural fluid in the appearance of lung scan. J Nucl Med 11:138–139, 1970.

90. Valdez VA, Crucitti TW, Herrera NE: Agenesis of right pulmonary artery. J Nucl Med Tech 7:40–42, 1979.

91. Vandevivere J, Spehl M, Dab I: Bronchiectasis in childhood. Ped Radiol 9:193–198, 1980.

92. Wagner HN Jr: Nuclear Medicine. New York: H.P. Publishing, 1975.

92A. Webber MM, Bennett LR, Cragin M, et al: Thrombophlebitis demonstration by scintiscanning. Radiology 92:620–623, 1969.

93. Welch MH, Richardson RH, Whitecomb WH, et al: The lung scan in alpha-one antitrypsin deficiency. J Nucl Med 10:687–690, 1969.

94. White RI, James AE, Wagner HN: The significance of unilateral absence of pulmonary artery perfusion by lung scanning. Am J Roentgenol 111:501–509, 1971.

95. Williams O, Lyall J, Vernon M, et al: Ventilation perfusion lung scanning for pulmonary emboli. Brit Med J 1:600–602, 1974.

95A. Wood MJ: Ventilation-perfusion mismatch. Clin Nucl Med 8:181, 1983.

96. Zieger LS, Moss EG: Ventilation and perfusion imaging in Swyer-James syndrome. Clin Nucl Med 2:109, 1977.

Chapter 52

Lung Ventilation—Xenon, Krypton[†]

EDWARD B. SILBERSTEIN

I. Poor or absent wash-in; delayed wash-out

   A. Common

The use of an asterisk * in this chapter indicates that this entity has been observed by the author but the case report has not been published.

†Demonstrated with Xe-133 or Xe-127; 13 second $t_{1/2}$ Kr-81m cannot demonstrate wash-out phase.

    1. Chronic obstructive lung disease (7, 12, 16)
        a. bullous emphysema (20)
        b. centrilobular emphysema (20)
        c. chronic bronchitis (12, 20)
    2. Asthma (17, 20)
    3. Tuberculosis and its sequelae (20, 26)
    4. Bronchogenic carcinoma (20, 23)
    5. Mucus plugs post-operatively (atelectasis) (12, 13)
    6. Pneumonia (3, 12)
    7. Pleural effusion (3)
    8. Artefact from xenon
        a. in liver (20)
        b. in stomach (20, 22)
    9. Pulmonary edema (12)
  10. Hypoventilation (usually a symmetric abnormality)
        a. central hypoventilation (Ondine's Curse) may be asymmetric with diaphragmatic pacing (21)

B. Uncommon
    1. Endobronchial foreign body (3, 5, 20)
    2. Bronchiectasis (20, 27)
    3. Cystic fibrosis (4, 20)
    4. Bronchial adenoma (14)
    5. Bronchial carcinoid (15)
    6. Fibrothorax (12)
    7. Mitral stenosis (left lung only) (6)
    8. Respiratory burn (1)
    9. Pneumothorax (8)
  10. Post-radiotherapy (2)

C. Rare
    1. Pulmonary sequestration (25)
    2. Swyer-James syndrome (24)
    3. Transient bronchoconstriction with pulmonary embolism (9, 18)
    4. Bronchopleural fistula (28)
    5. Emphysema from alpha-one antitrypsin deficiency (11)
    6. Pulmonary papillomatosis (10)

II. Non-pulmonary xenon concentration

A. Common
    1. Fatty infiltration of liver (20)
    2. Gastric retention (20, 22)
    3. Diffuse mild background in very obese patients*

B. Uncommon
    1. Liposarcoma (19)
    2. Bronchopleural fistula (28)

REFERENCES

1. Adiseshan N, Pegg SP, Hinckley VM: Radioxenon retention in the early diagnosis of respiratory burns. Clin Nucl Med 2:424–426, 1977.
2. Alderson PO, Bradley EW, Mendenhall KS, et al: Radionuclide evaluation of pulmonary function following hemithorax irradiation of normal dogs with ^{60}Co or fast neutrons. Radiology 130:425–433, 1979.
3. Alderson PO, Rujanavech N, Secker-Walker RH, et al: The role of ^{133}Xe ventilation studies in the scintigraphic detection of pulmonary embolism. Radiology 120:633–640, 1976.
4. Alderson PO, Secker-Walker RH, Strominger DB, et al: Quantitative assessment of regional ventilation and perfusion in children with cystic fibrosis. Radiology 111:151–155, 1974.
5. Apau RL, Saenz R, Siemsen JK: Bloodless lung due to bronchial obstruction. J Nucl Med 13:561–562, 1972.
6. Dawson A, Rocamora JM, Morgan JR: Relative ventilation and perfusion of left versus right lung in mitral stenosis. Am J Cardiol 34:284–287, 1974.
7. DeNardo GL, Goodwin DA, Ravasini R, et al: The ventilatory lung scan in the diagnosis of pulmonary embolism. NEJM 282:1334–1336, 1970.
8. Dhekne RD, Burdine JA: The diagnosis of pneumothorax by ventilation-perfusion imaging. Radiology 129:119–121, 1978.
9. Epstein J, Taylor A, Alazraki N, et al: Acute pulmonary embolus associated wtih transient ventilatory defect. J Nucl Med 16:1017–1020, 1975.
10. Espinola D, Rupani H, Camargo EE, et al: Ventilation-perfusion imaging in pulmonary papillomatosis. J Nucl Med 22:975–977, 1981.
11. Fallat RJ, Powell MR, Kueppers F, et al: [133]Xe ventilatory studies in alpha-one antitrypsin deficiency. J Nucl Med 14:5–13, 1973.
12. Farmelant MH, Trainor JC: Evaluation of a ^{133}Xe ventilation technique for diagnosis of pulmonary disorders. J Nucl Med 12:586–590, 1971.
13. Giudi JC, Komansky HJ, Gordon R: Ventilation scan: Use in the evaluation of occult airway obstruction. Chest 77:576, 1980.
14. Grant JL, Naylor RW, Crandell WB: Bronchial adenoma resection with relief of hypoxic pulmonary vasoconstriction. Chest 77:446–449, 1980.
15. Hepper NG, Payne WS, Sheps SG, et al: Unilateral hypoperfusion of the lung and carcinoid syndrome due to bronchial carcinoid tumor. Am Rev Respir Dis 115:351–357, 1977.
16. Kaplan E, Mayron LW, Gergans GA, et al: Pulmonary function and [81m]Kr scans in obstructive pulmonary disease. Int J Nucl Med Biol 8:39–51, 1981.
17. Kawakami K, Katsuyama N, Fukuda Y, et al: A Kr-81m inhalation method for detection of absence of uniform ventilation in asthma. Clin Nucl Med 6:463–467, 1981.
18. Kessler RM, McNeil BJ: Impaired ventilation in a patient with angiographically demonstrated pulmonary emboli. Radiology 114:111–112, 1975.
19. Kim EE, DeLand FH, Maruyama T, et al: Detection of lipoid tumors by xenon-133. J Nucl Med 19:64–66, 1978.
20. Liehn JC, Ferrand O, Jouet JB, et al: Regional pulmonary ventilation studies with multiple view late xenon washout images. Int J Nucl Med Biol 7:319–325, 1980.
21. Makhija MC, Bronfman HJ, Lange RC, et al: Ventilation patterns mimicking COPD in patients with diaphragmatic pacing for Ondine's curse. Radiology 129:111–116, 1978.
22. Marx WJ, Courtney JV, MacMahon H, et al: Xenon in the gastric fundus: Potential pitfall in ventilation scan interpretation. Am J Roetngenol 132:676–677, 1979.

23. Moser KM, Guisan M, Cuomo A, et al: Differentiation of pulmonary vascular from parenchymal diseases by ventilation-perfusion scintiphotography. Ann Int Med 75:597–604, 1971.
24. O'Dell CW, Taylor A, Higgins CB, et al: Ventilation-perfusion lung images in Swyer-James syndrome. Radiology 121:423–426, 1976.
25. Prosin MA, Mishkin FS: Radionuclide diagnosis of pulmonary sequestration. J Nucl Med 15:636–638, 1974.
26. Ramos M, Baumann HR, Muhlberger F: Perfusion and ventilation imaging in pulmonary tuberculosis. Clin Nucl Med 3:233–241, 1978.
27. Vandevivere J, Spehl M, Dab I, et al: Bronchiectasis in childhood. Ped Radiol 9:193–198, 1980.
28. Zelefsky MN, Freeman LM, Stern H: A simple approach to the diagnosis of bronchopleural fistula. Radiology 124:843–844, 1977.

Chapter 53

Lung Ventilation—Aerosol†

AMOLAK SINGH

I. Predominately central deposition

    A. Common

        1. Moderate or severe chronic obstructive disease of large airways (3, 4, 5, 6)

           a. following assisted ventilation in infants (1)

        2. Bronchial asthma with large airway constriction (2, 7)

        3. Early bronchitis (7)

        4. Normal airways (when aerosol particles $>2\ \mu$ or in uncooperative patient) (3, 4, 7, 10)

II. Irregular peripheral deposition

    A. Common

†Such as Tc-99m DTPA or Tc-99m radiocolloid.

    1. Chronic obstructive disease of small airways (4, 5, 6)
    2. Bronchiectasis and end stage bronchiolitis (7)
    3. Cigarette smokers (7)
    4. Atopic individuals with asthma and bronchitis (7)

III. Excessive central deposition with irregular peripheral deposition (mixed pattern)

  A. Common
    1. Chronic obstructive airway disease (6, 9)
    2. Chronic smokers with bronchitis (9)

IV. Localized deposition of aerosol

  A. Common
    1. Neoplasia
      a. bronchogenic carcinoma (2, 8)
      b. melanoma of larynx or trachea (2)
      c. squamous carcinoma of larynx (2)
    2. Tuberculous bronchostenosis (2, 6)
    3. Bronchiectasis (6)
    4. Retained secretions (3)
    5. Bronchial constriction (8)

V. Diminished aerosol deposition in both lower lung fields

  A. Uncommon
    1. Alpha-one antitrypsin deficiency (7)

VI. Unilateral lung deficit

  A. Uncommon
    1. Bronchogenic carcinoma (2)
  B. Rare
    1. Swyer-James syndrome (7)

REFERENCES

1. Gates GF, Dore EK, Markarian M, et al: Radionuclide imaging of airway obstruction following assisted ventilation. Am J Dis Child 130:122–127, 1976.
2. Itoh H, Ishii T, Suzuki T, et al: Radioscintigraphy in the diagnosis of upper airway obstruction. Radiology 123:135–140, 1977.
3. Poe ND, Cohen MB, Yanda RL: Application of delayed lung imaging following radioaerosol inhalation. Radiology 122:739–746, 1977.
4. Ramanna L, Tashkin DP, Taplin G, et al: Radioaerosol lung imaging in chronic obstructive lung disease. Chest 68:634–640, 1975.

5. Santolicandio A, Giuntini C: Patterns of deposition of labeled monodispersed aerosols in obstructive lung disease. J Nucl Med Allied Sci 23:115–127, 1979.
6. Secker-Walker RH: Pulmonary nuclear medicine in Gottschalk A, Potchen EJ (eds): Diagnostic Nuclear Medicine. Baltimore: Williams and Wilkins, 1976, pp. 341–398.
7. Taplin GV, Hayes M: Lung imaging with radioaerosols for the assessment of airway disease. Sem Nucl Med 10:243–251, 1980.
8. Taplin GV, Poe ND, Isawa T, et al: Radioaerosol and xenon gas inhalation and lung perfusion scintigraphy. Scand J Resp Dis Suppl 85:144–158, 1974.
9. Taplin GV, Tashkin DP, Chopra SK, et al: Early detection of chronic obstructive pulmonary disease using radionuclide lung imaging procedures. Chest 71:567–575, 1977.
10. Wasnich RD: A high-frequency ultrasonic nebulized system for radioaerosol delivery. J Nucl Med 17:707–710, 1976.

Part XI

Skeletal System

Chapter 54

Bone Localization†

JOHN G. McAFEE

EDWARD B. SILBERSTEIN

I. Regional hyperemia of extremities demonstrated on early "blood pool" images with skeletal agents (1)

  A. Common

    1. Trauma, with or without fracture

    2. Osteomyelitis

    3. Cellulitis

    4. Arthritis

      a. synovial visualization (162A)

    5. Hemangioma

    6. Arterio-venous fistula

  B. Less common

    1. Primary bone tumors

    2. Sickle cell crisis with infarction

    3. Sympathetic dystrophy

      a. denervation

      b. sciatica

II. Single localized area of increased uptake in the skeleton

  A. Common

The use of an asterisk * in this chapter indicates that this entity has been observed by one of the authors but the case report has not been published.

† Demonstrated with Tc-99m pyrophosphate or diphosphonates.

1. Normal variants—asymmetry of shoulders, segments of sternum (143)
2. Metastatic carcinoma (lung, breast, prostate, large bowel) (3, 116, 117, 145)
3. Bone surgery including grafts, prostheses, thoracotomy, biopsy, amputation stump (116, 117, 143)
4. Fracture within the preceding 18–24 months (84)
   a. vertebral compression (117)
   b. stress fracture (159)
   c. non-union (30)
   d. acute plastic bowing (88)
   e. spontaneous femoral osteonecrosis (54)
5. Periodontal abscess (90)
6. Tooth extraction (90)
7. Monoarticular degenerative joint disease (117)
8. Paget's disease (116, 117, 148)
9. Pyogenic osteomyelitis and bone abscess (45, 117, 118)
10. Monoarticular rheumatoid arthritis (118)

B. Less common
   1. Metastatic tumor (116, 117, 145)
      a. carcinoma of cervix
      b. carcinoma of kidney
      c. carcinoma of thyroid
      d. carcinoma of bladder
      e. carcinoma of pancreas
      f. carcinoma of stomach
      g. melanoma
      h. neuroblastoma
      i. lymphoma
      j. lymphoepithelioma
      k. rhabdomyosarcoma
      l. thymoma (16)
      m. pinealoma (146)
   2. Primary bone and marrow tumors (117, 121, 153)
      a. osteosarcoma (50)
      b. Ewing's tumor
      c. osteochondroma (32)
      d. myeloma (116, 162) and plasmacytoma (35)
      e. osteoid osteoma (134)
   3. Meningioma (6, 86)
   4. Normal bone adjacent to malignant bone tumors (50)
   5. Aseptic necrosis (23)
      a. bone infarct in sickle cell disease (52)
      b. osteitis pubis (93, 136)
      c. condensing osteitis of clavicle (122, 138)

      d. frostbite (76)

      e. Legg-Perthes' disease (133)

      f. Osgood-Schlatter disease (92)

6. Monoarticular arthritis

      a. gout (117)

      b. pseudogout (111)

      c. chondrocalcinosis (20)

      d. Reiter's syndrome (68)

      e. septic arthritis (111)

      f. Whipple's disease (63)

7. Periostitis of undetermined cause (153)

8. Calcaneal periostitis (plantar fasciitis) (113)

9. Discitis (42)

10. Spondylolysis (44)

11. Tietze's syndrome (107)

C. Rare

    1. Primary bone tumors

      a. fibrosarcoma (121)

      b. chondrosarcoma (121)

      c. osteoblastoma (benign) (83, 142)

      d. fibroma (1, 13, 20)

      e. enchondroma (121)

      f. histiocytic lymphoma of bone (121)

      g. giant cell tumor (121)

      h. eosinophilic granuloma (118)

      i. leiomyoma of periosteum (21)

      j. histiocytosis X (121)

      k. xanthoma (121)

      l. ameloblastoma (95)

      m. chondroblastoma (121, 149)

    2. Non-pyogenic osteomyelitis

      a. tuberculosis (106)

      b. coccidioidomycosis (116, 128)

      c. brucellosis (21A)

    3. Sarcoidosis (118)

    4. Scurvy (41)

    5. Fibrous dysplasia (121)

    6. Pseudofracture in osteomalacia (20)

    7. Hemophiliac arthropathy (20)

    8. Pellegrini-Stieda disease (148)

    9. Gaucher's disease (17)

   10. Bone island (58, 162)

   11. "Brown cell tumor" from hyperparathyroidism (105)

   12. Sclerotic pedicle (Wilkinson syndrome) (132)

13. Single or aneurysmal bone cyst (81, 121)

III. Multiple areas of increased uptake in the skeleton (may be caused by almost any disorder noted in Section II above)
- A. Common
    1. Metastatic tumors, particularly carcinomas of lung, breast, kidney, thyroid, prostate, neuroblastoma (3, 59, 116, 117)
    2. Fractures within preceding 18–24 months (84)
        a. "battered child syndrome" (57)
    3. Degenerative osteoarthritis (19)
    4. Other arthritides (articular and juxta-articular distribution) (31, 155)
        a. ankylosing spondylitis (73)
        b. acute rheumatic fever (161)
        c. rheumatoid arthritis (155)
        d. psoriatic arthritis (155)
        e. Reiter's disease (155)
        f. gout (155)
        g. pseudogout (155)
        h. Behçet's syndrome (31)
    5. Paget's disease (20)
    6. Lymphomas (47)
    7. Leukemia (47)
    8. Aseptic necrosis, especially of femoral heads (29, 52)
- B. Less common
    1. Pyogenic osteomyelitis (117)
    2. Multiple myeloma (116, 162)
    3. Bone infarcts
        a. sickle cell disease (52)
    4. Histiocytosis X (47)
    5. Eosinophilic granuloma (4)
    6. Polyostotic fibrous dysplasia (152)
    7. Metastatic or multifocal bone tumors
        a. osteosarcoma (47)
        b. Ewing's tumor (116)
        c. osteochondromata (exostoses) (32)
    8. Osteomalacia with pseudofractures (123)
    9. Hyperparathyroidism (28, 72)
- C. Rare
    1. Non-pyogenic osteomyelitis
        a. tuberculosis (109A)
        b. coccidioidomycosis (5, 116)
    2. Neurofibromatosis*
    3. Pseudofractures in metabolic bone disease
        a. renal osteodystrophy (40)

       b. hyperparathyroidism (28, 72)

       c. osteomalacia (28, 37, 72, 123)

   4. Multiple enchondromatosis (Ollier's disease) (1)

   5. Metastatic carcinoid tumors (33)

   6. Osteopetrosis (98)

   7. Sarcoidosis (120)

   8. Scurvy (41)

   9. Gaucher's disease (17)

  10. Secondary syphilis (144)

  11. Leprosy (49)

  12. Melorheostosis (156)

  13. Hemophiliac arthropathy (20)

  14. Mafucci's syndrome*

  15. Hypervitaminosis A (114)

  16. Regional migratory osteoporosis (54, 96)

  17. Caffey's disease (infantile cortical hyperostosis) (53)

  18. Tumorous phosphaturic osteomalacia

       a. from multiple bone hemangiomata (24)

  19. Disseminated bone necrosis (139)

IV. Localized increase in uptake of skeletal agents in the skull

  A. Common

   1. Hyperostosis frontalis interna (118)

   2. Metastatic tumors (34)

   3. Craniotomy, and other surgical procedures (6)

   4. Sinusitis and mastoiditis (20)

   5. Trauma, with or without fracture, including "battered child syndrome" (57)

   6. Paget's disease (34)

   7. Paranasal sinus malignancies (10)

  B. Less common

   1. Hyperparathyroidism (72)

   2. Craniofacial fibrous dysplasia (34)

   3. Meningioma (34)

   4. "Ivory" osteoma (20)

   5. Premature craniosynostosis (sutural distribution) (43)

       a. infantile hypophosphatasia (131)

   6. Multiple myeloma (162)

   7. Histiocytosis X (47)

   8. Osteomyelitis (10)

   9. Post cytotoxic chemotherapy (22)

  10. Calvarial depression from delivery (130)

  C. Rare

   1. Neurofibromatosis*

  2. Sarcoidosis (120)
  3. Secondary syphilis (144)
  4. Mucormycosis at base of skull (163)
  5. Engelmann's disease (progressive diaphyseal dysplasia) (129)
  6. Caffey's disease (infantile cortical hyperostosis) (53)
  7. Dural calcification (12)

V. Increased uptake of skeletal agents in teeth and jaws (2, 27, 147)

  A. Common
    1. Ill-fitting dentures
    2. Tooth extraction
    3. Periodontal abscess, periodontitis, apical granuloma
    4. Post root-canal treatment
    5. Pulpitis, gingivitis
    6. Fractures
    7. Surgical trauma
    8. Bone grafts
    9. Free pertechnetate adsorbed to lingual squamous epithelium
  B. Less common
    1. Simple or multilocular cysts
    2. Odontogenic keratocysts
    3. Osteomyelitis
        a. actinomycosis
    4. Mandibular and maxillary tumors
        a. fibroma
        b. odontoma
        c. enchondroma
        d. osteoma
        e. lymphoma
    5. Bone invasion from oral or paranasal sinus malignancies
    6. Paget's disease
    7. Fibrous dysplasia
    8. Hyperparathyroidism (72)
    9. Impaction
  C. Rare
    1. Ameloblastoma (95)
    2. Caffey's disease (infantile cortical hyperostosis) (53)
    3. Periodontitis worsening post irradiation (10A)

VI. Bilateral increased uptake in sacroiliac joints

  A. Common
    1. Rheumatoid (ankylosing) spondylitis (73)
  B. Less common

    1. Reiter's disease (73)
    2. Crohn's disease (18)
    3. Ulcerative colitis (18)
    4. Psoriatic arthropathy (73)
    5. Metastases (41A)

VII. Unilateral increased uptake in sacroiliac joint

  A. Common
    1. Metastases from many tumors (41A)
    2. Pyogenic sacroiliitis (87)
  B. Uncommon
    1. Artefact from overlying colostomy (65A)

VIII. Localized increased uptake of skeletal agents in hips

  A. Common
    1. Degenerative or post-traumatic osteoarthritis (31)
    2. Rheumatoid arthritis (155)
    3. Aseptic necrosis (29, 52)
    4. Fracture and post-surgical (84)
    5. Osteomyelitis (117)
    6. Metastases (3, 59, 116, 117)
    7. Transient synovitis of hip joint in children (1)
    8. Septic arthritis (114)
  B. Less common
    1. Regional migratory osteoporosis (61, 96)
    2. Myositis ossificans (15)
    3. Tuberculosis*
  C. Rare
    1. Amyloidosis (151)
    2. Multiple enchondromata (121)
    3. Villonodular synovitis*
    4. Conversion defect of femoral neck (115)
    5. Congenital dislocation of the hips (104)

IX. Localized increased uptake surrounding hip or knee prosthesis (46, 154)

  A. Common
    1. Normal for 6–9 months following prosthetic surgery
    2. Loosening
    3. Infection
    4. Fracture or dislocation
    5. Heterotopic calcification (15)
  B. Less common

1. Delayed healing of trochanteric osteotomy
2. Trochanteric bursitis

X. Increased uptake of skeletal agents in extensive areas involving one or both extremities and/or hands and feet (136)

A. Uncommon
  1. Pulmonary osteoarthropathy, especially in terminal phalanges (19, 136)
  2. Obstruction to venous and/or lymphatic return (82)
  3. Primary hyperparathyroidism (72)
  4. Renal osteodystrophy (158)
  5. Hyperthyroidism (36, 126, 135)
  6. Reflex sympathetic dystrophy (71)
      a. hemiplegia (71, 101)
      b. immobilization (101)
  7. Shin splints (125)
  8. Within 2–3 months of radiotherapy (9)
  9. Following intra-arterial chemotherapy (124A)

B. Rare
  1. Hypoparathyroidism (72)
  2. Pseudohypoparathyroidism (72)
  3. Thyroid acropachy (110)
  4. Mastocytosis (urticaria pigmentosa) (138)
  5. Pachydermoperiostosis (60)
  6. Acro-osteolysis from polyvinyl chloride (91)
  7. Engelmann's disease (progressive diaphyseal dysplasia) (20, 129)
  8. Acromegaly (36, 119)
  9. Vitamin A toxicity (114)
  10. Post-sympathectomy (119)
  11. Symmetric osteomyelitis (100)
  12. Dysbaric osteonecrosis (79)
  13. Intra-arterial injection (2A)

XI. Increased uptake in patellae

A. Common
  1. Arthritides of knee joints (69)

B. Less common
  1. Bilateral fracture (69)
  2. Bursitis (69)
  3. Metastatic disease (69)
  4. Paget's disease (69)
  5. Osteomyelitis (69)
  6. Hyperparathyroidism, primary or secondary (72)

      7. Pulmonary osteoarthropathy (69)

      8. Post-knee surgery (69)

      9. Pellegrini-Stieda disease (peritendinitis calcarea of the medial collateral ligament of the knee joint) (148)

XII. Cortical circumferential uptake in long bones (''double stripe'' sign)

  A. Common

      1. Pulmonary osteoarthropathy (20)

      2. Paget's disease (20)

      3. Stress fracture (125)

XIII. Generalized increase in skeletal uptake

  A. Common pattern of metabolic bone disease (37)

      1. Increased uptake in the axial skeleton including calvaria, mandible, and sternum

      2. Accumulation in the metaphyses of long bones

      3. Increased costochondral junction uptake

      4. Decreased renal uptake

  B. Common

      1. Renal osteodystrophy (usually combines osteomalacia and secondary hyperparathyroidism) (158)

      2. Primary or secondary hyperparathyroidism (28, 158)

      3. ''Saturation'' metastatic carcinoma, especially from prostatic or breast (38)

      4. Pulmonary osteoarthropathy (prominent in extremities) (67)

  C. Less common

      1. Osteomalacia (39, 158)

         a. renal

         b. vitamin D deficiency

         c. related to mesenchymal tumors (24)

      2. Systemic lupus erythematosus (157)

      3. Scleroderma (157)

      4. Hyperthyroidism (157)

      5. Hypervitaminosis D (39)

      6. Leukemia (18)

      7. Aplastic anemia (18)

      8. Waldenström's macroglobulinemia (18)

      9. Myelofibrosis (70)

      10. Acromegaly (36)

  D. Rare

      1. Malnutrition (157)

         a. scurvy (41)

      2. Osteopetrosis (98)

    3. Mastocytosis (urticaria pigmentosa) (138)
    4. Engelmann's disease (diaphyseal dysplasia) (20)
    5. Lipid (cholesterol) granulomatosis (Chester-Erdheim disease) (8)
    6. Hyperphosphatasemia (64)

XIV. Abnormal radionuclide skeletal images with minimal or absent radiographic changes (for references cf. above)

  A. Common
    1. Metastatic malignancy
      a. myeloma
    2. Early osteomyelitis
    3. Early Paget's disease (148)
    4. Early aseptic necrosis (78)
      a. Legg-Perthe's disease
      b. osteochondritis dissecans (78)
      c. sickle cell disease (25, 52)
    5. Fractures, especially ribs, hands and feet, stress fractures (159), and fractures in young children (59)
    6. Radiation therapy portals (124)

  B. Uncommon
    1. Arthritides, including osteoarthritis, septic arthritis, hemarthrosis, sacroiliitis (31)
    2. Lymphoma
    3. Renal osteodystrophy
    4. Pulmonary osteoarthropathy
    5. Lower extremities in hemiplegia or paraplegia (101)

  C. Rare
    1. Primary hyperparathyroidism
    2. Myelofibrosis
    3. Leukemic infiltration

XV. Focal defects in skeletal images (photon-deficient areas)

  A. Common
    1. Surgical defects*
    2. Shielding artefacts from external or internal dense objects (56)
      a. barium
      b. cardiac pacemakers
      c. breast prosthesis
      d. orthopedic prosthesis
      e. dental work
      f. coins
      g. pendants
    3. Malignancies with bone destruction or intraosseous vascular obstruction (151)

        a. metastatic carcinoma (137)
- **(1)** unknown primary
- **(2)** breast carcinoma
- **(3)** lung carcinoma
- **(4)** bladder carcinoma

        b. metastatic neuroblastoma (47, 66)
        c. osteosarcoma (51)
        d. fibrosarcoma (81A)

    4. Aseptic necrosis (48, 56, 76, 127), traumatic or atraumatic
        a. sickle cell disease (59)
    5. Radiation therapy fields (127)
    6. Cyst (127)

B. Less common
    1. Acute pyogenic osteomyelitis (106)
    2. Cavernous hemangioma of bone (160)
    3. In a child's extremity due to reflex sympathetic dystrophy, improving with sympathetic nerve block (80)

C. Rare
    1. Chronic renal failure with areas of myelofibrosis (102)
    2. Brown tumors associated with hyperparathyroidism (14)
    3. Gaucher's disease (17)
    4. Parietal thinning (103)
    5. Congenital or acquired absence of a pedicle (spondylolysis) (44, 141)

XVI. Localized filling defect in femoral head

A. Common
    1. Hip prosthesis
    2. Aseptic necrosis, early
        a. Legg-Perthe's disease (25)
        b. homozygous sickle cell disease (59)
        c. secondary to septic arthritis (1)
    3. Subcapital fracture with ischemia of proximal fragment (1)

B. Less common
    1. Ischemia of femoral head epiphysis in children secondary to hip joint effusion (7)
    2. Slipped femoral capital epiphysis (7)
    3. Metastasis (48)

C. Rare
    1. Gaucher's disease (17)

XVII. Generalized decrease in skeletal uptake

A. Common
    1. Severe osteoporosis (75)

    2. Radiopharmaceutical failure (16A)

    3. Poor hydration (119A)

B. Rare

    1. Hemochromatosis and transfusion iron-overload (159)

    2. Advanced renal osteodystrophy*

    3. Advanced osteopetrosis*

    4. Thalassemia major (150)

    5. Rhabdomyolysis with muscle uptake greatly exceeding the skeleton (119)

XVIII. Skeletal lesions demonstrated with radiogallium but not with skeletal agents

    A. Common

        1. Acute osteomyelitis, especially early and in neonatal period (59, 62)

        2. Acute septic arthritis (59)

    B. Less common

        1. Ewing's tumor*

XIX. Skeletal lesions demonstrated with skeletal agents but not with radiogallium

    A. Common

        1. Skeletal metastases (59)

        2. Long-standing, inactive osteomyelitis (62)

XX. Positive radiographic findings with negative skeletal radionuclide images

    A. Common

        1. Idiopathic or post menopausal osteoporosis*

        2. Multiple myeloma (162)

        3. Purely destructive metastatic carcinoma*

        4. Benign cortical defects in children (59)

        5. Fracture less than 48 hours old (20)

        6. Simple bone cyst (1)

        7. Metastatic neuroblastoma (47, 66)

        8. Bone island (26)

        9. Multiple exostoses (32)

      10. Thoracic scoliosis (112)

    B. Less common

        1. Spinal disc-space infection (94)

        2. Histiocytosis X (47)

        3. Coccidioidomycosis (5)

    C. Rare

        1. Osteopoikilosis (156)

        2. Osteopathia striata (156)

REFERENCES

1. Alderson PO, Gilday DL, Wagner HN, Jr.: Atlas of Pediatric Nuclear Medicine. St. Louis: C. V. Mosby Co., 1978.
2. Alexander JM: Radionuclide bone scanning in the diagnosis of lesions of the maxillofacial region. J Oral Surg 34:249–256, 1976.
2A. Andrews GA, Theocheung JL, Andrews E, et al: Unintentional intra-arterial injection of bone-imaging agent. Clin Nucl Med 5:499–501, 1980.
3. Antoniades J, Croll MN, Walner RJ, et al: Bone scanning in carcinomas of the colon and rectum. Dis Colon Rectum 19:139–143, 1976.
4. Antonmattei S, Tetalman MR, Lloyd, T: The multiscan appearance of eosinophilic granuloma. Clin Nucl Med 4:53–55, 1979.
5. Armbuster TG, Georgen TG, Resnick D, et al: Utility of bone scanning in disseminated coccidioidomycosis: case report. J Nucl Med 18:450–454, 1977.
6. Arzoumanian A, Rosenthall L: The combined use of radiopertechnetate and ^{99m}Tc-polyphosphate in distinguishing cerebral and calvarial lesions. J Assoc Canadienne Rad 25:178–183, 1974.
7. Ash JM: The bone scan as an aid to therapy in paediatric disease. Brit J Radiol 52:249–250, 1979.
8. Atkins, HL, Kloppe JF, Ansari AN, et al: Lipid (cholesterol) granulomatosis (Chester-Erdheim disease) and congenital megacalices. Clin Nucl Med 3:324–327, 1978.
9. Bekier A: Extraosseous accumulation of Tc-99m pyrophosphate in soft tissue after radiation therapy. J Nucl Med 19:225–226, 1978.
10. Bergstedt HF, Carenfelt C, Lind MG: Facial bone scintigraphy. Acta Rad Diagnostica 20:458–464, 1979.
10A. Bergstedt HF, Lind MG: Facial bone scintigraphy III. Effects of radiation therapy. Acta Rad Diagnostica 20:75–80, 1979.
11. Blau M, Ganatra R, Bender MA: F-18 fluoride for bone imaging. Sem Nucl Med 2:31–37, 1972.
12. Bobba RV, Fink-Bennett D: A dural calcification presenting as a solitary lesion on radionuclide bone scan. Clin Nucl Med 3:35, 1978.
13. Brenner RJ, Hattner RS, Lilien DL:Scintigraphic features of nonosteogenic fibroma. Radiology 131:727–730, 1979.
14. Brown WT, Lyons KP, Winer RL: Changing manifestations of brown tumors on bone scan in renal osteodystrophy. J Nucl Med 19:1146–1148, 1978.
15. Campeau RJ, Hall MF, Miale A Jr.: Detection of total hip arthroplasty complications with Tc-99m pyrophosphate. J Nucl Med 17:526–531, 1976.
16. Cancroft E, Montorfano D, Goldfarb CR: Metastases to bone from malignant thymoma detected by technetium phosphate and gallium-67 scintigraphy. Clin Nucl Med 3:312–314, 1978.
16A. Chaudhuri TK: Liver uptake of ^{99m}Tc-diphosphonate. Radiology 119:485–486, 1976.
17. Cheng TH, Holman BL: Radionuclide assessment of Gaucher's disease. J Nucl Med 19:1333–1336, 1978.
18. Cheng TH, Holman BL: Increased skeletal-renal uptake ratio. Radiology 136:455–459, 1980.
19. Christensen SB, Arnold CC: Distribution of ^{99m}Tc phosphate compounds in osteoarthritic femoral heads. J Bone Joint Surg 62A:90–96, 1980.
20. Citrin DL, McKillop JH: Atlas of Technetium Bone Scans. Philadelphia: W.B. Saunders, 1978.

21. Conklin JJ, Camargo EE, Wagner HN: Bone scan detection of peripheral periosteal leiomyoma. J Nucl Med 22:97, 1981.

21A. Coulaud JP, Mechali D, Morau G: La scintigraphie osseuse et le diagnostic de la tuberculose osteo-articulaire du transplante. Ann-Med Int 133:261–265, 1982.

22. Creutzig H, Dach W: The "sickle-sign" in bone scintigraphy. Eur J Nucl Med 6:99–101, 1981.

23. Dalinka MK, Alavi A, Forsted DH: Aseptic (ischemic) necrosis of the femoral head. JAMA 238:1059–1061, 1977.

24. Daniels RA, Weisenfeld I: Tumorous phosphaturic osteomalacia. Am J Med 67:155–159, 1979.

25. Danigelis JA, Fisher RL, Ozonoff MB, et al: ^{99m}Tc polyphosphate bone imaging in Legg-Perthe's disease. Radiology 115:407–413, 1975.

26. Davies JAK, Hall FM, Goldberg RP, et al: Positive bone scan in a bone island. J Bone Joint Surg 61A:943–945, 1979.

27. D'Avignon MB, Baum S: Increased jaw radioactivity on bone imaging. Sem Nucl Med 12:219, 1982.

28. DeLong JF, Davis HG: Bone scan findings in a patient with hyperparathyroidism and a large cystic parathyroid adenoma in the mediastinum. Clin Nucl Med 2:114–118, 1977.

29. DeRossi G, Focacci C, Maini CL, et al: The particular usefulness of radioisotope methods in some benign bone diseases. Eur J Nucl Med 4:203–206, 1979.

30. Desai A, Alavi A, Dalinka M, et al: Role of bone scintigraphy in the evaluation and treatment of nonunited fractures. J Nucl Med 21:931–934, 1980.

31. Desaulniers M, Fuks A, Hawkins D, et al: Radiotechnetium polyphosphate joint imaging. J Nucl Med 15:417–423, 1974.

32. Epstein DA, Levin EJ: Bone scintigraphy in hereditary multiple exostoses. Am J Roentgenol 130:331–333, 1978.

33. Feldman JM, Plank JW: ^{99m}Tc pyrophosphate bone scans in patients with metastatic carcinoid tumors. J Nucl Med 18:71–80, 1977.

34. Fitzer PM: Radionuclide angiography—brain and bone imaging in craniofacial fibrosis dysplasia (CFD): case report. J Nucl Med 18:709–712, 1977.

35. Floyd JL: Prather JL: Vascular plasmacytoma. Clin Nucl Med 2:243–244, 1977.

36. Fogelman I, Hay ID, Citrin DJ, et al: Semi-quantitative analysis of the bone scan in acromegaly. Br J Radiol 53:874–877, 1980.

37. Fogelman I, McKillop JH, Bessent RG, et al: The role of bone scanning in osteomalacia. J Nucl Med 19:245–248, 1978.

38. Fogelman I, McKillop JH, Boyle IT, et al: Absent kidney sign associated with symmetrical and uniformly increased uptake of radiopharmaceutical by the skeleton. Eur J Nucl Med 2:257–259, 1977.

39. Fogelman I, McKillop JH, Cowden E, et al: Bone scan findings in hypervitaminosis D: case report. J Nucl Med 18:1205–1207, 1977.

40. Fogelman I, McKillop JH, Greig WR, et al: Pseudofracture of the ribs detected by bone scanning. J Nucl Med 18:1236–1237, 1977.

41. Front D, Hardoff R, Levy J, et al: Bone scintigraphy in scurvy. J Nucl Med 19:916–917, 1978.

41A. Front D, Hardoff R, Robinson E: Bone scintigraphy in primary tumors of the head and neck. Cancer 42:111–117, 1978.

42. Gates GF: Scintigraphy of discitis. Clin Nucl Med 2:20–25, 1977.

43. Gates GF, Dore EK: Detection of premature craniosynostosis with ^{18}F. J Nucl Med 14:397–398, 1973.

44. Gelfand MJ, Strife JL, Kereiakes JG: Radionuclide bone imaging in spondylolysis of the lumbar spine in children. Radiology 140:191–195, 1981.
45. Gelfand MJ, Silberstein EB: Radionuclide imaging: Use in diagnosis of osteomyelitis in children. JAMA 237:245–247, 1977.
46. Gelman MI, Coleman RE, Stevens PM, et al: Radiography, radionuclide imaging and arthrography in the evaluation of total hip and knee replacement. Radiology 128:677–682, 1978.
47. Gilday DL, Ash J, Reilly BJ: Radionuclide skeletal survey for pediatric neoplasms. Radiology 123:399–406, 1977.
48. Goergen TG, Alazraki NP, Halpern SE, et al: "Cold bone lesions": a newly recognized phenomenon of bone imaging. J Nucl Med 15:1120–1124, 1974.
49. Goergen TG, Resnick D, Lomonaco A, et al: Radionuclide bone-scan abnormalities in leprosy: case report. J Nucl Med 17:788–790, 1976.
50. Goldman AB, Braunstein P: Augmented radioactivity on bone scans of limbs bearing osteosarcomas. J Nucl Med 16:423–424, 1975.
51. Goris ML, Basso LV, Etcubanas E: Photopenic lesions in bone scintigraphy. Clin Nucl Med 5:299–301, 1980.
52. Grayson ND, Kassel EE: Serial bone-scan changes in recurrent bone infarction. J Nucl Med 17:184–186, 1976.
53. Greer LW, Friedman AC, Madewell JE: Periosteal reaction of the femur in infant with fever. JAMA 245:1765–1766, 1981.
54. Greyson ND, Lotem MM, Gross AE, et al: Radionuclide evaluation of spontaneous femoral osteonecrosis. Radiology 142:729–735, 1982.
55. Greyson ND, Pang S: The variable bone scan appearance of nonosteogenic fibroma of bone. Clin Nucl Med 6:242–245, 1981.
56. Gupta SM, Panduranga A, Buckley M, et al: Significance of photon-deficient areas in radionuclide bone scans. J Nucl Med Tech 8:208–210, 1980.
57. Haase GM, Ortiz VN, Sfakianakis G: The value of radionuclide bone scanning in the early recognition of deliberate child abuse. J Trauma 20:873–875, 1980.
58. Hall FM, Goldberg RP, Davies JAK, et al: Scintigraphic assessment of bone islands. Radiology 135:737–742, 1980.
59. Harcke HT Jr.: Bone imaging in infants and children. J Nucl Med 19:324–329, 1978.
60. Hattner RS: Skeletal scintigraphy in pachydermoperiostosis. Eur J Nucl Med 6:477–479, 1981.
61. Helfgott S, Tannenbaum H, Rosenthall L: Radiophosphate imaging of regional migratory osteoporosis. Clin Nucl Med 4:330–332, 1979.
62. Helson L, Watson RC, Benua RS, et al: F-18 radioisotope scanning of metastatic bone lesions in children with neuroblastoma. Am J Roentgenol 115:191–199, 1972.
63. Ho G, Claunch BC, Sadovnikoff N: Scintigraphic evidence of transient unilateral sacroiliitis in a case of Whipple's disease. Clin Nucl Med 5:548–550, 1980.
64. Iancu TC, Almagor G, Friedman E, et al: Chronic familial hyperphosphatemia. Radiology 129:669–676, 1978.
65. Janousek J, Preston DF, Martin NL, et al: Bone scan in melorheostosis. J Nucl Med 17:1106–1108, 1976.
65A. Jones AE, Ghaed N, Dunson GL, et al: Clinical evaluation of orally administered fluorine-18 for bone scanning. Radiology 107:129–131, 1973.
66. Kaufman RA, Thrall JH, Keyes JW Jr., et al: False negative bone scans in neuroblastoma metastatic to the ends of long bones. Am J Roentgenol 130:131–135, 1978.
67. Kay CJ, Rosenberg MA: Positive ^{99m}Tc-polyphosphate bone scan in case of secondary

hypertrophic osteoarthropathy. J Nucl Med 15:312–313, 1974.

68. Khalkali I, Stadalnik RC, Wiesner KB, et al: Bone imaging of the heel in Reiter's syndrome. Am J Roentgenol 132:110–112, 1979.

69. Kipper MS, Alazraki NP, Feiglin DH: The "hot" patella. Clin Nucl Med 7:28–32, 1982.

70. Kim EE, DeLand FH: Myelofibrosis presenting as hypermetabolic bone disease by radionuclide imaging in a patient with asplenia. Clin Nucl Med 3:406–408, 1978.

71. Kozin F, Soin JS, Ryan LM, et al: Bone scintigraphy in the reflex sympathetic dystrophy syndrome. Radiology 138:437–443, 1981.

72. Krishnamurthy GT, Brickman AS, Blahd WH: Technetium-99m-Sn-pyrophosphate pharmacokinetics and bone image changes in parathyroid disease. J Nucl Med 18:236–242, 1977.

73. Lentle BC, Russell AS, Percy JS, et al: Scintigraphic findings in ankylosing spondylitis. J Nucl Med 18:524–528, 1977.

74. Lentle BC, Russell AS, Percy JS, et al: The scintigraphic investigation of sacroiliac disease. J Nucl Med 18:529–533, 1977.

75. Levine SB, Haines JE, Larson SM, et al: Reduced skeletal localization of ^{99m}Tc-diphosphonate in two cases of severe osteoporosis. Clin Nucl Med 2:318–321, 1977.

76. Lisbona R, Rosenthall L: Assessment of bone viability by scintiscanning in frostbite injuries. J Trauma 16:989–992, 1976.

77. Lisbona R, Rosenthall L: Observations on the sequential uses of ^{99m}Tc-phosphate complex and ^{67}Ga imaging in osteomyelitis, cellulitis and septic arthritis. Radiology 123:123–129, 1977.

78. Lotke PA, Ecker ML, Alavi A: Painful knees in older patients — radionuclide diagnosis of possible osteonecrosis with spontaneous resolution. J Bone Joint Surg 59A:617–621, 1977.

79. MacLeod MA, Pearson RR, McEwan AJB, et al: Bone scintigraphy in dysbaric related osteopathy. Nucl Med Communic 2:236–241, 1981.

80. Majd M: Personal communication, 15 April, 1982.

81. Makhija MC: Bone scanning in aneurysmal bone cyst. Clin Nucl Med 6:500–501, 1981.

81A. Makhija MC: Fibrosarcoma: Photopenic lesion on a bone scan. Clin Nucl Med 8:265–266, 1983.

82. Manoli RS, Soin JS: Unilateral increased radioactivity in the lower extremities on routine ^{99m}Tc-pyrophosphate bone imaging. Clin Nucl Med 3:374–378, 1978.

83. Martin NL, Preston DF, Robinson RG: Osteoblastomas of the axial skeleton shown by skeletal scanning: case report. J Nucl Med 17:187–189, 1976.

84. Matin P: The appearance of bone scans following fractures, including immediate and long-term studies. J Nucl Med 20:1227–1231, 1979.

85. McCombs RK, Olson WH: Positive ^{18}F bone scan in a case of osteoid osteoma: case report. J Nucl Med 16:465–466, 1975.

86. McQuade S, Higgins HP: ^{99m}Tc-polyphosphate in diagnosing meningiomas of the sphenoid wing. J Nucl Med 15:1205–1206, 1974.

87. Miller JH, Gates GF: Scintigraphy of sacroiliac pyarthrosis in children. JAMA 238:2701–2704, 1977.

88. Miller JH, Osterkamp JA: Scintigraphy in acute plastic bowing of the forearm. Radiology 142:742, 1982.

89. Milstein DM, Nusynowitz ML: Cranial cholesteatoma: Unusual ^{99m}Tc-Sn polyphosphate and ^{99m}Tc-pertechnetate scintiphotos. Clin Nucl Med 4:240–241, 1979.

90. Moon NF, Dworkin HJ, LaFluer PD: The clinical use of sodium fluoride F-18 in bone photoscanning. JAMA 204:116–122, 1968.
91. Murray IPC: Bone scanning in occupational acro-osteolysis. Skel Radiol 3:149–154, 1978.
92. Namey TC, Daniel WW: Scintigraphic study of Osgood-Schlatter disease following delayed clinical presentation. Clin Nucl Med 5:551–553, 1980.
93. Nissenkorn I, Servadio C, Lubin E: The treatment of osteitis pubis with heparin. J Urol 125:528–529, 1981.
94. Norris S, Ehrlich MG, Keim DE, et al: Early diagnosis of disc-space infection using gallium-67. J Nucl Med 19:384–386, 1978.
95. Olson WH, McCombs RK: Positive (^{99m}Tc) diphosphonate and ^{67}Ga-citrate scans in ameloblastoma: case report. J Nucl Med 18:348–349, 1977.
96. O'Mara RE, Pinals RS: Bone scanning in regional migratory osteoporosis: case report. Radiology 97:579–581, 1970.
97. Papavasilious C, Kostamis P, Angelakis P, et al: Localization of Sr-87m in extraosseous tumor. J Nucl Med 12:265–268, 1971.
98. Park H-M, Lambertus J: Skeletal and reticuloendothelial imaging in osteopetrosis: case report. J Nucl Med 18:1091–1095, 1977.
99. Parker JA, Jones AG, Davis MA, et al: Reduced uptake of bone seeking radiopharmaceuticals related to iron excess. Clin Nucl Med 1:267–268, 1976.
100. Parker M, Cowan RJ: Symmetrical osteomyelitis of the lower extremities. Clin Nucl Med 4:303, 1979.
101. Prakash V, Kamel NJ, Lin MS, et al: Increased skeletal localization of ^{99m}Tc-diphosphonate in paralyzed limbs. Clin Nucl Med 1:48–50, 1976.
102. Quint PA, Klingensmith WC, Datu JA: Multiple regions of absent bone mineral and marrow function in a patient with chronic renal failure. Radiology 130:751–752, 1979.
103. Rao BK, Lieberman LM: Parietal thinning: a cause for photopenia on bone scan. Clin Nucl Med 5:313, 1980.
104. Rao BK, Lieberman LM: Bilateral congenital dislocation of hips: diagnosis on a bone scan. Clin Nucl Med 5:556–557, 1980.
105. Rosenthall L, Kaye M: Technetium-99m-pyrophosphate kinetics and imaging in metabolic bone disease. J Nucl Med 16:33–45, 1975.
106. Russin LD, Staab EV: Unusual bone scan findings in acute osteomyelitis: case report. J Nucl Med 17:617–619, 1976.
107. Sain AK: Bone scan in Tietze's syndrome. Clin Nucl Med 3:470–471, 1978.
108. Samuels LD: Diagnosis of malignant bone disease with strontium. Can Med Assoc J 104:411–413, 1971.
109. Samuels LD: Skeletal scintigraphy in children. Sem Nucl Med 2:89–107, 1972.
109A. Scoggin CH, Schwarz MI, Dixon BW, et al: Tuberculosis of the skull. Arch Int Med 136:1154–1156, 1976.
110. Seigel RS, Thrall JH, Sisson JC: ^{99m}Tc-pyrophosphate scan and radiographic correlation in thyroid acropathy: case report. J Nucl Med 17:791–793, 1976.
111. Seto H, Tonami N, Hisada K: Utility of combined ^{99m}Tc-phosphate and ^{67}Ga imaging in the diagnosis of septic arthritis. Clin Nucl Med 3:1–3, 1978.
112. Sevastikoglou JA, Aaro S, Elmstedt E, et al: Bone scanning of the spine and thorax in idiopathic thoracic scoliosis. Clin Orth Rel Res 149:172–175, 1980.
113. Sewell JR, Black CM, Chapman AH, et al: Quantitative scintigraphy in diagnosis and management of plantar fasciitis (calcaneal periostitis). J Nucl Med 21:633–636, 1980.

114. Shayvitz BA, Siegel NJ, Pearson HA: Megavitamins for minimal brain dysfunction: a potentially dangerous therapy. JAMA 238:1749–1750, 1977.
115. Shigeno C, Fukunaga M, Morita R, et al: Accumulation of ^{99m}Tc-methylene diphosphonate in a so-called conversion defect of the femoral neck. Eur J Nucl Med 6:421–423, 1981.
116. Shirazi PH, Rayudu VS, Fordham EW: F-18 bone scanning: Review of indications and results of 1,500 scans. Radiology 112:361–368, 1974.
117. Shirazi PH, Rayudu VS, Fordham EW: Review of solitary F-18 bone scan lesions. Radiology 112:369–372, 1974.
118. Silberstein EB: Causes of abnormalities reported in nuclear medicine testing. J Nucl Med 17:229–232, 1976.
119. Silberstein EB, Bove K: Visualization of alcohol-induced rhabdomyolysis. J Nucl Med 20:127–129, 1979.
119A. Silberstein EB, Saenger EL, Tofe AJ, et al: Imaging of bone metastases with ^{99m}Tc-Sn-EHDP (diphosphonate), ^{18}F and skeletal radiography. Radiology 107:551–555, 1973.
120. Silver HM, Shirkhoda A, Simon DB: Symptomatic osseous sarcoidosis with findings on bone scan. Chest 73:238–240, 1978.
121. Simon MA, Kirchner PT: Scintigraphic evaluation of primary bone tumors. J Bone Joint Surg 62A:758–764, 1980.
122. Simpson AJ: Positive bone scintigraphy in condensing osteitis of the clavicle. Clin Nucl Med 3:204, 1978.
123. Singh BN, Spies SM, Mehta SP, et al: Unusual bone scan presentation in osteomalacia: symmetrical uptake—a suggestive sign. Clin Nucl Med 3:292–295, 1978.
124. Sorkin SJ, Horii SC, Passalaqua A, et al: Decreased activity on bone scan following therapeutic radiation: a source of possible error. Clin Nucl Med 3:67, 1978.
124A. Sorkin SJ, Horii SC, Passalaqua A, et al: Augmented activity on bone scan following local chemoperfusion. Clin Nucl Med 2:451, 1977.
125. Spencer RP, Levinson ED, Baldwin RD, et al: Diverse bone scan abnormalities in ''shin splints.'' J Nucl Med 20:1271–1272, 1979.
126. Spencer RP, Daty JA: Bilateral lower limb uptake of bone scanning agents. Sem Nucl Med 10:314–316, 1980.
127. Stadalnik RC: ''Cold spot''—bone imaging. Sem Nucl Med 19:2–3, 1979.
128. Stadalnik RC, Goldstein E, Hoeprich PD, et al: Diagnostic value of gallium and bone scans in evaluation of extrapulmonary coccidioidal lesions. Am Rev Resp Dis 121:673–676, 1980.
129. Sty JR, Babbitt DP, Starshak RJ: Bone scintigraphy demonstrating Engelmann's disease. Clin Nucl Med 3:69–70, 1978.
130. Sty JR, Babbitt DP: Bone scintigraphy: derby hat deformity. Clin Nucl Med 5:554–555, 1980.
131. Sty JR, Boedecker RA, Babbitt DP: Skull scintigraphy in infantile hypophosphatasia. J Nucl Med 20: 305–306, 1979.
132. Sty JR, Starshak RJ, Babbitt D: Bone scintigraphy: the sclerotic pedicle. Clin Nucl Med 5:558, 1980.
133. Sutherland AD, Savage JP, Paterson DC, et al: The nuclide bone-scan in the diagnosis and management of Perthe's disease. J Bone Joint Surg 62B:300–306, 1980.
134. Swee RG, McLeod RA, Beabout JW: Osteoid osteoma. Radiology 130:117–123, 1979.
135. Sy WM: Bone scan in primary hyperparathyroidism. J Nucl Med 15:1089–1091, 1974.
136. Sy WM, Bay R, Camera A: Hand images: normal and abnormal. J Nucl Med 18:419–424, 1977.

137. Sy WM, Westring DW, Weinberger G: "Cold" lesions on bone imaging. J Nucl Med 16:1013–1016, 1975.
138. Sy WM, Bonventre MV, Camera A: Bone scan in mastocytosis: case report. J Nucl Med 17:699–701, 1976.
139. Szasz I, Morrison RT, Lyster DM, et al: Bone scintigraphy in massive disseminated bone necrosis. Clin Nucl Med 6:97–100, 1981.
140. Teates CD, Brown AC, Williamson BRJ, et al: Bone scans in condensing osteitis of the clavicle. So Med J 71:736–751, 1978.
141. Tessler F, Lander P, Lisbona R: Congenital absence of a pedicle with photon deficiency on bone scan. Clin Nucl Med 6:498–499, 1981.
142. Thompson SK: Benign osteoblastoma of the spine. J Royal Coll Surg 25:271–275, 1980.
143. Thrall JH, Ghaed N, Geslien GE, et al: Pitfalls in Tc-99m-polyphosphate skeletal imaging. Am J Roentgenol 121:739–747, 1974.
144. Tight RR, Warner JG: Skeletal involvement in secondary syphilis detected by bone scanning. JAMA 235:2326–2327, 1976.
145. Tofe AJ, Francis MD, Harvey WJ: Correlation of neoplasms with incidence and localization of skeletal metastases: an analysis of 1355 diphosphonate bone scans. J Nucl Med 15:986–989, 1975.
146. Tonami N, Seto H, Maeda T, et al: Increased concentration of ^{99m}Tc-methylene diphosphonate and ^{67}Ga-citrate in extracranial bone metastases from pinealoma. Clin Nucl Med 3:467–469, 1978.
147. Tow DE, Garcia DA, Jansons D, et al: Bone scan in dental disease. J Nucl Med 19:845–847, 1978.
148. Turner JW, Syed IB, Spencer RP: Two unusual causes of peripatellar nonmetastatic positive bone scans in patients with malignancies: case report. J Nucl Med 17:693–695, 1976.
149. Ulreich S, Swartz G, Steir S, et al: Benign chondroblastoma of talus demonstrated by skeletal scanning. Clin Nucl Med 3:62–63, 1976.
150. Valdez VA, Jacobstein JG: Decreased bone uptake of technetium-99m polyphosphate in thalassemia major. J Nucl Med 21:47–49, 1980.
151. Vieras F, Herzberg DL: Focal decreased skeletal uptake secondary to metastatic disease. Radiology 118:121–122, 1976.
152. Wagman E, Hsieh E, Schwinger A: A case of polyostotic fibrous dysplasia demonstrated by bone scan using ^{99m}Tc-stannous polyphosphate. Clin Nucl Med 1:215–216, 1976.
153. Wanken JF, Eyring EJ, Samuels LD: Diagnosis of pediatric bone lesions: Correlation of clinical, roentgenographic, Sr-87m scan, and pathologic diagnoses. J Nucl Med 14:803–806, 1973.
154. Weiss PE, Mall JC, Hoffer PB, et al: ^{99m}Tc-methylene diphosphonate bone imaging in the evaluation of total hip prostheses. Radiology 133:727–728, 1979.
155. Weissberg DL, Resnick D, Taylor A, et al: Rheumatoid arthritis and its variants: Analysis of scintiphotographic, radiographic, and clinical examinations. Am J Roentgenol 131:665–673, 1978.
156. Whyte MP, Murphy WA, Siegel BA: ^{99m}Tc-pyrophosphate bone imaging in osteopoikilosis, osteopathia striata and melorheostosis. Radiology 127:439–443, 1978.
157. Wiegmann T, Kirsh J, Rosenthall L, et al: The relationship between bone uptake of ^{99m}Tc-pyrophosphate and hydroxyproline in blood and urine. J Nucl Med 17:711–714, 1976.
158. Wiegmann T, Rosenthall L, Kaye M: Technetium-99m-pyrophosphate bone scans in hyperparathyroidism. J Nucl Med 18:231–235, 1977.

159. Wilcox JR, Moniot A, Green JP: Bone scanning in the evaluation of exercise-related stress injuries. Radiology 123:699–703, 1977.

160. Winter PF, Perl LJ: Cold areas in bone scanning. J Nucl Med 17:755, 1976.

161. Wolff JA, Tuomanen EI, Greenberg ID: Radionuclide joint imaging: acute rheumatic fever simulating septic arthritis. Pediatrics 65:339–341, 1980.

162. Woolfenden JM, Pitt MJ, Durie BGM, et al: Comparison of bone scintigraphy and radiography in multiple myeloma. Radiology 134:723–728, 1980.

162A. Yon JW, Spicer KM, Gordon L: Synovial visualization during Tc-99m MDP bone scanning in septic arthritis of the knee. Clin Nucl Med 8:249–251, 1983.

163. Zwas ST, Czerniak P: Head and brain scan findings in rhinocerebral mucormycosis: case report. J Nucl Med 16:925–927, 1975.

Chapter 55

Non-Osseous Uptake†

JOHN G. McAFEE

EDWARD B. SILBERSTEIN

I. Artefacts

    A. Common

        1. Skin contamination

            a. urine (1)

            b. hyperhydrosis (2)

    B. Uncommon

        1. Injection sites (19)

        2. Liver and kidney uptake due to increase in circulating aluminum (71)

        3. Phimosis (58)

II. Malignant neoplasms concentrating skeletal agents in soft tissues

The use of an asterisk * in this chapter indicates that this entity has been observed by one of the authors but the case report has not been published.

† Skeletal agents such as Tc-99m pyrophosphate or diphosphonates.

A. Common
   1. Liver metastases
      a. colonic cancer (64, 116)
      b. squamous and oat cell lung carcinoma (75, 89)
      c. breast cancer (9)
   2. Malignant pleural effusions (147)
   3. Neuroblastoma (123)
      a. ganglioneuroblastoma (123)
   4. Primary and metastatic carcinomas
      a. breast (9, 39, 112, 114, 161)
      b. lung (114, 116)
      c. colon (64, 112)
   5. Osteogenic sarcoma, primary and metastatic (141)
B. Less common
   1. Primary carcinomas
      a. nasopharynx (112)
      b. stomach (151)
      c. cholangiocarcinoma of liver (64)
      d. ovary (54)
      e. thyroid (163)
      f. liver (116)
      g. renal (152)
      h. esophageal (173)
   2. Lymphomas (all cell types) (32, 161, 175)
      a. meningeal seeding (145)
   3. Malignant melanoma (162)
   4. Embryonal cell carcinoma (103)
   5. Chondrosarcoma (114)
   6. Pulmonary metastases
      a. osteosarcoma (136)
      b. seminoma (66)
   7. Cerebral metastases
      a. bronchogenic carcinoma (31)
      b. renal carcinoma (35)
   8. Peritoneal metastases
      a. endometrial carcinomas (24)
C. Rare
   1. Leukemic infiltrates (129)
   2. Fibrosarcoma (129)
   3. Abdominal wall metastatic carcinoma from rectum (30)
   4. Primary osteosarcoma of small bowel (141)
   5. Squamous penile carcinoma (90)
   6. Ewing's tumor (25)
   7. Malignant fibrous histiocytoma (125)
   8. Islet cell tumor of pancreas (94)

    9. Liposarcoma (33)
   10. Astrocytoma (103)
   11. Schwannoma, malignant (34)
   12. Synovioma (34)
   13. Hemangiopericytoma (34)
   14. Rhabdomyosarcoma (34)
   15. Calcified synovial sarcoma (69A)

III. Benign neoplasms concentrating skeletal agents in soft tissues

  A. Uncommon
    1. Neurofibroma (109)
    2. Meningioma (62)
    3. Intraductal papilloma of breast (69)
    4. Uterine leiomyoma (47, 98)
    5. Thyroid adenomas (143)
    6. Lipoma (33)
    7. Ovarian cystic teratoma (138)
    8. Ovarian cyst with hematoma*
    9. Angiolipoma (34)
   10. Myxoma (34)
   11. Neurilemoma (34)
   12. Lymphangiomyoma (34)
   13. Hamartoma (34)
   14. Fibromatosis, aggressive (34)
   15. Cystosarcoma phyllodes (7)
   16. Desmoid tumor (84)

IV. Localized increased uptake of skeletal agents in intracranial and other soft tissues of the head

  A. Common
    1. Cerebral ischemic infarction (50, 62, 172)
  B. Less common
    1. Metastatic carcinoma (62)
    2. Primary cerebral neoplasms (35, 62)
      a. astrocytoma (103)
      b. meningioma (62)
      c. acoustic neuroma (62)
    3. Chronic subdural hematoma (62)
    4. Arteriovenous malformation (62)
    5. Focal cerebritis and abscess (62)
  C. Rare
    1. Cysticercosis (62)
    2. Nostril after trauma (57)

   3. Dural calcification (16)

V. Extraskeletal uptake of bone agents in the neck
   A. Common
      1. Normal tracheal and thyroid cartilages (149)
      2. Arterial calcifications*
   B. Less common
      1. Thyroid adenoma (143)
      2. Thyroid papillary adenocarcinoma (163)
      3. Medullary carcinoma of thyroid (139A)
      4. Calcified hemorrhagic cyst*
      5. Metastatic calcification of thyroid in hypercalcemia (5)
      6. Multinodular goiter with calcific degeneration (76)
      7. Trauma from nasogastric tube (60)
      8. Congenital fibromatosis (157)

VI. Uptake of skeletal agents in soft tissues of the thorax
   A. Heart—see Chapter 4—^{99m}Tc-pyrophosphate commonly employed to detect myocardial infarct (22)
   B. Diffusely increased uptake in the lungs (63)
      1. Common
         a. chronic renal disease with secondary hyperparathyroidism; dialysis (124, 169)
         b. primary hyperparathyroidism (36, 171)
         c. hypercalcemia due to extensive skeletal metastases (171)
         d. hypercalcemia due to multiple myeloma (18, 167)
      2. Less common
         a. hypervitaminosis D (171)
         b. prolonged therapy with phosphates, adrenocorticosteroids or calcium infusions (171)
         c. hypercalcemia with malignant melanoma (35)
         d. hypercalcemia with non-Hodgkin's lymphoma (177)
      3. Rare
         a. idiopathic alveolar microlithiasis (without hypercalcemia) (20)
         b. aspergillosis (121)
         c. tuberculosis (121)
         d. radiation pneumonitis (130)
         e. berylliosis (111)
   C. Pleura
      1. Common
         a. malignant pleural effusion (36, 147)
      2. Rare
         a. fibrothorax (119)

    D. Mediastinum (non-neoplastic)
        1. Sarcoid (114)
    E. Lymph node
        1. Following extensive extravasation in hand (28)

VII. Breast uptake of skeletal agents

    A. Common
        1. Normal breasts (35)
        2. Carcinoma (133)
    B. Less common
        1. Lactating breast (80)
        2. Calcified tissue around breast prosthesis (72)
        3. Gynecomastia (133), especially drug-induced (117)
            a. estrogens
            b. digitalis
            c. cimetidine
            d. spironolactone
        4. Abscess (94)
        5. Fibrosis (94)
        6. Chronic fibrocystic disease (94)
        7. Dysplasia (69) and mazoplasia (131)
        8. Fibroadenomatosis (69)
        9. Fat necrosis (69)
    C. Rare
        1. Intraductal papilloma (69)
        2. Intra-mammary bone (37)
        3. Amyloidosis (104)

VIII. Increased uptake of skeletal agents in soft tissues of abdomen and pelvis (GI tract, liver, gallbladder, kidneys, ureters, bladder and neoplasia are covered elsewhere)

    A. Common
        1. Urinary contamination of skin
    B. Uncommon
        1. Ascites (68)
    C. Rare
        1. Pregnant uterus in the first month of gestation (on blood pool only) (96)
        2. Benign ovarian cyst (99)

IX. Urinary tract (ureters, bladder) uptake

    A. Common
        1. Rupture with extravasation of urine (105)

  2. Dilatation of urinary collecting system—hydronephrosis, obstructive uropathy (95)
  3. Bladder diverticulum*
B. Uncommon
  1. Exstrophy of the bladder (118)
  2. Inguinal hernia (97)
  3. Traumatic renal laceration with extravasation (urinoma) (77)

X. Abnormally intense concentration in renal parenchyma

  A. Common
   1. Urinary tract obstruction, calyceal (focal uptake) or diffuse (10)
   2. Poor hydration*
  B. Uncommon
   1. Following chemotherapy
      a. cyclophosphamide (92)
      b. vincristine (92)
      c. doxorubicin (92)
      d. intra-arterial mitomycin (78)
   2. Radiation therapy fields (176)
   3. Hypercalcemia
      a. with renal failure (125)
      b. from metastatic tumor (27)
      c. hyperparathyroidism (160)
   4. Nephrocalcinosis (18)
   5. Renal vein thrombosis (79A)
  C. Rare
   1. Acute tubular necrosis (82)
      a. gentamicin toxicity (148)
      b. acute rhabdomyolysis (148)
   2. Iron overload states
      a. hemochromatosis or transfusion iron overload (113)
      b. sickle cell disease*
      c. thalassemia major (165)
      d. DiGuglielmo's erythroleukemia (19)
   3. Myelofibrosis (15)
   4. Hypervitaminosis A (55)
   5. Cirrhosis (78)
   6. Following radiographic contrast (sodium diatrizoate) (40)
   7. Renal artery stenosis (81)
   8. Calcification of intrarenal tumor
      a. myeloma (1)
      b. breast cancer (146)
      c. lung carcinoma (145)
      d. renal carcinoma (138, 145)

9. Artefactual from increased blood aluminum (71)
10. Paroxysmal nocturnal hemoglobinuria (145)
11. Acute pyelonephritis (145)
12. Crossed renal ectopia (122)
13. Communicating renal cortical cyst (154A)
14. Traumatic rhabdomyolysis with myoglobinuria (155A)

XI. Liver uptake

A. Common
1. Neuroblastoma (51)
2. Metastatic carcinoma (see Section II)
   a. colon (64)
   b. lung (109)
   c. breast (9)
3. Artefactual
   a. prior sulfur colloid liver scan*
   b. colloid from improper radiopharmaceutical preparation (114)

B. Less common
1. Metastases to liver
   a. malignant melanoma (35, 172)
   b. esophageal carcinoma (173)
2. Cholangiocarcinoma (64)
3. Amyloidosis (170)
4. Lymphoma*
5. Massive hepatic necrosis or infarct (93)
6. Hypercalcemia (46)
7. Hepatoma (78)
8. Thalassemia major (166)
9. After radiographic (sodium diatrizonate) contrast media (40)
10. Artefactual from increased blood aluminum (29)

XII. Spleen uptake

A. Common
1. Sickle cell disease (61)

B. Less common
1. Thalassemia major (70) and sickle-thalassemia (128)
2. Metastatic carcinoma (9)
3. Glucose-6-phosphate dehydrogenase deficiency (88)
4. Hemosiderosis with histiocytic lymphoma (175)
5. Hodgkin's disease
   a. with autoimmune hemolytic anemia (32)
6. Subcapsular hematoma (156)

XIII. Adrenal uptake

    A. Uncommon
        1. Wolman's disease (155)

XIV. Stomach uptake

    A. Common
        1. Artefact, due to Tc-99m pertechnetate in radiopharmaceutical preparation (45, 53)
        2. Hypercalcemia
            a. myeloma (167)
            b. Hodgkin's disease (73)
            c. milk-alkali syndrome (43)
        3. Renal failure (120, 124)
            a. dialysis patients (42)
    B. Uncommon
        1. Gastric carcinoma (151)
        2. Gastric bleeding (83)

XV. Intestine uptake

    A. Common
        1. Urinary diversion surgical procedures (101)
    B. Uncommon
        1. Neonatal necrotizing enterocolitis (135)
        2. Vesicoenteric fistula (48, 74)
        3. Intestinal (mesenteric) infarction (experimental in dogs) (8)
    C. Rare
        1. Normal intestine (38)

XVI. Gallbladder uptake (22A,38)

XVII. Peritoneum

    A. Rare
        1. Peritoneal metastases from endometrial carcinoma (13)

XVIII. Vessels (see Part I—Cardiovascular System)

    A. Common
        1. Aortic aneurysm (23, 161)
        2. Femoral artery calcification (150)

B. Uncommon
   1. Thrombophlebitis (100, 142)
   2. Monckeberg's sclerosis (161)

XIX. Increased soft tissue uptake of skeletal agents in the extremities

   A. Common
   1. Artefact
      a. contamination of skin from urine or hyperhidrosis (2, 67)
      b. injection site extravasation (67)
   2. Surgical trauma (114)
      a. scar 5 weeks post-operative (144)
      b. scar 2 years post-operative*
   3. Calcific tendinitis (13)
   4. Cellulitis (65)
   5. Septic arthritis (65)
   6. Osteomyelitis (65)
   7. Rheumatoid arthritis and synovitis (44)
   8. Arterial calcifications (161)
   9. Myositis ossificans, post-traumatic (112)
   10. Reflex sympathetic dystrophic syndromes
      a. shoulder-hand syndrome (79, 100)
      b. stroke syndrome (79)
      c. lumbar discogenic disease (26)
      d. peripheral neuropathy*
      e. post-lumbar sympathectomy (85)
   11. Skeletal muscle diseases (see Section XX)
   12. Radiation therapy fields (10, 65, 114)
   13. Malignant primary bone tumors (35)
   14. Lymphedema (100)
      a. scrotal lymphedema (117A)
   15. Synovitis (68)
   16. Bursitis (67)
   B. Less common
   1. Thrombophlebitis (100, 142)
   2. Abscess (31)
   3. Para-articular ossification due to paraplegia (para-osteoarthropathy, heterotopic bone) (35, 106)
   4. Calcifying hematoma (129)
   5. Neurofibroma, extraosseous (109)
   6. Calcinosis circumscripta or universalis (35, 115)
   C. Rare
   1. Gouty tophi (3)
   2. Pseudogout (68)

   3. Amyloidosis (169)
      a. testicular amyloidosis (157A)
   4. Neonatal subcutaneous fat necrosis (174)
   5. Pretibial myxedema and thyroid acropachy (132)
   6. Tumoral calcinosis (21, 49)
   7. Inadvertent arterial injection of skeletal agent (35)
   8. Filarial infestation (110)
   9. Pellegrini-Stieda's disease (peritendinitis calcarea of the medial collateral ligament of the knee joint) (164)
   10. Inflamed breast implant (72)
   11. Pseudoxanthoma elasticum (17, 91)
   12. Extravasated calcium solution (6)
   13. Lymph nodes draining extravasated ^{99m}Tc-pyrophosphate (28)
   14. Desmoid tumor (86)
   15. Xanthomatosis, extraosseous (140)

XX. Increased uptake of bone agents in skeletal muscle

   A. Common
      1. After strenuous exercise or seizures (12, 84)
      2. Myositis ossificans (158)
      3. Heterotopic ossification after prosthetic surgery (67)
   B. Less common
      1. Para-articular ossification secondary to paraplegia (35)
      2. Acute traumatic rhabdomyolysis
         a. crush injuries (12)
         b. post thrombectomy (19)
         c. electric shock (87)
         d. frostbite (126)
      3. Non-traumatic rhabdomyolysis
         a. alcoholic (19, 148)
      4. Polymyositis (11, 154)
      5. Dermatomyositis (134)
      6. Scleroderma (11, 134)
      7. McArdle syndrome (myophosphorylase deficiency) (159)
      8. Sickle cell disease (56)
      9. Duchenne muscular dystrophy (11)
      10. Steinert's disease (myotonia dystrophica) (11)
      11. Ischemic muscle (52)
      12. Injections
         a. iron-dextran (168)
         b. meperidine (19, 59)
         c. calcium heparinate (113A)
      13. Muscle hernia (139)

14. Following chemoperfusion (melphelan and actinomycin D) (153)
15. Post-radiotherapy (10)
16. Paroxysmal nocturnal hemoglobinuria*

REFERENCES

1. Adams KJ, Shuler SE, Witherspoon LP: A retrospective analysis of renal abnormalities detected on one scan. Clin Nucl Med 5:1–7, 1980.
2. Ajmani SK, Lerner SR, Pirchen FJ: Bone scan artifact caused by hyperhidrosis: case report. J Nucl Med 18:801–802, 1977.
3. Alarcon-Segovia D, Lazo C, Sepulveda J, et al: Uptake of ^{99m}Tc-labeled phosphates by gouty tophic. J Rheumatol 1:314–318, 1974.
4. Alevizaki CC, Georgiou E, Nikiforakis E, et al: Transient splenic uptake of ^{99m}Tc-MDP associated with hemolysis. Eur J Nucl Med 7:510–512, 1982.
5. Arbona GL, Antonimattei S, Tetalman MR, et al: Tc-99m diphosphonate distribution in a patient with hypercalcemia and metastatic calcifications. Clin Nucl Med 5:422, 1980.
6. Balsam D, Goldfarb CR, Stringer B, et al: Bone scintigraphy for neonatal osteomyelitis: simulation by extravasation of intravenous calcium. Radiology 135:185–186, 1980.
7. Baum SN, Lyons KP, Wu SY, et al: Atlas of Nuclear Medicine Imaging. New York: Appleton Century Crofts, 1980, pp. 203–204.
8. Barth KH, Alderson PO, Strandberg JH, et al: ^{99m}Tc-pyrophosphate imaging in experimental mesenteric infarction. Radiology 129:491–495, 1978.
9. Baumert JE, Lantieri RL, Horning S, et al: Liver metastases of breast carcinoma detected on ^{99m}Tc-methylene diphosphonate bone scan. Am J Roentgenol 134:389–391, 1980.
10. Bekior A: Extraosseous accumulation of Tc-99m pyrophosphate in soft tissue after radiation therapy. J Nucl Med 19:225–226, 1978.
11. Bellina CR, Bianchi R, Bombardieri S, et al: Quantitative evaluation of ^{99m}Tc-pyrophosphate muscle uptake in patients with inflammatory and noninflammatory muscle disease. J Nucl Med Allied Sci 22:89–96, 1978.
12. Blair RJ, Schroder ET, McAfee JG, et al: Skeletal muscle uptake of bone seeking agents in both traumatic and non-traumatic rhabdomyolysis with acute renal failure. J Nucl Med 16:515–516, 1975.
13. Blau M, Ganatra R, Bender MA: F-18 fluoride for bone imaging. Sem Nucl Med 2:31–37, 1972.
14. Bledin AG, Kim EE, Haynie TP: Bone scintigraphic findings related to unilateral mastectomy. Eur J Nucl Med 7:500–501, 1982.
15. Blei CL, Born ML, Rollo FD: Gallium bone scan in myelofibrosis: case report. J Nucl Med 18:445–447, 1972.
16. Bobba RV, Fink-Bennett D: A dural calcification presenting as a solitary lesion on radionuclide bone scan. Clin Nucl Med 3:35, 1978.
17. Bossuyt A, Verbeelen D: Accumulation of ^{99m}Tc pyrophosphate in the skin lesions of pseudoxanthoma elasticum. Clin Nucl Med 1:245, 1976.
18. Bossuyt A, Verbeelen D, Jonckheer MH, et al: Usefulness of ^{99m}Tc-methylene diphosphonate scintigraphy in nephrocalcinosis. Clin Nucl Med 4:333–334, 1979.
19. Brill DR: Radionuclide imaging of non-neoplastic soft tissue disorders. Sem Nucl Med 11:277–278, 1981.
20. Brown ML, Swee RG, Olson RJ, et al: Pulmonary uptake of ^{99m}Tc diphosphonate in alveolar microlithiasis. Am J Roentgenol 131:703–704, 1978.

21. Brown ML, Thrall JH, Cooper RA, et al: Radiography and scintigraphy in tumoral calcinosis. Radiology 124:757–758, 1977.

22. Bruno FP, Cobb FR, Rivas F: Evaluation of ^{99m}Tc- technetium stannous pyrophosphate as an imaging agent in acute myocardial infarction. Circulation 54:71–81, 1976.

22A. Bussaka H, Takahashi M: Abnormal accumulation of ^{99m}Tc-hydroxymethylene diphosphonate in the gall bladder. Jap J Nucl Med 19:817–821, 1982.

23. Campeau RJ, Gottlieb S, Kallos N: Aortic aneurysm detected by ^{99m}Tc-pyrophosphate imaging: case report. J Nucl Med 18:272–273, 1977.

24. Cannon JR Jr., Long RF, Berens SV, et al: Metastatic abdominal implants of endometrial carcinoma demonstrated on ^{99m}Tc-methylene diphosphonate bone scan. Clin Nucl Med 3:310–311, 1978.

25. Carlson DH, Simon H: Uptake of ^{99m}Tc-methylene diphosphonate in a case of extraskeletal Ewing's sarcoma. Clin Nucl Med 5:203, 1979.

26. Carlson DH, Simon H, Wegnre W: Bone scanning and diagnosis of reflex sympathetic dystrophy secondary to herniated lumbar disks. Neurology 27:781–783, 1977.

27. Chabria PB, Stankey RM, Pinsky ST: Extraskeletal uptake of ^{99m}Tc-Sn-pyrophosphate in hypercalcemia associated with carcinoma of the urinary bladder. Clin Nucl Med 2:87–88, 1977.

28. Chatterton BE, Vannitumlit M, Cook DJ: Lymph node visualization: an unusual artefact in the ^{99m}Tc pyrophosphate bone scan. Eur J Nucl Med 5:187–188, 1980.

29. Chaudhuri TK: Liver uptake of ^{99m}Tc-diphosphonate. Radiology 119:485–486, 1977.

30. Chaudhuri TK, Chaudhuri TK, Christie JH, et al: Tumor uptake of ^{99m}Tc-polyphosphate: its similarity with ^{87m}Sr-citrate and dissimilarity with ^{67}Ga citrate. J Nucl Med 15:458–459, 1974.

31. Chaudhuri TK, Chaudhuri TK, Gulesserian HP, et al: Extraosseous noncalcified soft tissue uptake of ^{99m}Tc-polyphosphate. J Nucl Med 15:1054–1056, 1974.

32. Chaudhuri TK, Chaudhuri TK, Suzuki Y: Splenic accumulation of Sr-87m in a patient with Hodgkin's disease. Radiology 105:617–618, 1972.

33. Chew FS, Hudson TM: Radionuclide imaging of lipoma and liposarcoma. Radiology 136:741–745, 1980.

34. Chew FS, Hudson TM, Enneking WF: Radionuclide imaging of soft tissue neoplasms. Sem Nucl Med 11:266–276, 1981.

35. Citrin DL, McKillop JH: Atlas of Technetium Bone Scans. Philadelphia: W.B. Saunders, 1978.

36. Cohen AM, Maxon HR, Goldsmith RE, et al: Metastatic pulmonary calcification in primary hyperparathyroidism. Arch Int Med 137:520–522, 1977.

37. Cole-Beuglet C, Kirk ME, Selevan R, et al: Bone within the breast. Radiology 119:643–644, 1976.

38. Conway JJ, Weiss SC, Khentigan J, et al: Gallbladder and bowel localization of bone imaging radiopharmaceuticals (abstract). J Nucl Med 20:622, 1979.

39. Costello P, Gramm HF, Steinberg D: Simultaneous occurrence of functional asplenia and splenic accumulation of diphosphonate in metastatic breast carcinoma. J Nucl Med 18:1237–1238, 1977.

40. Crawford JA, Gumerman LW: Alteration of body distribution of ^{99m}Tc-pyrophosphate by radiographic contrast. Clin Nucl Med 3:305–307, 1978.

41. Datz FL, Lewis SE, Conrad MR, et al: Pyomyositis diagnosed by radionuclide imaging and ultrasonography. So Med J 73:649–651, 1980.

42. DeGraaf P, Pauwek EKJ, Schicht M: Scintigraphic detection of gastric calcifications in dialysis patients. J Nucl Med 21:197, 1980.

43. Delcourt E, Baudoux M, Veve P: Tc-99m-MDP bone scanning detection of gastric calcification. Clin Nucl Med 5:546–547, 1980.
44. Desaulniers M, Fuks A, Hawkins D, et al: Radiotechnetium polyphosphate joint imaging. J Nucl Med 15:417–423, 1974.
45. Dhawan V, Yeh SD: Labeling efficiency and stomach concentration in methylene diphosphonate bone imaging. J Nucl Med 20:791–793, 1979.
46. Dudczak R, Angelberger P, Kletter K, et al: Transient accumulation of Tc-99m MDP in the liver. Eur J Nucl Med 5:189–191, 1980.
47. Ell PH, Breitfellner G, Meixner M: Technetium-99m-HEDP concentration in calcified myoma. J Nucl Med 17:323–324, 1976.
48. Engelstad B: Demonstration of a colovesical fistula on a bone scan. Clin Nucl Med 7:131, 1982.
49. Eugenidis N, Locher JR: Tumor calcinosis imaged by bone scanning: case report. J Nucl Med 18:34–35, 1977.
50. Fischer KC, Pendergrass HP, McKusick KA, et al: Increased brain scan specificity by the use of ^{99m}Tc-diphosphonate. J Nucl Med 15:490–495, 1974.
51. Fitzer PM: ^{99m}Tc-polyphosphate concentration in a neuroblastoma. J Nucl Med 15:904–906, 1974.
52. Floyd JL, Parther JH: ^{99m}Tc EHDP uptake in ischemic muscle. Clin Nucl Med 2:281, 1977.
53. Front D, Hardoff R, Mashour N: Stomach artifact in bone scintigraphy. J Nucl Med 19:974–975, 1978.
54. Gates GF: Ovarian carcinoma imaged by ^{99m}Tc pyrophosphate: case report. J Nucl Med 17:29–30, 1976.
55. Gelfand MJ, Lonon WD, Jost LA, et al: Chronic hypervitaminosis A. Orthopedic Review 10:93–97, 1981.
56. Gelfand MJ, Planitz MK: Uptake of ^{99m}Tc-diphosphonate in soft tissue in sickle cell anemia. Clin Nucl Med 2:355–356, 1977.
57. Glass EC, DeNardo GL, Hines HH: Immediate renal imaging and renography with ^{99m}Tc-methylene diphosphonate to assess renal blood flow, excretory function, and anatomy. Radiology 135:187–190, 1980.
58. Glassman AB, Selby JB: Another bone imaging agent false-positive: phimosis. Clin Nucl Med 5:34, 1980.
59. Go RT, Cook SA, Abu-Yousef M, et al: Etiology of soft tissue localization in radionuclide bone image. Scientific Exhibit, 28th Annual Meeting, Society of Nuclear Medicine, Las Vegas, Nevada, June, 1981.
60. Goldfarb CR, Shah PJ, Jay M: Extraosseous uptake of bone seeking tracers: an expected but unsuspected addition to the list. Clin Nucl Med 4:194–195, 1979.
61. Goy W, Crowe WJ: Splenic accumulation of ^{99m}Tc-diphosphonate in a patient with sickle cell disease: case report. J Nucl Med 17:108–109, 1976.
62. Grames GM, Jansen C, Carlsen FN, et al: The abnormal bone scan on intracranial lesions. Radiology 115:129–134, 1975.
63. Grames GM, Sauser DD, Jansen C, et al: Radionuclide detection of diffuse interstitial pulmonary calcification. JAMA 230:992–995, 1974.
64. Guiberteau MJ, Potsaid MS, McKusick KA: Accumulation of ^{99m}Tc- diphosphonate in four patients with hepatic neoplasm: case report. J Nucl Med 17:1060–1061, 1976.
65. Harcke HT Jr.: Bone imaging in infants and children: a review. J Nucl Med 19:324–329, 1978.

66. Hardy JG, Anderson GS, Newble GM: Uptake of ^{99m}Tc-pyrophosphate by metastatic extragenital seminoma. J Nucl Med 17:1105–1106, 1976.

67. Heck LL: Extraosseous localization of phosphate bone agents. Sem Nucl Med 10:311–313, 1980.

68. Heerfordt J, Vistisen L, Bohr H: Comparison of ^{18}F and ^{99m}Tc-polyphosphate in orthopedic bone scintigraphy. J Nucl Med 17:98–103, 1976.

69. Holmes RA, Manoli RS, Isitman AT: Tc-99m-labeled phosphates as indicator of breast pathology (abstract). J Nucl Med 16:536, 1975.

69A. Horne T, Mogle P, Finsterbush A, et al: Increased uptake of ^{99m}Tc-MDP in calcified synovial sarcoma. Eur J Nucl Med 8:75–76, 1983.

70. Howman-Giles RB, Gilday DL, Ash JM, et al: Splenic accumulation of Tc-99m diphosphonate in thalassemia major. J Nucl Med 19:976–977, 1978.

71. Jaresko GS, Zimmer AM, Pavel DG, et al: Effect of circulating aluminum on the biodistribution of Tc-99m-Sn-diphosphonate in rats. J Nucl Med Tech 8:160–161, 1980.

72. Jayabalan V, Berry S: Accumulation of ^{99m}Tc-pyrophosphate in breast prosthesis. Clin Nucl Med 2:452–453, 1977.

73. Jayabalan V, Dewitt B: Gastric calcification detected *in vivo* by ^{99m}Tc-pyrophosphate imaging. Clin Nucl Med 3:27–29, 1978.

74. Kida T, Togawa T: Vesicoenteric fistula discovered during routine bone scintigraphy. Clin Nucl Med 6:422–423, 1981.

75. Kim EE, Domstad PA, Choy YC, et al: Accumulation of Tc-99m phosphonate complexes in metastatic lesions from colon and lung carcinomas. Eur J Nucl Med 5:299–301, 1980.

76. Kim YC: Thyroid uptake in bone scan on a large multinodular, non-toxic goiter with calcific degeneration. Clin Nucl Med 5:561–562, 1980.

77. Kimmel RL, Sty JR: ^{99m}Tc-methylene diphosphonate renal images in a battered child. Clin Nucl Med 4:166–167, 1979.

78. Koizumi K, Tonami N, Hisada K: Diffusely increased Tc-99m-MDP uptake in both kidneys. Clin Nucl Med 6:362–365, 1981.

79. Kozin F, Soin JS, Ryan LM, et al: Bone scintigraphy in the reflex sympathetic dystrophy syndrome. Radiology 138:437–443, 1981.

79A. Lamki LM, Wyatt JK: Renal vein thrombosis as a cause of excess renal accumulation of bone seeking agents. Clin Nucl Med 8:267–268, 1983.

80. Landfarten S: Uptake of Tc-99m pyrophosphate by the lactating breast. J Nucl Med 18:943, 1977.

81. Lantieri RL, Lin MS, Martin W, et al: Increased renal accumulation of Tc-99m-MDP in renal artery stenosis. Clin Nucl Med 5:305–309, 1980.

82. Lavell KJ, Park HM, Moseman AM, et al: Quantitative evaluation of renal parenchymal Tc-99m HEDP uptake in experimental acute tubular necrosis. J Nucl Med 19:720–724, 1978.

83. Lee VW, Leiter BF, Weitzman F: Occult gastric bleeding demonstrated by bone scan and Tc-99m-DTPA renal scan. Clin Nucl Med 6:470–473, 1981.

84. Lentle B, Percy JS, Rigal WM, et al: Localization of Tc-99m pyrophosphate in muscle after exercise. J Nucl Med 19:223–224, 1978.

85. Lentle BC, Glazebrook GA, Percy JS, et al: Sympathetic denervation and the bone scan. Clin Nucl Med 2:276–278, 1977.

86. Lessig HJ, Devenney JE: Localization of bone-seeking agent within a desmoid tumor. Clin Nucl Med 4:164–165, 1979.

87. Lewis SE, Hunt JL, Baxter C, et al: Identification of muscle damage in acute electrical burn with technetium-99m pyrophosphate scintigraphy. J Nucl Med 20:646–647, 1979.

88. Lieberman CM, Hemingway DL: Splenic visualization in a patient with glucose-6-phosphate dehydrogenase deficiency. Clin Nucl Med 4:405–406, 1979.

89. Lowenthal IS, Tow DE, Chang YC: Accumulation of ^{99m}Tc-polyphosphate in two squamous cell carcinomas of the lung. J Nucl Med 16:1021–1022, 1975.

90. Lunia S, Chandrainouly BS, Chodos R, et al: Uptake of ^{99m}Tc-methylene diphosphonate in squamous cell carcinoma of the penis. Clin Nucl Med 5:204–205, 1979.

91. Lunia S, Chodos RB, Vedder DK: Localization of ^{99m}Tc-methylene diphosphonate in skin lesions of pseudoxanthoma elasticum. Clin Nucl Med 5:196–197, 1979.

92. Lutrin CL, McDougall IR, Goris ML: Intense concentration of technetium-99m pyrophosphate in the kidneys of children treated with chemotherapy drugs for malignant disease. Radiology 128:165–167, 1978.

93. Lyons KP, Kuperus J, Green HW: Localization of Tc-99m pyrophosphate in the liver due to massive liver necrosis: case report. J Nucl Med 18:550–552, 1977.

94. LeBovic J, Waxman AD, Siemsen JK: Localization of ^{99m}Tc pyrophosphate in an islet cell tumor of the pancreas. Clin Nucl Med 3:289–291, 1978.

95. Maher FT: Evaluation of renal and urinary tract abnormalities noted on scintiscans. Mayo Clin Proc 50:370–378, 1975.

96. Majd M: Personal communication. 15 April 1982.

97. Makhija MC: Bladder in the scrotum on a bone scan. Clin Nucl Med 6:550–551, 1981.

98. Makhija MC, Brodie M: Demonstration of extremely large pedunculated uterine fibroids on bone scan. Clin Nucl Med 6:384, 1981.

99. Mandell GA, Pizzica A, Zegel H, et al: Radionuclide diagnosis of hematoma of an ovarian cyst. J Nucl Med 22:930–931, 1981.

100. Manoli R, Soin JS: Unilateral increased radioactivity in the lower extremities on routine ^{99m}Tc-pyrophosphate bone imaging. Clin Nucl Med 3:374–378, 1978.

101. Mariani G, Levorato D, Tuoni M, et al: Incidental imaging of the large bowel in patients with uretero-sigmoidoscopy during bone scintigraphy with ^{99m}Tc-pyrophosphate. J Nucl Med Allied Sci 22:153–157, 1978.

102. Matsui K, Iio M, Chiba K, et al: Diagnostic aid for the differential diagnosis of brain tumor and CVD by using Tc-99m pyrophosphate. J Nucl Med 16:549–552, 1975.

103. Matsui K, Yamada H, Chiba K, et al: Visualization of soft tissue malignancies by using ^{99m}Tc-polyphosphate, pyrophosphate and diphosphonate (^{99m}Tc-P) (abstract). J Nucl Med 14:632–633, 1973.

104. McLellan GL, Stewart JH, Balachandran S: Localization of Tc-99m-MDP in amyloidosis of the breast. Clin Nucl Med 6:579–580, 1981.

105. Moinuddin M, Rockett JF: Ureteral rupture and bone scintigraphy. J Urol 120:365–366, 1978.

106. Muheim G, Donath A, Rossier AB: Serial scintigrams in the course of ectopic bone formation in paraplegic patients. Am J Roentgenol 118:865–869, 1973.

107. Nisbet AP, Maisey MN: Splenic accumulation of technetium-99m-methylene diphosphonate. Br J Radiol 55:454–455, 1982.

108. Nolan NG: Intense uptake of ^{99m}Tc-diphosphonate by an extraosseous neurofibroma. J Nucl Med 15:1207–1208, 1974.

109. Oren VO, Uszler JM: Liver metastases of oat cell carcinoma of lung detected on ^{99m}Tc-diphosphonate bone scan. Clin Nucl Med 3:355–358, 1978.

110. Oster Z: Appearance of filarial infestations on a bone scan. J Nucl Med 17:425–426, 1976.

111. Palmer PES, Stadalnik RC, Khalkhali I: Non-bony uptake of technetium-99m MDP in berylliosis. Br Med J 53:1195–1197, 1980.
112. Papavasilious C, Kostamia P, Angelakis P, et al: Localization of Sr-87 in extraosseous tumor. J Nucl Med 12:265–268, 1971.
113. Parker JA, Jones AG, Davis MA, et al: Reduced uptake of bone seeking radiopharmaceuticals related to iron excess. Clin Nucl Med 1:267–268, 1976.
113A. Planchon CA, Donadieu A-M, Perez R, et al: Calcium heparinate induced extraosseous uptake in bone scanning. Eur J Nucl Med 8:113–117, 1983.
114. Poulose KP, Reba RC, Eckelman WC: Estraosseous localization of ^{99m}Tc-Sn pyrophosphate. Br J Radiol 48:724–726, 1975.
115. Powers TA, Touyo JJ: Tc-99m-pyrophosphate bone scan in calcinosis universalis. Clin Nucl Med 5:302–304, 1980.
116. Que L, Wiseman J, Hales B: Small cell carcinoma of the lung: primary site and hepatic metastases both detected on Tc-99m-pyrophosphate bone scan. Clin Nucl Med 6:260–262, 1980.
117. Ram Singh PS, Pujara S, Logic JR: ^{99m}Tc-pyrophosphate uptake in drug induced gynecomastia. Clin Nucl Med 2:204, 1977.
117A. Rao BR, Hodgens DW: Soft tissue uptake of Tc-99m MDP in secondary scrotal lymphedema. J Nucl Med 24:275, 1983.
118. Rao BK, Weir JG, Lieberman LM: Exstrophy of the bladder: diagnosis on a bone scan. Clin Nucl Med 6:552–553, 1981.
119. Ravin CE, Hoyt TS, DeBlanc H: Concentration of ^{99m}Technetium polyphosphate in fibrothorax following pneumonectomy. Radiology 122:405–408, 1977.
120. Richards AG: Metastatic calcification and bone scanning. J Nucl Med 16:1087–1090, 1975.
121. Rohatgi PK, Simon DB, Goldstein RA, et al: Strontium-87m lung scan in pulmonary aspergillosis. Am J Roentgenol 129:879–882, 1977.
122. Ronai PM, Bigongiari LR, Preston DF: Pseudohydronephrosis on bone scan due to crossed renal ectopia. Urology 16:104–105, 1980.
123. Rosenfield N, Treves S: Osseous and extraosseous uptake of fluorine-18 and technetium-99m-polyphosphate in children with neuroblastoma. Radiology 111:127–133, 1974.
124. Rosenthal DI, Chandler HL, Azizi F, et al: Uptake of bone imaging agents by diffuse pulmonary metastatic calcification. Am J Roentgenol 129:871–874, 1977.
125. Rosenthall L: ^{99m}Tc-methylene diphosphonate concentration in soft tissue of malignant fibrous histiocytoma. Clin Nucl Med 3:58–61, 1978.
126. Rosenthall L, Kloiber R, Gagnon R, et al: Frostbite with rhabdomyolysis and renal failure. Am J Roentgenol 137:387–390, 1981.
127. Saha GB, Herzberg DL, Boyd CM: Unusual *in vivo* distribution of ^{99m}Tc-diphosphonate. Clin Nucl Med 2:303–305, 1977.
128. Sain A, Shain R, Silver L: Bone scan in sickle cell crisis. Clin Nucl Med 3:85, 1978.
129. Samuels LD: Skeletal scintigraphy in children. Sem Nucl Med 2:89–107, 1972.
130. Sarreck R, Sham R, Alexander LL, et al: Increased ^{99m}Tc-pyrophosphate uptake with radiation pneumonitis. Clin Nucl Med 4:403–404, 1979.
131. Schmitt GH, Holmes RA, Isitman AT, et al: A proposed mechanism for ^{99m}Tc-labeled polyphosphate and diphosphonate uptake by human breast tissue. Radiology 112:733–735, 1974.
132. Seigel RS, Thrall JH, Sisson JC: ^{99m}Tc-pyrophosphate scan and radiographic correlation in the thyroid acropachy: case report. J Nucl Med 17:791–793, 1976.
133. Serafini AN, Raskin MM, Zard LC, et al: Radionuclide breast scanning in carcinoma of

the breast. J Nucl Med 15:1149–1152, 1974.

134. Sfakianakis GN, Damoulaki-Sfakianakis E, Bass JC, et al: Tc-99m polyphosphate scanning in calcinosis universalis of dermatomyositis. J Nucl Med 16:568–571, 1975.

135. Sfakianakis GN, Oritz VN, Haase GM, et al: Tc-99m-diphosphonate abdominal imaging in necrotizing enterocolitis: a prospective study. J Nucl Med 19:691–692, 1978.

136. Sham R, Cortes EP, Mundia A, et al: Technetium-99m diphosphonate chest imaging: a valuable diagnostic and prognostic tool in metastatic osteosarcoma. J Nucl Med 16:568–570, 1975.

137. Sham R, Sain A, Silber L, et al: Localization of ^{99m}Tc-phosphate compounds in renal tumors. J Nucl Med 18:311–312, 1977.

138. Shigeno C, Fukunaga M, Morita R, et al: Accumulation of ^{99m}Tc-methylene diphosphonate within benign cystic teratoma of the ovary. Eur J Nucl Med 6:417–419, 1981.

139. Shigeno C, Fukunaga M, Yamamoto I, et al: Accumulation of ^{99m}Tc-pyrophosphate in a muscle hernia of the thigh. Eur J Nucl Med 6:425–428, 1981.

139A. Shigeno C, Fukunaga M, Yamamoto I: Accumulation of Tc-99m phosphorus compounds in medullary carcinoma of the thyroid. Clin Nucl Med 7:297–298, 1982.

140. Shigeno C, Morita R, Fukunaga M, et al: Scintigraphic visualization of extraosseous xanthomatosis. Eur J Nucl Med 7:434–436, 1982.

141. Shirazi PH, Rayudu GV, Fordham EW: Extraosseous osteogenic sarcoma of the small bowel demonstrated by ^{18}F scanning. J Nucl Med 14:295–296, 1973.

142. Shirazi PH, Rayudu GV, Fordham EW: F-18 bone scanning: review of indications and results of 1,500 scans. Radiology 112:361–368, 1974.

143. Siddiqui AR, Wellman HN, Park H-M, et al: Tc-99m diphosphonate imaging in the differential diagnosis of thyroid nodules. Clin Nucl Med 7:353–356, 1982.

144. Siddiqui AR, Stokka CL: Uptake of Tc-99m-methylene diphosphonate in a surgical scar. Clin Nucl Med 6:274, 1980.

145. Siddiqui AR: Increased uptake of technetium-99m-labeled bone imaging agents in the kidneys. Sem Nucl Med 12:101–103, 1982.

146. Siegal T, Or R, Matzner Y, et al: Spinal meningeal uptake of technetium-[99m]methylene diphosphonate in meningeal seeding by malignant lymphoma. Cancer 46:2413–2415, 1980.

147. Siegel ME, Walker WJ Jr., Campbell JL: Accumulation of ^{99m}Tc-diphosphonate in malignant pleural effusions. J Nucl Med 16:883–885, 1975.

148. Silberstein EB, Bove KE: Visualization of alcohol-induced rhabdomyolysis: a correlative radiotracer, histochemical and electron microscopic study. J Nucl Med 20:127–129, 1979.

149. Silberstein EB, Francis MD, Tofe AJ, et al: Distribution of ^{99m}Tc-Sn diphosphonate and free ^{99m}Tc-pertechnetate in selected soft and hard tissues. J Nucl Med 16:58–61, 1975.

150. Silberstein EB, Shafa M, Signer C, et al: Confirmation of femoral artery calcification by bone scintigraphy (abstract). J Nucl Med 23:P77, 1982.

151. Singh A, Rosenbloom M, Usher MS, et al: Extraosseous accumulation of ^{99m}Tc-phosphate tracers: case report and review of reported causes. J Can Assoc Radiol 28:219–221, 1977.

152. Singh BN, Rierson TW, Kesala BA, et al: 99m-Tc-diphosphonate uptake in renal cell carcinoma. Clin Nucl Med 2:95–99, 1977.

153. Sorkin SJ, Horii SC, Passalaqua A, et al: Augmented activity on bone scan following local chemoperfusion. Clin Nucl Med 2:451, 1977.

154. Spies SM, Swift TR, Brown M: Increased ^{99m}Tc-polyphosphate muscle uptake in a

patient with polymyositis: case report. J Nucl Med 16:1125–1127, 1975.

154A. Straub WH, Slasky BS: Accumulation of bone scanning agent in a communicating renal cortical cyst. Clin Nucl Med 7:378, 1982.

155. Sty JR, Starshak RJ: Scintigraphy in Wolman's disease. Clin Nucl Med 3:397, 1978.

155A. Sty JR, Starshak RJ: Abnormal Tc-99m MDP renal images associated with myoglobinuria. Clin Nucl Med 7:476, 1982.

156. Sty JR, Starshak RJ, Hubbard A: Accumulation of Tc-99m-MDP in the spleen of a battered child. Clin Nucl Med 7:292, 1982.

157. Sty JR, Starshak RJ, Oechler HW: Extraosseous uptake of Tc-99m-MDP in congenital fibromatosis. Clin Nucl Med 6:123, 1981.

157A. Sty JR, Starshak RJ: Tc-99m MDP scrotal image: Testicular amyloidosis. Clin Nucl Med 8:142, 1983.

158. Suzuki Y, Hisada K, Takeda M: Demonstration of myositis ossificans by Tc-99m-pyrophosphate bone scanning. Radiology 111:663–664, 1974.

159. Swift TR, Brown M: Tc-99m pyrophosphate labeling in McArdle syndrome. J Nucl Med 19:295–297, 1978.

160. Sy WM, Mottola MD, Lao RS, et al: Unusual bone images in hyperparathyroidism. Br J Radiol 50:740–744, 1977.

161. Thrall JH, Ghaed N, Geslien GE, et al: Pitfalls in Tc-99m-polyphosphate skeletal imaging. Am J Roentgenol 121:739–747, 1974.

162. Thrall JH, Ghaed N, Pinsky SM, et al: Pitfalls in the use of ^{99m}Tc-polyphosphate for bone scanning. J Nucl Med 14:460–461, 1973.

163. Tonami T, Sugilara M, Hisada K: Concentration of ^{99m}Tc-diphosphonate in calcified thyroid carcinoma. Clin Nucl Med 2:204, 1977.

164. Turner JW, Syed IB, Spence RP: Two unusual causes of peri-patellar non-metastatic positive bone scans in patients with malignancies. J Nucl Med 17:693–695, 1976.

165. Valdez VA, Jacobstein JG: Decreased bone uptake of technetium-99m polyphosphate in thalassemia major. J Nucl Med 21:47, 1980.

166. Valdez VA, Jacobstein JG: Visualization of the liver with ^{99m}Tc-EHDP in thalassemia major. Gastroint Radiol 6:175–176, 1981.

167. Valdez VA, Jacobstein JG, Perlmutter S, et al: Metastatic calcification in lungs and stomach demonstrated on bone scan in multiple myeloma. Clin Nucl Med 4:120–121, 1979.

168. Vanek JA, Bukowski RM: Hepatic uptake of Tc-99m-labeled diphosphonate in amyloidosis: case report. J Nucl Med 18:1086–1088, 1977.

169. Venkatesh N, Polcyn RE, Norback DH: Metastatic calcification: the role of bone scanning. Radiology 129:755–758, 1978.

170. VanAntwerp JD, Hall JN, O'Mara RE, et al: Bone scan abnormality produced by interaction of Tc-99m-diphosphonate with iron dextran. J Nucl Med 16:577, 1975.

171. VanAntwerp JD, O'Mara RE, Pitt MJ, et al: Technetium-99m-diphosphonate accumulation in amyloid. J Nucl Med 16:238–240, 1975.

172. Wenzel WW, Heast RG: Uptake of Tc-99m-stannous polyphosphate in an area of cerebral infarction. J Nucl Med 15:207–209, 1974.

173. Wilkinson RH, Gaedo JT: Concentration of Tc-99m methylene-diphosphonate in hepatic metastases from squamous cell carcinoma. J Nucl Med 20:303–305, 1979.

174. Williams JL, Capitanio MA, Harcke HT Jr.: Bone scanning in neonatal subcutaneous fat necrosis. J Nucl Med 19:861–863, 1978.

175. Winter PF: Splenic accumulation of ^{99m}Tc-diphosphonate. J Nucl Med 17:850, 1976.

176. Wistow BW, McAfee JG, Sagerman RH, et al: Renal uptake of Tc-99m methylene diphosphonate after radiation therapy. J Nucl Med 20:32–34, 1979.
177. Wychank S: ^{99m}Tc-methylene diphosphonate lung uptake in mixed small and large cell lymphoma. Eur J Nucl Med 7:47–48, 1982.
178. Yood RA, Skinner M, Cohen AS, et al: Soft tissue uptake of bone seeking radionuclide in amyloidosis. J Rheumatol 8:760–766, 1981.